Dermatology

Editor

JEFFREY P. CALLEN

MEDICAL CLINICS OF NORTH AMERICA

www.medical.theclinics.com

Consulting Editor
JACK ENDE

July 2021 • Volume 105 • Number 4

ELSEVIER

1600 John F. Kennedy Boulevard • Suite 1800 • Philadelphia, Pennsylvania, 19103-2899

http://www.theclinics.com

MEDICAL CLINICS OF NORTH AMERICA Volume 105, Number 4
July 2021 ISSN 0025-7125, ISBN-13: 978-0-323-89694-8

Editor: Katerina Heidhausen
Developmental Editor: Arlene Campos

Medical Clinics of North America (ISSN 0025-7125) is published bimonthly by Elsevier Inc., 360 Park Avenue South, New York, NY 10010-1710. Months of publication are January, March, May, July, September, and November. Business and editorial offices: 1600 John F. Kennedy Boulevard, Suite 1800, Philadelphia, PA 19103-2899. Periodicals postage paid at New York, NY, and additional mailing offices. Subscription prices are USD $304.00 per year (US individuals), $910.00 per year (US institutions), $100.00 per year (US Students), $381.00 per year (Canadian individuals), $965.00 per year (Canadian institutions), $200.00 per year for (foreign students), $100.00 per year for (Canadian students), $422.00 per year (foreign individuals), and $965.00 per year (foreign institutions). To receive student/resident rate, orders must be accompanied by name of affiliated institution, date of term, and the signature of program/residency coordinator on institution letterhead. Orders will be billed at individual rate until proof of status is received. Foreign air speed delivery is included in all Clinics' subscription prices. All prices are subject to change without notice. **POSTMASTER:** Send address changes to *Medical Clinics of North America*, Elsevier Health Sciences Division, Subscription Customer Service, 3251 Riverport Lane, Maryland Heights, MO 63043. **Customer Service: Telephone: 1-800-654-2452** (U.S. and Canada); **1-314-447-8871** (outside U.S. and Canada). **Fax: 314-447-8029. E-mail: journalscustomerserviceusa@elsevier.com** (for print support); **journalsonlinesupport-usa@elsevier.com** (for online support).

Reprints. For copies of 100 or more of articles in this publication, please contact the Commercial Reprints Department, Elsevier Inc., 360 Park Avenue South, New York, NY 10010-1710. Tel.: 212-633-3874; Fax: 212-633-3820; E-mail: reprints@elsevier.com.

Medical Clinics of North America is also published in Spanish by McGraw-Hill Interamericana Editores S. A., P.O. Box 5-237, 06500 Mexico, D.F., Mexico.

Medical Clinics of North America is covered in *MEDLINE/PubMed (Index Medicus), Current Contents, ASCA, Excerpta Medica, Science Citation Index,* and *ISI/BIOMED.*

PROGRAM OBJECTIVE

The goal of the *Medical Clinics of North America* is to keep practicing physicians up to date with current clinical practice by providing timely articles reviewing the state of the art in patient care.

TARGET AUDIENCE

All practicing physicians and other healthcare professionals.

LEARNING OBJECTIVES

Upon completion of this activity, participants will be able to:

1. Review dermatologic manifestations of various systemic conditions.
2. Explain how careful assessment can lead to diagnosis of systemic conditions in the presence of skin diseases.
3. Discuss new and emerging therapies in the treatment of psoriasis.

ACCREDITATION

The Elsevier Office of Continuing Medical Education (EOCME) is accredited by the Accreditation Council for Continuing Medical Education (ACCME) to provide continuing medical education for physicians.

The EOCME designates this journal-based CME activity for a maximum of 12 *AMA PRA Category 1 Credit*(s)™. Physicians should claim only the credit commensurate with the extent of their participation in the activity.

All other healthcare professionals requesting continuing education credit for this enduring material will be issued a certificate of participation.

DISCLOSURE OF CONFLICTS OF INTEREST

The EOCME assesses conflict of interest with its instructors, faculty, planners, and other individuals who are in a position to control the content of CME activities. All relevant conflicts of interest that are identified are thoroughly vetted by EOCME for fair balance, scientific objectivity, and patient care recommendations. EOCME is committed to providing its learners with CME activities that promote improvements or quality in healthcare and not a specific proprietary business or a commercial interest.

The planning committee, staff, authors and editors listed below have identified no financial relationships or relationships to products or devices they or their spouse/life partner have with commercial interest related to the content of this CME activity:

Afsaneh Alavi, MD; Cynthia X. Chan, BS; Sidharth Chand, BA; Regina Chavous-Gibson, MSN, RN; Mark D.P. Davis, MD; Boni Elewski, MD; Jack Ende, MD, MACP; Samuel Gnanakumar; Alex Hines, MD; Giuseppe Ingrasci, BS; Taylor A. Jamerson, BA; Jordan M. Jones, MD; Robert S. Kirsner, MD, PhD; Daniela Kroshinsky, MD, MPH; Kylee J.B. Kus, BS; Avery H. LaChance, MD, MPH; Zoe M. Lipman, BS; Justin W. Marson, MD; Tiffany T. Mayo, MD; Cindy England Owen, MD; Merlin Packiam; Ana Preda-Naumescu, BS; Sarem Rashid, BS; Renajd Rrapi, BA; Caralin Schneider, BA; Margaret L. Snyder, MD; Scott Stratman, BS; Ruth Ann Vleugels, MD, MPH, MBA; John A. Zic, MD; Kathryn A. Zug, MD

The planning committee, staff, authors and editors listed below have identified financial relationships or relationships to products or devices they or their spouse/life partner have with commercial interest related to the content of this CME activity:

Crystal Aguh, MD: consultant/advisor: DevaConcepts LLC, L'Oreal, Inc, LEO Pharma A/S, UCB: royalties/patents: UpToDate, Inc.

Jeffrey P. Callen, MD: consulltant/advisor: Principia Biopharma; stock ownership: 3M, Abbott, AbbVie, Allergan, Amgen Inc, Celgene Corporation, Gilead Sciences, Inc, Johnson & Johnson, Merck Sharp & Dohme Corp, Pfizer Inc, Procter & Gamble

Mark G. Lebwohl, MD: consultant/advisor: Aditum Bio, Almirall, AltruBio, AnaptysBio, Inc., Arcutis Biotherapeutics, Aristea Therapeutics, Arrive Technologies, Inc, Avotres Inc, BiomX, Boehringer Ingelheim International GmbH, Bristol-Myers Squibb Company, Cara Therapeutics, Castle Biosciences, Inc, CorEvitas, LLC, Dermavant Sciences, Inc, Dr. Reddy's Laboratories Ltd, Evelo Biosciences, Inc, Evommune, Inc, Forte Biosciences Inc, Helsinn Healthcare SA, Hexima, LEO Pharma Inc, Meiji Seika Pharma Co, Ltd, Mindera, Pfizer Inc, Seanergy Dermatology Ltd, Verrica Pharmaceuticals

Hensin Tsao, MD, PhD: consultant/advisor: Epiphany Dermatology, Lazarus AI; royalties/ patents: UpToDate

Gil Yosipovitch, MD: consultant/advisor: Pfizer Inc, Trevi Therapeutics, Galderma Laboratories, L.P., Regeneron Pharmaceuticals Inc., Sanofi, Novartis AG, LEO Pharma Inc, Kiniksa Pharmaceuticals, Ltd, Lilly; research funds: Pfizer Inc, Sun Pharmaceutical Industries Ltd., Kiniksa Pharmaceuticals, Ltd, Novartis AG

UNAPPROVED/OFF-LABEL USE DISCLOSURE

The EOCME requires CME faculty to disclose to the participants;

1. When products or procedures being discussed are off-label, unlabelled, experimental, and/or investigational (not US Food and Drug Administration [FDA] approved); and
2. Any limitations on the information presented, such as data that are preliminary or that represent ongoing research, interim analyses, and/or unsupported opinions. Faculty may discuss information about pharmaceutical agents that is outside of FDA-approved labelling. This information is intended solely for CME and is not intended to promote off-label use of these medications. If you have any questions, contact the medical affairs department of the manufacturer for the most recent prescribing information.

TO ENROLL

To enroll in the *Medical Clinics of North America* Continuing Medical Education program, call customer service at 1-800-654-2452 or sign up online at http://www.theclinics.com/home/cme. The CME program is available to subscribers for an additional annual fee of USD 324.00.

METHOD OF PARTICIPATION

In order to claim credit, participants must complete the following;

1. Complete enrolment as indicated above.
2. Read the activity.
3. Complete the CME Test and Evaluation. Participants must achieve a score of 70% on the test. All CME Tests and Evaluations must be completed online.

CME INQUIRIES/SPECIAL NEEDS

For all CME inquiries or special needs, please contact elsevierCME@elsevier.com.

MEDICAL CLINICS OF NORTH AMERICA

SERIES OF RELATED INTEREST

Primary Care: Clinics in Office Practice
https://www.primarycare.theclinics.com/
Dermatologic Clinics
https://www.derm.theclinics.com/

Contributors

CONSULTING EDITOR

JACK ENDE, MD, MACP
The Schaeffer Professor of Medicine, Department of Medicine, Perelman School of Medicine, University of Pennsylvania, Philadelphia, Pennsylvania

EDITOR

JEFFREY P. CALLEN, MD, FACP, MAAD, MACR
Professor of Medicine (Dermatology), Chief, Division of Dermatology, Department of Medicine, University of Louisville School of Medicine, Louisville, Kentucky

AUTHORS

CRYSTAL AGUH, MD
Assistant Professor, Department of Dermatology, Johns Hopkins School of Medicine, Baltimore, Maryland

AFSANEH ALAVI, MD
Senior consultant, Department of Dermatology, Mayo Clinic, Rochester, Minnesota

CYNTHIA X. CHAN, BS
Medical Student, Dartmouth Geisel School of Medicine, Hanover, New Hampshire

SIDHARTH CHAND, BA
Department of Dermatology, Massachusetts General Hospital, Boston, Massachusetts

MARK D.P. DAVIS, MD
Professor of Dermatology, Department of Dermatology, Mayo Clinic, Rochester, Minnesota

BONI ELEWSKI, MD
Professor and Chair, Department of Dermatology, The University of Alabama at Birmingham, Birmingham, Alabama

ALEX HINES, MD
Internal medicine resident, Department of Internal Medicine, Mayo Clinic, Rochester, Minnesota

GIUSEPPE INGRASCI, BS
Dr Phillip Frost Department of Dermatology and Miami Itch Center, University of Miami, Miami, Florida

TAYLOR A. JAMERSON, BA
Medical Student, University of Michigan Medical School, Ann Arbor, Michigan

JORDAN M. JONES, MD
PGY-2, Division of Dermatology, Department of Medicine, Louisville, Kentucky

ROBERT S. KIRSNER, MD, PhD
Department of Dermatology and Cutaneous Surgery, University of Miami Miller School of Medicine, Miami, Florida

DANIELA KROSHINSKY, MD, MPH
Department of Dermatology, Massachusetts General Hospital, Boston, Massachusetts

KYLEE J.B. KUS, BS
Department of Dermatology, Brigham and Women's Hospital, Harvard Medical School, Boston, Massachusetts; Oakland University William Beaumont School of Medicine, Rochester, Michigan

AVERY H. LACHANCE, MD, MPH
Director, Connective Tissue Disease Clinic, Department of Dermatology, Brigham and Women's Hospital, Harvard Medical School, Boston, Massachusetts

MARK G. LEBWOHL, MD
Department of Dermatology, Icahn School of Medicine at Mount Sinai, New York, New York

ZOE M. LIPMAN, BS
Dr Phillip Frost Department of Dermatology and Miami Itch Center, University of Miami, Miami, Florida

JUSTIN W. MARSON, MD
National Society for Cutaneous Medicine, New York, New York

TIFFANY T. MAYO, MD
Assistant Professor, Department of Dermatology, The University of Alabama at Birmingham, Birmingham, Alabama

CINDY ENGLAND OWEN, MD
Associate Clinical Professor, Division of Dermatology, Department of Medicine, Louisville, Kentucky

ANA PREDA-NAUMESCU, BS
School of Medicine, The University of Alabama at Birmingham, Alabama

SAREM RASHID
Department of Dermatology, Wellman Center for Photomedicine, Massachusetts General Hospital, Boston University School of Medicine, Boston, Massachusetts

RENAJD RRAPI, BA
Department of Dermatology, Massachusetts General Hospital, Boston, Massachusetts

CARALIN SCHNEIDER, BA
Department of Dermatology and Cutaneous Surgery, University of Miami Miller School of Medicine, Miami, Florida

MARGARET L. SNYDER, MD
Department of Dermatology, Icahn School of Medicine at Mount Sinai, New York, New York

SCOTT STRATMAN, BS
Department of Dermatology and Cutaneous Surgery, University of Miami Miller School of Medicine, Miami, Florida

HENSIN TSAO, MD, PhD
Department of Dermatology, Wellman Center for Photomedicine, Massachusetts General Hospital, Boston, Massachusetts

RUTH ANN VLEUGELS, MD, MPH, MBA
Director, Autoimmune Skin Disease Program, Department of Dermatology, Brigham and Women's Hospital, Harvard Medical School, Boston, Massachusetts

GIL YOSIPOVITCH, MD
Dr Phillip Frost Department of Dermatology and Miami Itch Center, University of Miami, Miami, Florida

JOHN A. ZIC, MD, MMHC
Professor of Dermatology, Director, Department of Dermatology, VU Cutaneous Lymphoma Clinic, Vanderbilt University Medical Center, Vanderbilt Dermatology, Nashville, Tennessee

KATHRYN A. ZUG, MD
Professor, Dartmouth Geisel School of Medicine, Hanover, New Hampshire; Department of Dermatology, Dartmouth-Hitchcock Medical Center, Lebanon, New Hampshire

Contents

Severe cutaneous adverse reactions to medications (SCARs) include drug reaction with eosinophilia and systemic symptoms, Stevens-Johnson syndrome, toxic epidermal necrolysis, and acute generalized exanthematous pustulosis. They are all non–immunoglobulin E mediated hypersensitivity reaction patterns, distinguished from simple cutaneous drug eruptions by immunologic pathogenesis and internal organ involvement. Herein the clinical features, diagnostic workup, and management considerations are presented for each of these major SCARs.

Alopecia is a dermatologic condition in which sudden or gradual loss of hair occurs on 1 or more areas of the body, most commonly the scalp. Hair loss can be acute or chronic in nature as a result of underlying inflammation, autoimmune processes, stressors, chemotherapy, or hairstyling practices. Alopecia can have substantial psychological consequences, having a negative impact on the quality of life in affected patients. The ability to both recognize and distinguish these condition holds great significance not only in providing adequate and timely treatment to improve outcomes but also meeting patient needs.

This is a comprehensive and current guide for the diagnosis, differential diagnosis, treatment, and management of eczematous dermatitis, with a focus on atopic dermatitis, irritant and allergic contact dermatitis, hand dermatitis including recurrent vesicular and hyperkeratotic types, asteatotic dermatitis, and nummular or discoid dermatitis. Diagnostic options highlighted are clinical history, physical examination, and patch testing. Therapeutic options highlighted are moisturizers, topical corticosteroids, topical calcineurin inhibitors, crisaborole, phototherapy, and systemic medications including biologics.

Psoriasis is a systemic inflammatory condition that negatively affects the quality of life and medical health of 125 million individuals globally. Although psoriasis has historically been viewed as a skin-limited disease and managed with topical agents (eg, coal tar, corticosteroids, and vitamin D analogues), the recontextualization of psoriasis as a systemic condition involving multiple organ systems has prompted the development of numerous immunomodulating, systemic agents with more targeted mechanisms of action. This article briefly discusses the indications and nuances of new and developing therapeutic agents for psoriasis management.

Melanoma accounts for approximately 1% of all skin cancers but contributes to almost all skin cancer deaths. The developing picture suggests that melanoma phenotypes are driven by epigenetic mechanisms that reflect a complex interplay between genotype and environment. Furthermore, the growing consensus is that current classification standards, notwithstanding pertinent clinical history and appropriate biopsy, fall short of capturing the vast complexity of the disease. This article summarizes the current understanding of the clinical picture of melanoma, with a focus on the tremendous breakthroughs in molecular classification and therapeutics.

Lower extremity ulcerations contribute to significant morbidity and economic burden globally. Chronic wounds, or those that do not progress through healing in a timely manner, are estimated to affect 6.5 million people in the United States alone causing, significant morbidity and economic burden of at least an estimated $25 billion annually. Owing to the aging population and increasing rates of obesity and diabetes mellitus globally, chronic lower extremity ulcers are predicted to increase. Here, we explore the pathophysiology, diagnosis, and management of the most (and least) commonly seen lower extremity ulcers.

Diabetes mellitus is a significant worldwide health concern and cutaneous manifestations are common. This review describes characteristic skin findings of diabetes, general skin findings related to diabetes, and findings related to diabetes treatment with a focus on clinical presentation, diagnosis, pathophysiology, epidemiology, and treatment. As the prevalence of diabetes continues to rise, cutaneous manifestations of diabetes mellitus likely will be encountered more frequently by physicians in all disciplines including dermatologists and primary care physicians. Accordingly, knowledge regarding the prevention, diagnosis, and management of cutaneous manifestations is an important aspect in the care of patients with diabetes.

Chronic pruritus (itch lasting ≥6 weeks) is a bothersome chief complaint that may present in a broad variety of diseases. Most itch-causing diagnoses fit into 1 of 5 categories (inflammatory, secondary to systemic disease, neuropathic, chronic pruritus of undetermined origin, and psychogenic itch) and this broad differential can be narrowed using key findings in the history and physical. In this article, we discuss which key findings are most pertinent for narrowing this differential and guiding further workup and treatment, as well as how to treat many itchy conditions.

Cellulitis is a common skin infection resulting in increasing hospitalizations and health care costs. There is no gold standard diagnostic test, making cellulitis a potentially challenging condition to distinguish from other mimickers. Physical examination typically demonstrates poorly demarcated unilateral erythema with warmth and tenderness. Thorough history and clinical examination can narrow the differential diagnosis of cellulitis and minimize unnecessary hospitalization. Antibiotic selection is determined by patient history and risk factors, severity of clinical presentation, and the most likely microbial culprit.

The cutaneous lymphomas are malignancies of T-cell and B-cell lymphocytes in which the skin is the primary organ of involvement. The cutaneous T-cell lymphomas include variants that can mimic the presentation of common skin diseases or arthropod bites. Mycosis fungoides, the most common cutaneous T-cell lymphoma, usually presents as fixed asymptomatic patches or plaques in sun-protected areas. The cutaneous B-cell lymphomas have fewer variants that often present as papules or nodules that can mimic nonmelanoma skin cancers. Some therapies for cutaneous lymphoma have unique side effects such as central hypothyroidism, hyperlipidemia, and peripheral neuropathy.

Connective tissue diseases (CTDs) encompass a broad spectrum of clinical presentations that involve multidisciplinary management. Cutaneous findings are common in CTD and careful examination of these features aids in appropriate diagnosis and subsequent evaluation. Thorough work-up of CTD is crucial to properly identify disease subtypes and systemic involvement. Management plans can be developed based on

Foreword

What Can We Learn from Our Dermatology Colleagues?

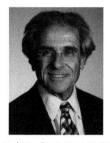

Jack Ende, MD, MACP
Consulting Editor

Dermatology training programs are very competitive. Their trainees are drawn from the best and brightest students in every medical school class. As a general internist, I find my dermatology colleagues to be among medicine's most gifted. Generalizations like this are often misguided, of course, but, more often than not, dermatologists are true to type. They are conscientious, thorough, insightful, and astute. But what makes them such effective clinicians? I believe it is something else.

They are astute observers, almost Sherlockian, if you will.

Interestingly, Sir Arthur Conan Doyle apparently found inspiration for his fictional detective, Sherlock Holmes, from a highly regarded physician, James Bell, whose skills as a diagnostician rested upon his remarkable ability as an observer. Bell, it turned out, was a surgeon. I believe he would have made a fine dermatologist.

Dermatologists rely on their well-honed skills as careful and contemplative observers. Yes, they depend significantly on the detailed information gleaned from biopsies. But they ground their diagnoses in the "big picture." Dermatologists are able to look at a field of seborrheic keratoses on an older patient's back and spot the "ugly duckling," which turns out to be the melanoma. They look at the sharply demarcated distribution of a red, raised rash and know straightaway it is a contact dermatitis, the so-called "outside job". They employ big-picture, gestalt-type questions like "is the patient sick?." "is he immunocompromised?." "is there an underlying systemic illness?" as branch points for diagnostic algorithms that can distinguish a drug reaction from an infection, a Kaposi sarcoma from a benign purpura, or an ulcer of pyoderma gangrenosum from a simple traumatic wound.

And the beauty of it all is that the best dermatologists make it look so easy.

Why is that? Because dermatologists are taught how to observe, and how to understand what they see. As medicine appropriately embraces highly technical, analytic methods, electrophysiologic mapping or flow cytometry, for example- clinicians should not forget the power of observation. The legendary Faith Fitzgerald, a master clinician if ever there was one, published an article decades ago called, "The Bedside Sherlock Holmes."[1] She provided a treasure trove of diagnostic pearls available if only the clinician keeps his or her eyes wide open and attends to what he or she sees. How long ago did the patient feel well enough to polish her nails? Answer: One day per millimeter from the nail bed. How long has the patient been hemiparetic? Answer: Look at the soles of the shoes. Are these findings conclusive? Hardly. But they can be the keys that unlock the diagnosis. Dermatologists may be our profession's consummate locksmiths.

In this issue of *Medical Clinics of North America*, "Dermatology," guest editor Dr Jeffrey P. Callen has assembled an outstanding cadre of dermatologists who provide clinical updates and diagnostic assistance for prevalent dermatology problems encountered by practitioners in both the office and the hospital. Let's keep our eyes wide open, try to observe as dermatologists observe, and learn from these experts.

Jack Ende, MD, MACP
The Schaeffer Professor of Medicine
Department of Medicine
Perelman School of Medicine of the
University of Pennsylvania
Philadelphia, PA 19104, USA

E-mail address:
jack.ende@uphs.upenn.edu

REFERENCE

1. Fitzgerald FT, Tierney LM. The bedside Sherlock Holmes. West J Med 1982;137:169–75.

Preface

Skin Signs of Systemic Diseases

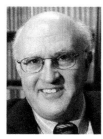

Jeffrey P. Callen, MD, FACP, MAAD, MACR
Editor

Cutaneous disease is frequent and may be reflective of internal disease. Whole texts have been devoted to discussion of the dermatologic manifestations that are reflective of systemic diseases. In many instances, the presence of skin diseases heralds an underlying systemic disease, and thus, careful assessment may lead to the recognition and diagnosis of an underlying systemic condition. In addition, there are skin lesions and diseases that are important for ALL physicians to recognize.

When I was invited to serve as editor of this issue of *Medical Clinics of North America* and told that I could select only 12 topics for discussion, I elected to request input from potential readers. To that end, I sent e-mails to my colleagues who lead the internal medicine training program at the University of Louisville as well as several to local practitioners in Louisville. Their requests for updates were surprisingly uniform in their focus. The top requests are those that you will read in this issue.

There is no particular order to the topics that are covered in this issue. I did have the pleasure of inviting colleagues with whom I have worked with on multiple occasions throughout the past 40+ years of my involvement in academic medicine. The lead authors are well-known experts in the area in which they have written, and the process of reading and editing their submissions was a most pleasant process.

Med Clin N Am 105 (2021) xvii–xviii
https://doi.org/10.1016/j.mcna.2021.04.013
0025-7125/21/© 2021 Published by Elsevier Inc.

I am hopeful that the readers of this issue will find the information contained in these articles to be of use as they care for patients in their practices, and that the result is improved health for patients.

Jeffrey P. Callen, MD, FACP, MAAD, MACR
Division of Dermatology
Department of Medicine
University of Louisville
School of Medicine
3810 Springhurst Boulevard
Louisville, KY 40241, USA

E-mail address:
jeffreycallen01@gmail.com

Recognition and Management of Severe Cutaneous Adverse Drug Reactions (Including Drug Reaction with Eosinophilia and Systemic Symptoms, Stevens-Johnson Syndrome, and Toxic Epidermal Necrolysis)

Cindy England Owen, MD*, Jordan M. Jones, MD

KEYWORDS

- SCAR • Cutaneous drug reaction • DRESS • SJS • TEN • AGEP

KEY POINTS

- Identifying and discontinuing the culprit medication is essential to management of all severe cutaneous adverse reactions (SCARs). Additional therapies and supportive care are often included based on extent of disease.
- Genetic predisposition to SCARs based on HLA genotype is most strongly seen with drug reaction with eosinophilia and systemic symptoms (DRESS) but has also been witnessed in Stevens-Johnson syndrome (SJS)/toxic epidermal necrolysis (TEN). Acute generalized exanthematous pustulosis (AGEP) does not demonstrate a significant genetic/medication link.
- On average, DRESS presents 2 to 6 weeks, SJS/TEN 3 to 4 weeks, and AGEP within days after culprit medication administration.
- Mortality of all SCARs ranges from 4% for AGEP, 2% to 6% for DRESS, and up to 48% for TEN.

The authors have nothing to disclose.
Division of Dermatology, Department of Medicine, 3810 Springhurst Boulevard, Suite 200, Louisville, KY 40241, USA
* Corresponding author.
E-mail address: Cindy.owen@louisville.edu

Med Clin N Am 105 (2021) 577–597
https://doi.org/10.1016/j.mcna.2021.04.001
medical.theclinics.com

INTRODUCTION

Severe cutaneous adverse reactions to medications (SCARs) are dose-dependent manifestations of hypersensitivity phenotypes. Drug reaction with eosinophilia and systemic symptoms (DRESS), Steven-Johnson syndrome (SJS), toxic epidermal necrolysis (TEN), and acute generalized exanthematous pustulosis (AGEP) are among the most commonly recognized SCARs, and are all non–immunoglobulin E (IgE)-mediated reaction patterns. Immunologic pathogenesis and internal organ involvement distinguish SCARs from simple cutaneous drug hypersensitivity reactions.[1] The following sections detail relevant clinical and diagnostic features of each of these 3 SCARs, along with management and prognostic considerations.

DRUG REACTION WITH EOSINOPHILIA AND SYSTEMIC SYMPTOMS/DRUG-INDUCED HYPERSENSITIVITY SYNDROME

Epidemiology

DRESS, also known as drug-induced hypersensitivity syndrome (DIHS), was first reported in 1996 to describe patients who developed a cutaneous eruption accompanied by adenopathy, internal organ involvement, and peripheral eosinophilia in response to medication.[2] The estimated population risk for DRESS is 0.9 to 2 per 100,000 patients per year.[3] For high-risk medications, the incidence is between 1 in 1000 and 1 in 10,000 drug exposures.[4] There is generally no predilection between male and female individuals, with an average age of 47.8 years (with a wide reported range of 3–84 years).[5]

Risk Factors

Proposed mechanisms that increase risk for patients include mutated drug detoxification enzymes (leading to accumulation of reactive metabolites), agents that induce CYP450 activity and result in decreased glutathione levels, and immunosuppression.[4] Reactivation of human herpesvirus (HHV) family members, specifically HHV-6, has been associated with DRESS.[6] In one cohort of 24 patients with DIHS, vitamin D3 levels were found to be significantly lower than in non-DIHS controls.[7]

The aromatic antiepileptic drugs (AEDs) are commonly implicated in DRESS; phenytoin was the first drug linked to this reaction pattern, but a number of other associated drugs have since been reported.[4] Other aromatic AEDs with DRESS risk include carbamazepine, phenobarbital, zonisamide, and lamotrigine.[8] Lamotrigine in particular has been reported to present differently from other DIHS cases, with milder elevations in alanine aminotransferase (ALT), lower percentage of atypical lymphocytes, and lower levels of lactate dehydrogenase (LDH).[9] The risk of DRESS with the first or second prescription of an aromatic AED is reported to be 2.3 to 4.5 in 10,000 cases.[10]

DRESS has often been associated with the sulfonamide class of medications, namely the long-acting agents sulfamethoxazole, sulfadiazine, and sulfasalazine, but importantly for many clinicians, there are only 2 case reports to date of furosemide resulting in DRESS.[11] Antibiotics in general are not considered high-risk medications for DRESS, but there have been 32 case reports identified of vancomycin-induced DIHS, with higher degree of renal impairment than non–vancomycin-induced cases.[12]

Other reported medications are dapsone, minocycline, cyclosporine, captopril, diltiazem, terbinafine, azathioprine, and allopurinol.[4] Allopurinol particularly is associated with longer onset time to symptoms, greater eosinophilia, and higher incidence of renal involvement. Abacavir and nevirapine are also known to result in DRESS, although human leukocyte antigen (HLA) predisposition is more associated with the former.[13,14] Immune checkpoint inhibitors have recently been identified as rare causes of DRESS syndrome.[15] **Table 1** identifies the most commonly implicated medications: those identified as "very probable" culprits in the RegiSCAR study (international registry of severe cutaneous adverse reactions to drugs).[16]

Pharmacogenetic Associations

HLA-I molecules are major histocompatibility complex proteins that function to present peptides to CD8+ T cells in humans.[14] Although the exact manner of hypersensitivity induction is under investigation, various HLA-I genotypes are regarded as "necessary but not sufficient" for developing DRESS with specific medications, as listed in **Table 2**.[24]

Table 2 is not exhaustive of all reported HLA associations, but summarizes some of the most widely recognized pharmacogenetic links. Not all medications known to cause DRESS have strong HLA linkages, and even those with known MHC predispositions may cause DRESS in other populations, therefore the diagnosis should remain in the differential for all populations, even if not classically considered "high risk" by genotype.

Clinical Features

Clinical manifestations of DRESS present on average 2 to 8 weeks after drug exposure.[9] The presentation is classically a fever greater than 38°C that may precede a morbilliform rash by up to 2 weeks.[4] The rash usually affects more than 50% body surface area and often demonstrates follicular accentuation (**Figs. 1** and **2**). Facial edema is seen in most cases, sometimes accompanied by pruritic facial erythema that spares the periorbital region (**Figs. 3** and **4**).[1] Mucosal involvement (cheilitis, oral erosions, or tonsillitis) is present in up to 50% of cases. Symptoms persist for weeks after discontinuation of the responsible drug.

Other required features are lymphadenopathy and internal organ involvement; hepatic abnormalities are typically reported, with aspartate aminotransferase (AST)/ALT/LDH elevations (greater than twice the upper limit of normal by some criteria) marking liver dysfunction.[2,6,10] Interstitial nephritis, interstitial pneumonitis, and

Table 1
Associated very probable culprit medications in drug reaction with eosinophilia and systemic symptoms[16]

Medication Class	Implicated Medications
Antiepileptic drugs	Carbamazepine Phenytoin Lamotrigine Oxcarbazepine Phenobarbital
Sulfonamides	Sulfasalazine Dapsone Sulfamethoxazole-trimethoprim Sulfadiazine
Antibiotics	Vancomycin Minocycline Amoxicillin Ampicillin/sulbactam
Uricosurics	Allopurinol

Table 2
HLA-I genotypes and medication associations in drug reaction with eosinophilia and systemic symptoms

Medication	HLA-I Genotype	Population
Abacavir	HLA-B*57:01	White[17]
Allopurinol	HLA-B*58:01	Han Chinese[18]
Carbamazepine	HLA-A*31:01	Japanese[a][19]
Dapsone	HLA-B*13:01	Chinese[20]
Phenytoin	HLA-A*24:02	Spanish Romani[21]
Vancomycin	HLA-A*32:01	European ancestry[22]

[a] Some studies report generalized increased risk across multiple ethnicities.[22] HLA DR3 and DQ2 (major histocompatibility complex II) haplotypes have also been reported in association with DRESS related to carbamazepine, without ethnic predilection.[23]

carditis also have also been reported as systemic manifestations, and some guidelines allow for any single internal organ involvement to satisfy diagnostic criteria for DRESS.[2,10]

A common misconception may be that eosinophilia is required to make the diagnosis of DRESS. Rather, although eosinophilia was historically reported, it is estimated to be present in at most 60% to 70% of DRESS cases.[6] Other hematologic abnormalities that may be present instead of eosinophilia are leukocytosis, lymphocytosis, or lymphocytopenia; presence of atypical lymphocytes; or thrombocytopenia.[2,6,10]

Evaluation

The evaluation of a suspected DRESS case hinges on laboratory tests and identifying the suspected culprit drug. Basic laboratory tests—complete blood count (CBC) with differential, complete metabolic panel (CMP), and urinalysis will reveal hematologic derangements and most renal and hepatic involvement. Coagulation studies, cardiac enzymes, human immunodeficiency virus (HIV) screening, erythrocyte sedimentation rate (ESR), and C-reactive protein (CRP) are also recommended to estimate the severity of disease. Swabs from lesions sent for virology and bacterial culture may

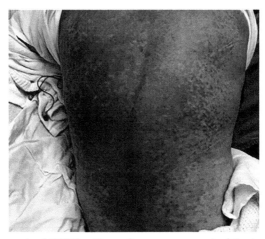

Fig. 1. Morbilliform rash of DRESS with confluence over most of the back.

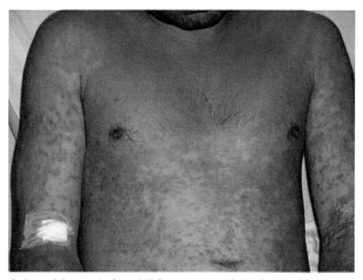

Fig. 2. Cephalocaudal spread of morbilliform DRESS rash on the trunk.

be considered to rule out alternative diagnoses or superinfection. Biopsy is not required, as histopathologic findings are variable, but if vesicles or bullae are present, biopsy taken adjacent to a blister may be useful to rule out an immunobullous disorder. Laboratory tests to rule out other potential causes of morbilliform eruptions may include antinuclear antibody, blood culture, hepatitis A/B/C virus serology, and chlamydia/mycoplasma antigens.[1]

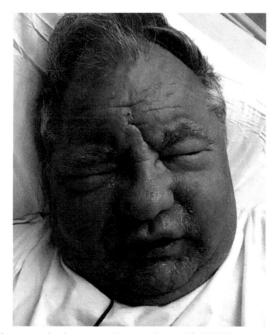

Fig. 3. Facial erythema and edema seen in a patient with DRESS.

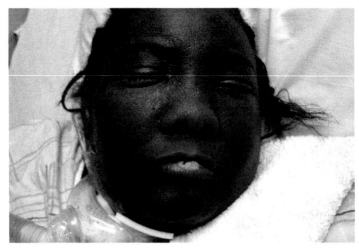

Fig. 4. DRESS with facial edema and erythema notably sparing the periorbital region. (*Courtesy*, Jeffrey P. Callen, MD.)

HHV-6 reactivation 2 to 3 weeks after onset of rash (marked by rise in HHV-6 IgG titers) has been demonstrated to be prevalent in most patients despite variable phenotypes or treatment.[6]

Diagnosis/Differential Diagnosis

Although there is not one confirmatory test or procedure for the diagnosis of DRESS/DIHS, there are 3 commonly cited sets of diagnostic criteria in the literature that may be referenced, summarized in **Table 3**.

Table 3
Proposed diagnostic criteria for drug reaction with eosinophilia and systemic symptoms/drug-induced hypersensitivity syndrome (DRESS/DIHS)

Bocquet et al,[2] 1996	RegiSCAR[10]	J-SCAR[a6]
All 3 criteria needed	Must fulfill 6 criteria: required components marked +	DIHS meets all 7, atypical DIHS meets first 5 criteria
1. Cutaneous eruption 2. Adenopathy ≥ 2 cm OR Hepatitis with transaminases > 2× upper limit of normal OR interstitial nephritis OR interstitial nephritis OR carditis 3. Eosinophilia > 1.5 × 10⁹/L OR atypical lymphocytes	1. Hospitalization + 2. Suspected drug related reaction + 3. Acute skin rash + 4. Fever >38°C 5. Enlarged lymph nodes in 2 sites 6. Involvement of at least one internal organ 7. Blood abnormalities	1. Maculopapular rash arising >3 wk after drug 2. Prolonged symptoms after discontinuation 3. Fever >38°C 4. Liver abnormalities 5. Leukocyte abnormalities 6. Lymphadenopathy 7. Human herpesvirus-6 reactivation

[a] Japanese study group of severe cutaneous adverse reactions to drugs.

DRESS should be discerned from other causes of fever and morbilliform or maculopapular rash. The differential diagnosis includes infectious processes, other types of cutaneous drug reactions, angioimmunoblastic T-cell lymphoma, Sezary syndrome, acute cutaneous lupus erythematosus, and hypereosinophilic syndrome. As summarized by Muzumdar and colleagues,[25] the following infectious processes may be considered, listed with distinguishing factors from DRESS/DIHS.

- Measles: cough, coryza, and conjunctivitis triad and cephalocaudal spread of rash not characteristic of DRESS
- Rubella: adenopathy and rash that starts on the face may be confusing for DRESS, but will have soft palate petechiae (Forchheimer spots) and positive serology
- Parvovirus: more prominent arthralgias and arthritis than in DRESS
- Meningococcemia: will feature prominent nuchal rigidity, altered mental status
- Mononucleosis: cervical lymphadenopathy, hepatosplenomegaly, and rash may be on the differential for DRESS, but the rash in mononucleosis appears much more rapidly after the onset of symptoms and resolves more quickly, 1 to 6 days after appearance

Exanthematous drug eruptions differ from DRESS in that they have shorter onset from drug exposure to rash (5–14 days) with low-grade fever, mucous membranes are not typically involved, and they lack visceral involvement.[25] AEDs with the greatest risk of rashes include phenytoin, carbamazepine, oxcarbazepine, and lamotrigine. Rashes associated with these agents typically start and resolve within 1 week of medication administration, and they lack systemic symptoms.[26]

MANAGEMENT

Once the diagnosis of DRESS has been made, it is critical to stop the suspected medication, taking into consideration the typically long latency between drug administration and onset of symptoms. Mild cases may be managed with potent topical steroid, but most will require systemic corticosteroids. In cases with significant renal or pulmonary involvement, oral prednisone 1 mg/kg or prednisone equivalent is given daily, tapered over 6 to 8 weeks.[1] The benefit of systemic corticosteroids in patients with isolated liver injury is unproven.[27] In recalcitrant cases, cyclosporine or other steroid-sparing immunosuppressive medications may be considered. Janus kinase inhibitors, intravenous immunoglobulin (IVIG), plasmapheresis, rituximab, and valganciclovir have all been reported though routine use is not recommended.[28]

Prognosis/Long-Term Sequelae

The mortality of DRESS is estimated between 2% and 10%, and typically results from fulminant hepatitis, for which transplantation is the only effective treatment option.[4,29] Other causes of mortality may be related to reactivation of HHV-6/7, Epstein-Barr virus, or provocation of autoimmune sequelae.[1] Certain drugs have been associated with specific late disease manifestations: allopurinol, dapsone, and carbamazepine have all been reported to cause kidney injury evidenced by hematuria and proteinuria without clinical symptoms. Minocycline is tied to lung pathology, as well as myocarditis presenting up to 4 months after cessation of medication (also seen with ampicillin).[4]

Other long-term consequences of DRESS are autoimmune disease: type 1 diabetes mellitus, graft-versus-host disease–like lesions, thyroid involvement, and systemic lupus erythematosus manifest in 10% of all patients, whether or not they were treated with steroids at diagnosis.[30]

STEVENS-JOHNSON SYNDROME/TOXIC EPIDERMAL NECROLYSIS
Epidemiology

SJS and TEN are rare, life-threatening SCARs, characterized by extensive bullae formation and sloughing of skin and mucosal surfaces. SJS and TEN represent different points on the spectrum of cutaneous involvement:

- SJS: less than 10% of total body surface area (BSA).
- SJS/TEN overlap: between 10% and 30% BSA.
- TEN: greater than 30% BSA.[31]

Incidence of SJS is reported to be 8 to 9 cases per million per year, with TEN occurring less frequently, between 1 and 2 cases per million per year.[32]

Risk Factors

Independent risk factors for developing SJS/TEN include hematologic malignancies, HIV (treated or untreated), systemic fungal infections, liver disease, and kidney disease. Increased risk has also been demonstrated in patients between 1 and 10 years and older than 70 years old.[33]

Highly associated culprit medications include antibacterial sulfonamides (sulfamethoxazole), antiepileptics (carbamazepine, phenytoin, phenobarbital, and lamotrigine), oxicam-type nonsteroidal anti-inflammatory drugs, nevirapine, and allopurinol.[14,31,33] As a class, aromatic antiepileptics represent the highest absolute risk, constituting 35% of all SJS/TEN cases, but as a single agent, allopurinol is the most commonly reported medication, identified in 20% of cases.[34] This risk is particularly increased for patients taking 200 mg or more of allopurinol daily.[35] Herbal remedies and biologic agents (CTLA-4 antagonists, PD-1 antibody nivolumab, epidermal growth factor receptor antagonist cetuximab, and V600E BRAF inhibitor vemurafenib) have all been identified in case reports as responsible for SJS/TEN, although not to the same degree as the more commonly prescribed medications listed previously.[33]

Importantly, certain medications have been demonstrated to have no increased risk for SJS/TEN; those include nonantibiotic sulfonamides (thiazide and furosemide diuretics, sulfonylureas), beta-blockers, angiotensin-converting enzyme inhibitors, calcium channel blockers, nonpantoprazole proton pump inhibitors, statins, oxicam-type analgesics (meloxicam), metformin, or oral contraceptives. Sertraline, a selective serotonin reuptake inhibitor, has been proposed in some instances to be a triggering medication, but this has not been consistent across all studies.[31,33,34]

Pharmacogenetic Associations

As with DRESS, certain HLA genotypes have been established as significant risks for developing SJS/TEN related to medications, the most widely reported of which are shown in **Table 4**.[36]

HLA-A*0206 has also been associated with cold medicine-triggered SJS/TEN with ocular complications, although not in a particular patient population.[33] As noted in **Table 3**, HLA-B*15:02, particularly in Han Chinese patients, is linked to SJS/TEN with multiple medications. As with DRESS, attention should be taken when prescribing any of these highly associated medications, and HLA genotyping should be routinely performed if the patient shares any genetically at-risk ancestry.

Table 4
HLA-I genotypes and medication associations in Stevens-Johnson syndrome/toxic epidermal necrolysis

Medication	HLA-I Genotype	Population
Sulfamethoxazole	HLA-B*38	European
Sulfamethoxazole-Trimethoprim	HLA-B*15:02-V*0801	Thai
Methazolamide	HLA-B*59:01 HLA-CW*1:02	Korean, Japanese
Lamotrigine	HLA-B*15:02	Han Chinese
Phenytoin	HLA-B*15:02	Han Chinese, Thai
Allopurinol	HLA-B*58:01	Han Chinese, Caucasian, Thai, Japanese
Carbamazepine[a]	HLA-B*15:02 HLA-A*31:01 HLA-B*15:11	Han Chinese (B*15:02)[14,31]
Aromatic antiepileptics (oxcarbazepine, phenytoin, lamotrigine)	HLA-B*15:02	Multiple/nonspecific[33]

[a] HLA alleles reported to have a protective effect in Asian patients treated with carbamazepine include HLA-B*4001, B*4601, B*5801.[36]

Clinical Features

Most cases of SJS/TEN present less than 8 weeks after initiation of the culprit medication, with a median time of less than 3 to 4 weeks for new drugs.[31] An abbreviated time to symptom onset (4.1 days) is seen in those with prior exposure to the medication.[35] Early lesions present as dusky, purpuric, atypical targetoid macules (in comparison to the typical raised targetoid lesions of erythema multiforme [EM] major), starting on the face, trunk, and upper extremities (**Figs. 5** and **6**).[33,37,38] Blisters arise anywhere

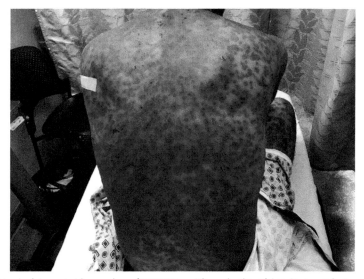

Fig. 5. Atypical targetoid macules of SJS/TEN, with early sloughing in some lesions.

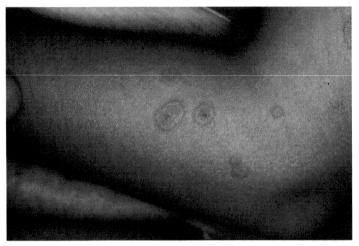

Fig. 6. Raised, typical targetoid lesions of EM. (*Courtesy,* Jeffrey P. Callen, MD.)

on the macules, and as the disease progresses, rupture easily and lead to sloughing of the skin surface (**Fig. 7**). In some cases, SJS/TEN presents as diffuse erythema progressing to blisters and erosions. Blisters will demonstrate a positive Nikolsky sign, where lateral shearing pressure on the surface of a bulla results in sloughing. Erosive involvement of mucosal surfaces, particularly oral and conjunctival, is characteristic,

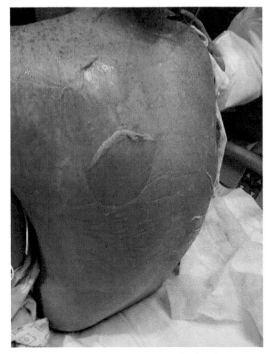

Fig. 7. Diffuse erythema and sheet-like sloughing on the back in TEN.

whereas the absence of any mucosal involvement should prompt consideration of a different diagnosis.[39] Oral lesions will often have gray-white pseudomembranes and crusting (**Fig. 8**), and ocular findings start with hyperemia, excessive tearing, and photophobia, but progress to corneal ulceration and anterior uveitis (**Fig. 9**).[37] Both undetached and detached erythematous skin is included in the calculation of total percent BSA involvement.[35] Systemic signs preceding cutaneous lesions are inconsistent, but when present, may include reports of pain on the skin, headache, sore throat, cough, myalgias, and malaise, generally between 1 to 3 days before cutaneous findings.[40]

There is no single laboratory abnormality that defines SJS/TEN. Patients are very ill, and will often demonstrate tachycardia and fever, which may make it more difficult to detect if/when sepsis from skin or peripheral line infection is lingering. Fever (>38°C), lymphopenia, and multiple metabolic derangements are also consistently noted.[37,38] Certain laboratory values have been identified as potential prognostic markers (elevated serum urea, glucose, decreased serum bicarbonate) but independently do not make the diagnosis.[41]

Histologic features taken of affected but noneroded skin will demonstrate subepidermal blistering, apoptotic keratinocytes, and full-thickness epidermal necrosis, with minimal inflammatory infiltrate. Importantly, when autoimmune blistering diseases are in the differential, biopsy of perilesional skin for direct immunofluorescence studies should be obtained.[33]

Evaluation

Evaluation of a suspected SJS/TEN case after careful history to elicit medication administration timelines and a thorough physical examination to determine extent of skin disease should also include basic laboratory tests, particularly CBC and CMP to use in prognostic calculations. Other laboratory tests/studies that are generally obtained in the workup of any SCAR are coagulation factors, ESR, CRP, HIV screening, and plain chest radiograph.[1] Biopsy helps to confirm a case and rule out other causes

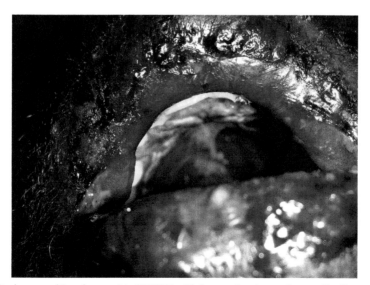

Fig. 8. Oral mucosal involvement in SJS/TEN with hemorrhagic crusting on the lips and gray-white pseudomembrane formation on the hard palate.

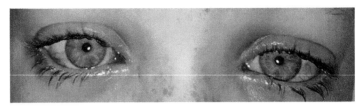

Fig. 9. Conjunctival injection in SJS/TEN.

of extensive blistering.[31] When fever, autonomic instability, or significant leukocytosis are present, there should be a low threshold for obtaining blood cultures, as sepsis from a skin or line infection is the most common complication seen in these patients.[1] Bacterial swabs from line insertion sites have not been shown to have high utility on their own, as they do not demonstrate strong positive predictive value for bloodstream infections, but some suggest collecting superficial swabs in conjunction with blood and urine cultures to corroborate the evidence if infection is present.[42]

Diagnosis/Differential Diagnosis

The differential diagnosis of SJS/TEN may be broad, with consideration to various diseases given based on the extent of skin blistering and sloughing. Commonly, the following diagnoses are included in the differential, with distinguishing factors provided[31,33,40]:

- EM major (EM with mucosal involvement): raised targetoid lesions predominate on the extremities and do not involve more than 10% BSA. Triggered by an infection rather than a medication.
- Staphylococcal scalded skin syndrome: lacks mucosal involvement, features an intraepidermal split on histopathology, compared with the subepidermal split seen in SJS/TEN.
- Generalized bullous fixed drug eruption: as the name implies, lesions recur in the same locations on repeated exposure to the culprit medication, should involve less than 10% BSA, and have less severe systemic symptoms compared with SJS/TEN.
- Autoimmune blistering diseases (pemphigus vulgaris, bullous pemphigoid, IgA linear dermatosis, paraneoplastic pemphigus): will all demonstrate various positive findings on direct and indirect immunofluorescent studies, which will be nonreactive in SJS/TEN.
- Toxic shock syndrome: features both raised and flat atypical targetoid lesions without bullae or vesicles, with nonerosive mucosal involvement.

In 1 retrospective review of inpatient dermatology consults for suspected SJS/TEN, a diagnosis other than SJS/TEN was ultimately given to 71.6% of patients. In addition to the preceding diagnoses, other mimickers identified included morbilliform drug rash, viral exanthem, DRESS, AGEP, and urticaria multiforme. The presence of positive Nikolsky sign, atypical targetoid lesions, fever, and lymphopenia together more strongly suggest SJS/TEN.[38]

Management

Stopping the culprit medication is paramount to management of SJS/TEN. Construction of a medication administration chart may be considered to help delineate the timeline of various drugs against symptom evolution, especially in cases of polypharmacy. The prodrome of headache, sore throat, cough, myalgias, and malaise that can occur up to 3 days before skin eruption should be taken into consideration when constructing the medication timeline to avoid assigning causality to a medication started for prodrome symptoms. The algorithm of drug causality for epidermal necrosis (ALDEN) has also been developed to help in determining the culprit drug, but again should be used as an adjunctive tool, along with the history and disease timeline.[31] Any medications not critical to acute management should be discontinued, including any herbal supplements the patient may be taking.

Although there is not one single treatment that is agreed on as the gold standard for SJS/TEN, supportive care and therapy targeted to minimizing long-term sequelae are imperative. Patients should ideally be in a burn unit or intensive care facility, with room temperatures maintained between 30 and 32°C. Wound care services should focus on covering erosions with nonadherent dressings, and as able, avoiding placement of cannulas/peripheral lines in active blistering areas.[1] With extensive sloughing of epidermis, monitoring for fluid losses and balancing nutritional status is important. Fluid replacement requirements are approximately one-third of the amount needed for burn patients. If oropharyngeal mucosal involvement is severe enough to significantly limit oral intake, nasogastric tube–administered nutrition should be initiated.[31,40] Prevention and prompt treatment of infection are of paramount importance, but prophylactic antibiotics are not recommended. Ophthalmology should be consulted for management of ocular disease to prevent long-term complications. In patients with vulvovaginal involvement, early evaluation and treatment by gynecology is imperative to prevent adhesions.

Adjuvant systemic therapy is typically considered within the first 24 to 48 hours of treatment. Treatment considerations in the literature vary between systemic corticosteroids, tumor necrosis factor (TNF) alpha inhibitors, cyclosporine, and IVIG.

- Corticosteroids have not consistently demonstrated survival advantage over other options in various studies, and still confer risks of infection (including *Candida* sepsis) and complications that would not be seen with supportive care alone.[40]
- Etanercept (a TNF alpha inhibitor) has shown greater improvement in skin and oral mucosa, with decreased incidence of gastrointestinal hemorrhage compared with corticosteroid-treated patients in 1 randomized controlled trial.[1,43] The same study reported successful halting of disease progression in 1 case when given 1 dose of etanercept (50 mg subcutaneous [SQ]) with IVIG 20 g daily for 3 days.[43] Another dosing schedule is etanercept 50 mg (25 mg if patient weight is <65 kg) SQ twice weekly until lesions demonstrate reepithelialization.[44] Among TNF inhibitors, etanercept may have advantages over infliximab, including subcutaneous rather than IV infusion administration, with lower risk of active tuberculosis and invasive fungal infections.[43]
- In one meta-analysis, IVIG did not demonstrate a mortality benefit when compared with predicted mortality calculated on SCORTEN (SCORe of Toxic Epidermal Necrosis) criteria; in comparison, cyclosporine, given at 3 to 5 mg/kg per day, has shown favorable outcomes in mortality and when compared with corticosteroids, along with shorter time to reepithelialization and shorter hospital stays.[1,31,45]
- Combination therapies (IVIG with corticosteroids, IVIG with TNF inhibitors) have not yet been studied in large enough cohorts to determine significant benefit of any over the other, but may be considered in cases recalcitrant to single-agent therapy.[40]

Prognosis/Long-Term Sequelae

On the spectrum of disease, SJS carries the more favorable prognosis, with estimated mortality of 5%. As extent of disease progresses, so does mortality: 30% for SJS/TEN overlap, up to 50% for TEN.[46] The SCORTEN criteria were proposed for predicting mortality based on 7 independent risk factors for death in patients with SJS/TEN: age, malignancy, tachycardia, degree of epidermal detachment at presentation, and serum values of urea, glucose, and bicarbonate. The total score ranges from 0 to ≥5, with probability of death increasing with score (**Table 5**).[41] SCORTEN calculations have been reported to be most prognostically accurate on the third day of hospitalization, and many recommend calculating prognosis on both days 1 and 3.[40]

The primary cause of mortality is multiorgan failure from sepsis, often from skin or peripheral line infection.[1,47] Hypovolemia from fluid losses can also contribute to acute morbidity.[31] Blisters and erosions typically heal without significant scarring. Cutaneous complications, however, occur in 23% to 100% of patients with SJS/TEN, with eruptive melanocytic nevi between 3 weeks and 3 years following the acute episode, along with dyspigmentation, milia, pruritus, and xerosis in areas of healed blistering.[32] Nail shedding with abnormal regrowth and hair loss (telogen effluvium) are common sequelae.

Involvement of mucosal surfaces can lead to strictures (oral, ocular, genitourinary), with the most common disabling long-term complication stemming from ocular sequelae. Problems may range from dryness to conjunctival and bulbar scarring causing symblepharon, ectropion/entropion, or trichiasis, with risk of vision loss after profound ulceration and scarring.[31,32] Many of these patients will need artificial tears and scleral lenses to decrease risk of trauma long-term.[32] Despite the potential severity of ocular complications, up to 75% of patients who experience some form of mucosal involvement will have complete healing by 2 months, increasing to more than 95% at 1 year.[32]

Long-term data show a mortality rate of up to 34% at 1 year. The greatest risk factors for mortality outside of the acute illness phase are old age and medical comorbidities, which can be useful factors to consider when counseling patients on prognosis.[32,47]

Table 5
SCORe of Toxic Epidermal Necrosis (SCORTEN) calculation and predicted mortality

Category	SCORTEN Parameters	Points
Age	> 40 y	1
Malignancy	Point given if present/detected	1
Tachycardia	Heart rate >120 beats per minute	1
% Body surface area (BSA) involvement	Initial epidermal detachment of >10% BSA	1
Hyperuricemia	Urea > 28 mg/dL	1
Hyperglycemia	Glucose >252 mg/dL	1
Serum bicarbonate	Bicarbonate <20 mEq/L	1

SCORTEN Total Points	Predicted Mortality (%)
0–1	3.2
2	12.1
3	35.8
4	58.3
5–7	90

ACUTE GENERALIZED EXANTHEMATOUS PUSTULOSIS
Epidemiology

AGEP was historically thought to represent a subset of generalized pustular psoriasis, but received recognition as a distinct entity in 1968, and was given its current name in 1980.[48,49] It has a reported incidence of 1 to 5 cases per million per year, slightly higher than SJS/TEN.[50] Medications constitute most culprits in AGEP, although a small portion have been attributed to acute infections, spider bites, and iodine-based intravenous contrast media. Most cases occur in patients 27 to 74 years of age, with a mean age of 56 years; women slightly outnumber men.[51,52]

Risk Factors

Despite its early associations as a potential pustular psoriasis variant, no significant difference between patients with AGEP and controls has been found regarding personal or family history of psoriasis, or history of psoriasis treatment.[52] No specific chronic conditions are typically associated with developing AGEP, but a number of acute infections have been reported as triggers in a minority (10%) of cases.[49] These infrequent causes include parvovirus B19, cytomegalovirus, coxsackie B4, *Mycoplasma pneumoniae, Escherichia coli,* and *Chlamydia pneumoniae.*[48,49]

The vast majority (more than 90%) of AGEP cases are attributable to medications; of those, beta-lactam antibiotics are the most common.[50] Other frequently reported medications include aminopenicillins, quinolones, sulfonamides, ketoconazole, fluconazole, terbinafine, diltiazem, hydroxychloroquine, and pristinamycin (a macrolide antibiotic not used in the United States).[48,51,52]

Pharmacogenetic Associations

Unlike the other SCARs reviewed here, AGEP has not been significantly linked to variations in HLA genotypes. Individuals with mutations in the interleukin-36 receptor antagonist gene may have increased susceptibility to AGEP; this same mutation is also seen in those with generalized pustular psoriasis. Lip and/or oral involvement is more likely to be seen with this mutation.[48,49]

Clinical Features

AGEP presents with sudden onset of hundreds of sterile, nonfollicular, pinhead-sized pustules on an erythematous base.[53] The face and intertriginous regions are first involved, followed by rapid and diffuse spread to encompass the rest of the body (**Fig. 10**).[52,54] During healing, desquamation of involved areas is characteristic (**Fig. 11**).[48] Pruritus and erythema may precede pustules, and acral and facial edema are common.[51] Mucosal involvement is reported in 20% to 25% of patients, and when present, is limited to a single mucosal surface (typically oral), in contrast to other SCARs that may involve multiple mucosal regions simultaneously.[49]

Systemic involvement occurs in an estimated 17% to 20% of patients, and includes fever, leukocytosis, eosinophilia, hypocalcemia, elevated absolute neutrophil count and CRP. Transaminase elevation (in either a hepatocellular or cholestatic pattern), reversible reduction in creatinine clearance, and pleural effusion have also been reported.[48,49]

Typical cases of AGEP have symptom onset within 48 hours of medication administration, with antibiotics associated with shorter latent period (1 day), up to 11 days in non–antibiotic-mediated cases.[52] The course is typically self-limiting, and on withdrawal of the culprit medication, symptoms resolve within a week.[48]

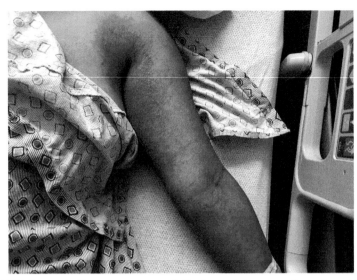

Fig. 10. AGEP demonstrating numerous nonfollicular pustules on erythematous skin extending from the axilla.

Evaluation

As with other SCARs, there is not a single laboratory test that is diagnostic of AGEP. Rather, the cutaneous eruption in the appropriate clinical setting (recent medication administration) is suggestive of the diagnosis. Routine laboratory tests (CBC with differential, CMP, serum albumin, and CRP) should be followed to detect potential

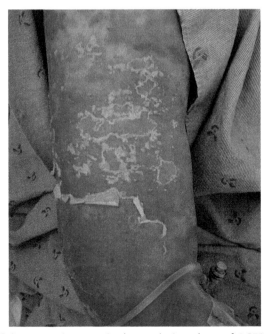

Fig. 11. Superficial desquamation seen in the resolution phase of AGEP.

systemic involvement. Significant neutrophilia and CRP elevation together may be indicators of hepatic, pulmonary, renal, or bone marrow involvement.[53] Bacterial and fungal swabs taken of pustule contents may also help to rule out other considerations in the differential, as pustules in AGEP are sterile and should not grow in culture (unless superinfection is present).

Biopsy results are not pathognomonic for AGEP but may add supporting evidence or aid in the exclusion of other conditions in the differential diagnosis. Typical histologic features in AGEP are intracorneal, subcorneal, and intraepidermal pustules with papillary dermal edema, along with superficial, interstitial, and mid-dermal infiltrate with an abundance of neutrophils.[48]

Diagnosis/Differential Diagnosis

EuroSCAR proposed a set of diagnostic criteria in 2007, and an AGEP validation score has subsequently been assigned to these criteria.[49,51] The broad categories of assessed criteria are the following:

- Morphology (pustules, erythema, distribution pattern, postpustular desquamation)
- Clinical course (rapid onset and resolution, fever, elevation in polymorphonuclear neutrophils)
- Histologic findings consistent with AGEP

Points are assigned or subtracted for each criterion based on whether or not the findings are typical or atypical for AGEP.[55] Scores may range from 0 to 12, with a total between 8 to 12 points considered definitive for AGEP.[49]

The differential diagnosis for AGEP is listed as follows, with features that help distinguish each entity.[48,49]

- Bacterial folliculitis: displays folliculocentric pustules, bacterial culture positive on pustule contents
- Bullous impetigo: more common in young children with pustules and vesicles most common on the head, neck, and intertriginous areas. Erosions develop honey-colored crust and cultures show *Staphylococcus aureus*
- Subcorneal pustular dermatosis (Sneddon-Wilkinson disease): recurrent crops of pustules in flexural regions, lacking systemic symptoms, possibly related to an underlying gammopathy
- Fungal infections: fungal growth on cultures of pustule contents
- Pustular psoriasis: demonstrates slower onset, pustules more likely to coalesce; histology will also show psoriasiform acanthosis, not seen in AGEP[49]
- DRESS: starts on the face (not intertriginous regions), with a longer latent and resolution period.

Management

Consistent with the theme of SCARs, the mainstay of treatment in AGEP is to remove the offending medication. Once the triggering drug is discontinued, symptoms typically resolve within a week, and the course is typically uncomplicated.[52] Supportive care often includes moist dressings and topical steroids. Oral steroid courses have been used in attempts to hasten disease clearance, but evidence of a significant reduction in duration is lacking.[48,51] Topical antibiotics may be used to prevent superinfection, which is one of the main risks for complication in an otherwise straightforward course.[50]

Prognosis/Long-Term Sequelae

AGEP has the lowest mortality of all SCARs, at 2% to 5%.[56] Death is typically due to end-organ dysfunction and disseminated intravascular coagulation.[48] Most cases, though, resolve uneventfully, with fever and cutaneous superinfection the most common complications. Unlike DRESS and SJS/TEN, long-term sequelae are not characteristic, and once the offending medication is removed, the overwhelming majority of patients do very well.[49]

CLINICS CARE POINTS

- SCARs (AGEP, DRESS, SJS/TEN) are rare diseases triggered by medications.

- Identifying and discontinuing the culprit medication is essential to management of all SCARs. Additional therapies and supportive care are often included based on extent of disease.

- Genetic predisposition to SCARs based on HLA genotype is most strongly seen with DRESS but has also been witnessed in SJS/TEN. AGEP does not demonstrate a significant genetic/medication link.

- On average, DRESS presents 2 to 6 weeks, SJS/TEN 3 to 4 weeks, and AGEP within days after culprit medication administration.

- Mortality of all SCARs ranges from less than 5% for AGEP, 2% to 10% for DRESS, and up to 50% for TEN.[1,29,56]

REFERENCES

1. Ardern-Jones MR, Mockenhaupt M. Making a diagnosis in severe cutaneous drug hypersensitivity reactions. Curr Opin Allergy Clin Immunol 2019;19(4): 283–93.
2. Bocquet H, Bagot M, Roujeau JC. Drug-induced pseudolymphoma and drug hypersensitivity syndrome (Drug Rash with Eosinophilia and Systemic Symptoms: DRESS). Semin Cutan Med Surg 1996;15(4):250–7.
3. Wolfson AR, Zhou L, Li Y, et al. Drug Reaction with Eosinophilia and Systemic Symptoms (DRESS) syndrome identified in the electronic health record allergy module. J Allergy Clin Immunol Pract 2019;7(2):633–40.
4. Husain Z, Reddy BY, Schwartz RA. DRESS syndrome: part I. Clinical perspectives. J Am Acad Dermatol 2013;68(5):693, e691-614; [quiz 706-698].
5. Fernando SL. Drug-reaction eosinophilia and systemic symptoms and drug-induced hypersensitivity syndrome. Australas J Dermatol 2014;55(1):15–23.
6. Shiohara T, Iijima M, Ikezawa Z, et al. The diagnosis of a DRESS syndrome has been sufficiently established on the basis of typical clinical features and viral reactivations. Br J Dermatol 2007;156(5):1083–4.
7. Ben M'Rad M, Leclerc-Mercier S, Blanche P, et al. Drug-induced hypersensitivity syndrome. Medicine 2009;88(3):131–40.
8. Kumari R, Timshina DK, Thappa DM. Drug hypersensitivity syndrome. Indian J Dermatol Venereol Leprol 2011;77(1):7–15.
9. Tashiro Y, Azukizawa H, Asada H, et al. Drug-induced hypersensitivity syndrome/drug reaction with eosinophilia and systemic symptoms due to lamotrigine differs from that due to other drugs. J Dermatol 2019;46(3):226–33.

10. Watanabe H. Recent advances in drug-induced hypersensitivity syndrome/drug reaction with eosinophilia and systemic symptoms. J Immunol Res 2018; 2018:1–10.
11. James J, Sammour YM, Virata AR, et al. Drug Reaction with Eosinophilia and Systemic Symptoms (DRESS) syndrome secondary to furosemide: case report and review of literature. Am J Case Rep 2018;19:163–70.
12. Madigan LM, Fox LP. Vancomycin-associated drug-induced hypersensitivity syndrome. J Am Acad Dermatol 2019;81(1):123–8.
13. Hiransuthikul A, Rattananupong T, Klaewsongkram J, et al. Drug-induced hypersensitivity syndrome/drug reaction with eosinophilia and systemic symptoms (DIHS/DRESS): 11 years retrospective study in Thailand. Allergol Int 2016; 65(4):432–8.
14. Fan WL, Shiao MS, Hui RC, et al. HLA association with drug-induced adverse reactions. J Immunol Res 2017;2017:3186328.
15. Coleman EL, Olamiju B, Leventhal JS. The life-threatening eruptions of immune checkpoint inhibitor therapy. Clin Dermatol 2020;38(1):94–104.
16. Kardaun SH, Sekula P, Valeyrie-Allanore L, et al. Drug reaction with eosinophilia and systemic symptoms (DRESS): an original multisystem adverse drug reaction. Results from the prospective RegiSCAR study. Br J Dermatol 2013;169(5): 1071–80.
17. Redwood AJ, Pavlos RK, White KD, et al. HLAs: key regulators of T-cell-mediated drug hypersensitivity. Hla 2018;91(1):3–16.
18. Hung SI, Chung WH, Jee SH, et al. Genetic susceptibility to carbamazepine-induced cutaneous adverse drug reactions. Pharmacogenet Genomics 2006; 16(4):297–306.
19. Kashiwagi M, Aihara M, Takahashi Y, et al. Human leukocyte antigen genotypes in carbamazepine-induced severe cutaneous adverse drug response in Japanese patients. J Dermatol 2008;35(10):683–5.
20. Liu H, Wang Z, Bao F, et al. Evaluation of prospective HLA-B*13:01 screening to prevent dapsone hypersensitivity syndrome in patients with leprosy. JAMA Dermatol 2019;155(6):666–72.
21. Mullan KA, Anderson A, Illing PT, et al. HLA-associated antiepileptic drug-induced cutaneous adverse reactions. Hla 2019;93(6):417–35.
22. Konvinse KC, Trubiano JA, Pavlos R, et al. HLA-A*32:01 is strongly associated with vancomycin-induced drug reaction with eosinophilia and systemic symptoms. J Allergy Clin Immunol 2019;144(1):183–92.
23. Pirmohamed M, Lin K, Chadwick D, et al. TNFalpha promoter region gene polymorphisms in carbamazepine-hypersensitive patients. Neurology 2001;56(7): 890–6.
24. Criado PR, Criado RF, Avancini JM, et al. Drug reaction with Eosinophilia and Systemic Symptoms (DRESS)/Drug-induced Hypersensitivity Syndrome (DIHS): a review of current concepts. An Bras Dermatol 2012;87(3):435–49.
25. Muzumdar S, Rothe MJ, Grant-Kels JM. The rash with maculopapules and fever in adults. Clin Dermatol 2019;37(2):109–18.
26. Mani R, Monteleone C, Schalock PC, et al. Rashes and other hypersensitivity reactions associated with antiepileptic drugs: a review of current literature. Seizure 2019;71:270–8.
27. Ichai P, Laurent-Bellue A, Saliba F, et al. Acute liver failure/injury related to drug reaction with eosinophilia and systemic symptoms: outcomes and prognostic factors. Transplantation 2017;101(8):1830–7.

28. Cho YT, Chu CY. Treatments for severe cutaneous adverse reactions. J Immunol Res 2017;2017:1503709.
29. Chen YC, Chiu HC, Chu CY. Drug reaction with eosinophilia and systemic symptoms: a retrospective study of 60 cases. Arch Dermatol 2010;146(12):1373–9.
30. Kano Y, Tohyama M, Aihara M, et al. Sequelae in 145 patients with drug-induced hypersensitivity syndrome/drug reaction with eosinophilia and systemic symptoms: survey conducted by the Asian Research Committee on Severe Cutaneous Adverse Reactions (ASCAR). J Dermatol 2015;42(3):276–82.
31. Mockenhaupt M. Stevens-Johnson syndrome and toxic epidermal necrolysis: clinical patterns, diagnostic considerations, etiology, and therapeutic management. Semin Cutan Med Surg 2014;33(1):10–6.
32. Lee HY, Walsh SA, Creamer D. Long-term complications of Stevens-Johnson syndrome/toxic epidermal necrolysis (SJS/TEN): the spectrum of chronic problems in patients who survive an episode of SJS/TEN necessitates multidisciplinary follow-up. Br J Dermatol 2017;177(4):924–35.
33. Lerch M, Mainetti C, Terziroli Beretta-Piccoli B, et al. Current perspectives on Stevens-Johnson syndrome and toxic epidermal necrolysis. Clin Rev Allergy Immunol 2018;54(1):147–76.
34. Frey N, Bodmer M, Bircher A, et al. Stevens-Johnson syndrome and toxic epidermal necrolysis in association with commonly prescribed drugs in outpatient care other than anti-epileptic drugs and antibiotics: a population-based case-control study. Drug Saf 2019;42(1):55–66.
35. Miliszewski MA, Kirchhof MG, Sikora S, et al. Stevens-Johnson syndrome and toxic epidermal necrolysis: an analysis of triggers and implications for improving prevention. Am J Med 2016;129(11):1221–5.
36. Wang Q, Sun S, Xie M, et al. Association between the HLA-B alleles and carbamazepine-induced SJS/TEN: a meta-analysis. Epilepsy Res 2017;135:19–28.
37. Duong TA, Valeyrie-Allanore L, Wolkenstein P, et al. Severe cutaneous adverse reactions to drugs. Lancet 2017;390(10106):1996–2011.
38. Weinkle A, Pettit C, Jani A, et al. Distinguishing Stevens-Johnson syndrome/toxic epidermal necrolysis from clinical mimickers during inpatient dermatologic consultation-A retrospective chart review. J Am Acad Dermatol 2019;81(3):749–57.
39. Wolf R, Parish JL, Parish LC. The rash that presents as target lesions. Clin Dermatol 2019;37(2):148–58.
40. Schneider JA, Cohen PR. Stevens-Johnson Syndrome and toxic epidermal necrolysis: a concise review with a comprehensive summary of therapeutic interventions emphasizing supportive measures. Adv Ther 2017;34(6):1235–44.
41. Bastuji-Garin S, Fouchard N, Bertocchi M, et al. SCORTEN: a severity-of-illness score for toxic epidermal necrolysis. J Invest Dermatol 2000;115(2):149–53.
42. Richard EB, Hamer D, Musso MW, et al. Variability in management of patients with SJS/TEN: a survey of burn unit directors. J Burn Care Res 2018;39(4):585–92.
43. Wang R, Zhong S, Tu P, et al. Rapid remission of Stevens-Johnson syndrome by combination therapy using etanercept and intravenous immunoglobulin and a review of the literature. Dermatol Ther 2019;32(4):e12832.
44. Wang CW, Yang LY, Chen CB, et al. Randomized, controlled trial of TNF-α antagonist in CTL-mediated severe cutaneous adverse reactions. J Clin Invest 2018;128(3):985–96.
45. Shokeen D. Cyclosporine in SJS/TEN management: a brief review. Cutis 2016;97(3):E17–8.

46. Chung WH, Wang CW, Dao RL. Severe cutaneous adverse drug reactions. J Dermatol 2016;43(7):758–66.
47. Torres-Navarro I, Briz-Redón Á, Botella-Estrada R. Accuracy of SCORTEN to predict the prognosis of Stevens-Johnson syndrome/toxic epidermal necrolysis: a systematic review and meta-analysis. J Eur Acad Dermatol Venereol 2020; 34(9):2066–77.
48. Szatkowski J, Schwartz RA. Acute generalized exanthematous pustulosis (AGEP): a review and update. J Am Acad Dermatol 2015;73(5):843–8.
49. Feldmeyer L, Heidemeyer K, Yawalkar N. Acute generalized exanthematous pustulosis: pathogenesis, genetic background, clinical variants and therapy. Int J Mol Sci 2016;17(8).
50. DaCunha M, Moore S, Kaplan D. Cephalexin-induced acute generalized exanthematous pustulosis. Dermatol Rep 2018;10(2):7686.
51. Ross CL, Shevchenko A, Mollanazar NK, et al. Acute generalized exanthematous pustulosis due to terbinafine. Dermatol Ther 2018;31(4):e12617.
52. Sidoroff A, Dunant A, Viboud C, et al. Risk factors for acute generalized exanthematous pustulosis (AGEP)-results of a multinational case-control study (Euro-SCAR). Br J Dermatol 2007;157(5):989–96.
53. Schmitz B, Sorrells T, Glass JS. Acute generalized exanthematous pustulosis caused by pantoprazole. Cutis 2018;101(5):e22–3.
54. Castner NB, Harris JC, Motaparthi K. Cyclosporine for corticosteroid-refractory acute generalized exanthematous pustulosis due to hydroxychloroquine. Dermatol Ther 2018;31(5):e12660.
55. Botelho LFF, Picosse FR, Padilha MH, et al. Acute generalized exanthematous pustulosis induced by cefepime: a case report. Case Rep Dermatol 2010; 2(2):82–7.
56. Saissi EH, Beau-Salinas F, Jonville-Béra AP, et al. [Drugs associated with acute generalized exanthematic pustulosis]. Ann Dermatol Venereol 2003;130(6–7): 612–8.

An Approach to Patients with Alopecia

Taylor A. Jamerson, BA[a], Crystal Aguh, MD[b],*

KEYWORDS

- Alopecia • Hair loss • Nonscarring alopecia • Scarring alopecia • Cicatricial alopecia

KEY POINTS

- Hair loss is exceedingly common in the United States, affecting both men and women.
- The clinical distinction between nonscarring and scarring hair loss arguably is one of the most important steps in making an accurate diagnosis.
- Although nonscarring alopecia generally is more prevalent, with several treatment options for restoration of hair growth, scarring alopecia often results in permanent hair loss and therapies are targeted at preventing progressive hair loss.

INTRODUCTION

Alopecia is a common and distressing medical condition affecting a majority of men and women worldwide by middle age. The psychosocial impact of hair loss can be substantial on patients. Not only are psychiatric disorders, such as depression and anxiety, exceedingly common among patients with hair loss compared with the general population, but also these individuals report a loss of confidence, heightened self-consciousness, and low self-esteem.[1,2]

Considering the significant emotional and physical burden of alopecia, it is essential for clinicians to regard hair loss as more than a cosmetic issue. Alopecia often can be a sign of various systemic conditions, such as autoimmune disease, anemia, nutritional deficiency, and chronic infection. A lack of thorough clinical evaluation or appropriate treatment can contribute to not only patient dissatisfaction but also, importantly, the identification of medically significant conditions.

A detailed patient history and physical examination are key to making distinctions between various forms of alopecia and should focus on establishing time of onset, recent stressors, changes in medications, hairstyling and hair care practices, and family history of hair loss. For simplicity, alopecia can be categorized primarily into 2 subtypes: nonscarring (noncicatricial) and scarring (cicatricial).

[a] University of Michigan Medical School, 1050 Wall Street, Apartment 2D, Ann Arbor, MI 48105, USA; [b] Department of Dermatology, Johns Hopkins University School of Medicine, 10710 Charter Drive, Shared Suite 420, Baltimore, MD 21044, USA
* Corresponding author.
E-mail address: cagi1@jhmi.edu

Med Clin N Am 105 (2021) 599–610
https://doi.org/10.1016/j.mcna.2021.04.002
0025-7125/21/© 2021 Elsevier Inc. All rights reserved.

medical.theclinics.com

NONSCARRING ALOPECIA

The term, *nonscarring alopecia*, refers to the patency of the follicular unit, which remains intact during the progression of hair loss. These processes can be focal, involving patches of hair loss, or diffuse, involving the entire scalp. Systemic immunologic processes can be an underlying cause of nonscarring hair loss and involve other areas of the body, including the face, extremities, axillae, and genitalia. An accurate diagnosis of nonscarring alopecias often can be made without the need for a scalp biopsy, and treatment centers on the restoration of hair growth.

Androgenetic Alopecia

Androgenetic alopecia (AGA), also referred to as male or female pattern hair loss, is the most prevalent form of progressive hair loss, affecting 70% of men and 50% of women by the age of 50.[3] Although more common in patients over the age of 50, it can present with varying age of onset and disease severity.[4] AGA is thought to be a polygenetic condition caused by the interaction of environmental factors and several genes, leading to increased 5α-reductase activity, an enzyme responsible for converting free testosterone into dihydrotestosterone (DHT).[4] The resulting elevation in DHT leads to a gradual shortening of the anagen phase, or growth phase, of the hair cycle and miniaturization of the hair follicle.[5]

In men, AGA often manifests as thinning along the scalp vertex and bitemporal hairline with relative sparing of the occipital scalp but also can present with recession of the frontal hairline.[6] Hair loss sometimes occurs rapidly with extensive involvement in men, and the end stage of this condition can give the scalp a smooth or shiny appearance, mimicking end-stage fibrosis, reminiscent of cicatricial alopecia. Contrarily, woman rarely progress to near baldness or complete baldness and instead have thinning on the crown and frontal scalp with characteristic widening of the frontal part, described as resembling the pattern of a Christmas tree.[7] In women presenting with early-onset AGA in the teen years and early 20s, a work-up for hormonal irregularities, such as polycystic ovarian syndrome, can be useful, especially if signs of hirsutism are present.[8]

Topical minoxidil is considered a first-line therapy for AGA in both men and women.[9] Although its mechanism of action is unclear, it partially works by reversing miniaturization of the hair follicle and lengthening the anagen phase of the hair cycle.[10] It is readily available over the counter as a foam or solution in 2% (primarily for women) and 5% concentrations (primarily for men), with the latter showing higher efficacy for both men and women.[11] The foam, which unlike the solution does not contain propylene glycol, is less likely to lead to an irritant contact dermatitis and is suitable for those who wash their hair frequently enough to avoid buildup of the product on the hair.[12] For women of African descent with tightly curled or coiled hair requiring less frequent washing, a solution may be preferred, because it is less likely to build up within the hair shaft over time. To minimize the risk of an irritant contact reaction from the solution's alcohol base, patients are advised to apply a light oil to the hair following application.

For patients who fail or are unable to tolerate topical minoxidil, additional treatment options include oral antiandrogen agents, such as finasteride and spironolactone. In contrast to topical agents, recommended oral therapy differs for men and women. In men, finasteride works by blocking the activity of type 2 5α-reductase and has demonstrated promising results when initiated early, at a dose of 1 mg once daily.[13] Patients should be counseled on the potential side effects, including impotence, sexual dysfunction, and the rare development of post-finasteride syndrome, defined as persistent physical, sexual, and mental adverse effects sustained even after discontinuation of finasteride.[14] Initiation of finasteride in women has not been found efficacious.[15,16] Instead, spironolactone has demonstrated efficacy when used as an adjunct treatment in women due to its antiandrogen effects on hair follicles in the scalp.[17,18] This treatment option is effective in particularly premenopausal women with hormonal abnormalities and is recommended at a starting dose of 50 mg daily, titrated up to doses ranging from 100 mg daily to 200 mg daily.[19] Oral antiandrogen agents are contraindicated in women who are pregnant or planning to become pregnant, because they can cause abnormalities of male fetal genitalia.[20]

Telogen Effluvium

Telogen effluvium is a form of temporary, nonscarring hair loss without predisposition to specific demographics.[21] It is a reactive process, with common triggers, listed in **Table 1**, leading to an abnormality of normal hair cycling.[22] Hair follicle activity goes through 3 cyclical phases: anagen, catagen, and telogen. In normal adults, an estimated 85% to 90% of hairs on the scalp are in the anagen phase, 10% to 15% in the telogen phase, and 1% in the catagen phase.[23] Telogen effluvium results when hair follicles prematurely enter the telogen phase of the hair cycle or when the telogen phase is shortened, leading to excessive shedding of these hairs 2 months to 3 months following the inciting event or stressor.[24] Recent reports have linked telogen effluvium with prior SARS-CoV-2 infections and at least 1 study has noted an increased incidence in minority communities that have been heavily affected by COVID-19 infections.[25]

Patients typically present with sudden, diffuse hair shedding. A hair pull test can be performed, where a small section of approximately 50 to 100 terminal hair strands is grasped from the scalp and gently tugged. A positive hair pull test yields more than 10% of pulled hairs from any given area in the scalp[26]; however, this test can be unreliable if patients present after the acute shedding has resolved or even shortly after washing the hair.[27] Telogen effluvium is considered a diagnosis of exclusion. Thus,

Table 1 Hairstyling risk stratification for traction alopecia		
High Risk	**Moderate Risk**	**Low Risk**
• Tight braids, dreadlocks, or sisterlocks • Application of braids to chemically relaxed • Tight ponytails or buns worn frequently • Application of hair extensions or weaves to chemically relaxed hair • Wigs glued into place around the hairline • Any style resulting in pain, stinging, tenting. pimples, or crusting 1–2 d within application	• Loosening of braids, dreadlocks, or sisterlocks • Application of braids to natural hair • Permanent waving • Application of hair extensions or weaves to natural hair • Wigs worn with nylon or cotton-lined wig caps	• Natural or unprocessed hair • Low-hanging, loose ponytails or buns • Wigs worn with a satin-lined or velvet-lined wig cap

Adapted from Haskin A, Aguh C. All hairstyles are not created equal: What the dermatologist needs to know about black hairstyling practices and the risk of traction alopecia (TA). *J Am Acad Dermatol* (2016) 75(3):606-11; with permission.

patient evaluation requires a detailed patient history to establish time course of hair loss, stressful events, and changes in medications (up to 6–12 weeks prior to onset of hair loss) in order to rule out other causes of hair loss. It also can be useful to obtain thyroid and iron studies when no apparent triggers for telogen effluvium are evident in the patient history.[27]

Considered a self-limited condition, telogen effluvium typically resolves spontaneously within 6 months of onset.[21] Providing reassurance and expectant management is appropriate in most settings. If a potential underlying cause is identified in work-up, such as stress or iron deficiency, the condition should be treated and managed accordingly to reverse hair loss.

Alopecia Areata

Alopecia areata (AA) is a nonscarring hair loss that affects approximately 2% of the general population in their lifetime.[28] In this T-cell–mediated autoimmune condition, autoantibodies directed against the hair follicle are thought to target several structures in the anagen-phase hair follicle, leading to transient hair loss.[28] AA also has been associated with other comorbid conditions, including thyroid disease, rheumatoid arthritis, lupus erythematosus, psoriasis, vitiligo, and inflammatory bowel disease.[29]

AA presents with various patterns of hair loss. Patch-type AA is characterized by small, well-circumscribed alopecic patches (**Fig. 1**), whereas ophiasis pattern presents with symmetric, bandlike hair loss involving the occipital, parietal, and temporal scalp (**Fig. 2**).[30] More extensive forms of AA include the totalis subtype (AT), characterized by complete or near-complete loss of hair on the scalp, and the universalis subtype (AU), which presents as total hair loss involving the scalp and body, including the eyebrows, eyelashes, axillary hair, pubic hair, extremity hair, and beard or chest hair in men.[31] On trichoscopic examination of the scalp, the presence of exclamation point hairs (dystrophic hairs with a short, broken hair shaft, and a narrow club-shaped hair root), and preservation of the hair follicle, sometimes seen as black dots in alopecic patches, are highly characteristic of AA.[32]

The prognosis for hair regrowth often is variable in patients. Younger age at the time of onset, more extensive disease involvement, and rapid onset of hair loss are associated with poorer outcomes.[33] For limited disease involvement (less than 50% of the scalp), treatment options include topical and intralesional corticosteroids, topical minoxidil, and phototherapy. For more extensive disease (ie, totalis and universalis),

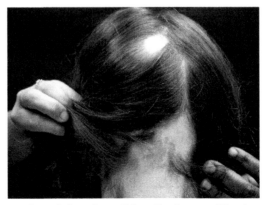

Fig. 1. AA—hairless patches of alopecia on this patient's nape. (*Courtesy of* Jeffrey P. Callen, MD.)

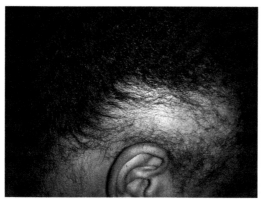

Fig. 2. Oophiasis pattern of AA. (*Courtesy of* Jeffrey P. Callen, MD.)

anti-inflammatory agents, such as systemic corticosteroids, intramuscular corticosteroids, methotrexate, and cyclosporine, have been used with variable and often disappointing results.

Recently, the Janus kinase–signal transducer and activator of transcription (JAK-STAT) signaling pathway has been implicated in the pathogenesis of AA.[34] Key genes within this pathway are expressed in hair cycling phases.[35] JAK-STAT inhibition not only is effective in reducing inflammatory signaling but also is thought to stimulate the activation and proliferation of stem cells of the hair follicle.[35] For this reason, JAK inhibitors have emerged as a promising treatment of more severe or therapy-resistant AA. Response rates in patients with AT and AU treated with oral tofacitinib or ruxolitinib have been reported to be upwards of 75%, with the side-effect profile including increased risk of infection, viral reactivation, and a theoretic yet undocumented risk for malignancy.[36,37]

Traction Alopecia

Traction alopecia, although highly prevalent among patients of African descent,[38] can present in any individual as a result of repetitive or extended tension on the hair follicles. It often is linked to specific hairstyling practices, such as the installation of tight weaves or braids (especially in chemically relaxed hair) and styling of the hair in tight ponytails or buns (**Table 2**).[39,40] Excess tension on the hair follicles is thought

Table 2 Causes of telogen effluvium[69]	
Immediate anagen release	• Medication changes • Emotional or physiologic stress • Severe illness • Major surgery • Anemia • Hypothyroidism • Crash dieting • Eating disorders
Delayed anagen release	• Pregnancy and childbirth • Discontinuation of oral contraceptives
Immediate telogen release	• Minoxidil

to lead to inflammation and miniaturization or dormancy of hair follicles.[41] Although traction alopecia is regarded primarily as a noncicatricial alopecia, over time, repeated trauma to the scalp can lead to permanent cicatricial hair loss in the affected areas.

Traction alopecia largely presents along the frontal or bitemporal region of the hairline. Exceptions to this generalization can be seen, however, based on hairstyling practice. For example, in Sikh Indian men, where keeping of the hair (kesh) and wearing of a turban are religious customs requiring long hair of the scalp and beard to be pulled tightly or knotted, traction alopecia instead can occur along the occipital scalp and beard area.[42] Early signs of impending traction alopecia include pain, stinging, pimples, tenting (raising of the skin on the scalp), and crusting in the scalp and occur within days of the hairstyling event.[40,41] Eventually, if the traction-causing hairstyle remains in place, highly characteristic features of this condition may develop, such as the fringe sign or retention of fine miniaturized hairs at the anterior margin of the hairline with hair loss posterior to the fringe.[41]

Encouraging the wearing of low-risk hairstyles often is an important first step in achieving hair regrowth and preventing progressive damage. Preferred hairstyling options include wearing the hair in a loose ponytail or bun and wigs lined with a silk or a satin cap.[43] In addition, the warning signs and symptoms of excess tension, such as pimples, stinging, pain, or crusting, should be reviewed in depth with patients. Concomitant use of medical treatments, such as topical minoxidil, 5% foam or solution; intralesional corticosteroids; and topical or oral antibiotics, may be appropriate, especially if there is evidence of active inflammation in the scalp. Full restoration of hair growth can be expected to occur within months in patients with early involvement who discontinue harmful styling habits. In advanced cases where permanent hair loss has occurred, hair transplantation can be curative.

SCARRING ALOPECIA

Scarring alopecias, also referred to as cicatricial alopecias, generally are considered to represent irreversible hair loss. These conditions are rare and cause complete destruction of the hair follicle due to underlying inflammation, loss of sebaceous glands, and eventual replacement of healthy subcutaneous tissue with fibrous tracts.[44] Stem cells, necessary to regenerate the follicular unit, are thought to be destroyed in the inflammatory process.[45] A punch biopsy of the affected area often is useful for establishing both diagnosis and prognosis. Treatments largely are aimed at eliminating inflammation and prevention of future hair loss as opposed to hair regrowth, yet recent evidence suggests that regeneration of hairs not yet fully destroyed may be possible.[45]

Lichen Planopilaris

Lichen planopilaris (LPP) is primary lymphocytic cicatricial alopecia that affects primarily adult women.[46] Although the exact cause of LPP is not well understood, the prevailing theory proposes mechanisms involving peroxisome proliferator–activated receptor gamma down-regulation[47] and interferon gamma dysfunction.[48] The damage from persistent inflammation around the follicular isthmus and infundibulum, which anatomically are close to pluripotent stem cells, is thought to account for resulting permanent hair loss.[49]

LPP clinically is characterized by follicular hyperkeratosis, perifollicular erythema, and loss of follicular ostia (**Fig. 3**).[49] Classic LPP typically presents with hair loss in

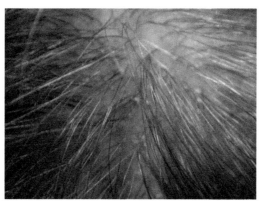

Fig. 3. LPP—note the follicular keratotic papules. (*Courtesy of* Jeffrey P. Callen, MD.)

the vertex and parietal areas of the scalp and can have focal or extensive involve-ment.[50] With disease progression, smaller alopecic patches can become confluent and form a reticulated pattern of alopecia. Associated symptoms may include a burning sensation, tenderness, or pain in the involved areas of the scalp. In addition, affected individuals with LPP also may experience noncicatricial body hair loss.[51] Near-total alopecia of the arms and legs has been documented in several patients with LPP years prior to the presentation of scalp findings.[52]

Several strategies have been proposed in the treatment of LPP based on small studies, case series, and case reports with varying outcomes, some even contradic-tory. There currently is no gold standard approach to treating LPP and often treatment strategies center on physician personal experience.[53] Generally however, application of a superpotent topical steroid, such as clobetasol propionate, in addition to intrale-sional corticosteroids, can be considered a first-line treatment.[53] Although some liter-ature cites the use of systemic oral corticosteroids as a second-line therapy for failed response to topicals, the relapse rate following complete taper has been reported to be as high as 80%.[53] Instead, oral hydroxychloroquine is recommended with the op-tion to switch to cyclosporine or mycophenolate mofetil if symptoms persist after 2 months to 4 months of therapy.[51,53]

Frontal Fibrosing Alopecia

Frontal fibrosing alopecia (FFA) often presents in postmenopausal women in the sixth or seventh decade of life, although women of African descent have been reported to have an earlier age of onset at approximately the fourth decade of life.[54,55] It is consid-ered a clinical variant of LPP due to shared histologic characteristics of lymphocytic inflammation concentrated around the follicular isthmus and infundibulum, although the clinical presentations differ.[49,56] Recent reports of exogenous factors, such as sunscreen use causing FFA, have not been supported by significant evidence and re-mains controversial.[57,58]

FFA presents with slow, progressive recession of the anterior hairline, appearing as a bandlike scarring alopecia. Often, isolated hairs are spared within the band of hair loss, a clinical finding referred to as the lonely hair sign.[59] The triad of characteristic findings has been described as (1) perifollicular erythema and hyperkeratosis; (2) pale, atrophic skin; and (3) decreased or complete loss of the eyebrows, which occurs in approximately 70% of affected individuals.[49,52] This is in contrast to LPP, which can present with multifocal involvement on the scalp and involves the loss of eyebrows less often than in FFA.[56] Nonetheless, treatments of FFA and LPP largely are the same and are detailed previously.

Central Centrifugal Cicatricial Alopecia

Central centrifugal cicatricial alopecia (CCCA) is a primary scarring alopecia that occurs almost exclusively in women of African descent.[60] Although the exact cause of CCCA is poorly understood, it is thought to be multifactorial, with genetics,[61] autoimmunity, and infection among several potential contributing factors.[62] There also have been reports of increased prevalence of uterine leiomyomas and diabetes among women with CCCA, suggesting possible systemic involvement in disease pathogenesis.[63,64] Hairstyling practices also have been suggested as possible causes of CCCA in the past; however, to date, no particular styling practice has been linked to its onset, casting this theory into doubt.

CCCA is characterized by clinical hair loss that begins in the crown or vertex scalp with the presence of subclinical inflammation, making it unique among other scarring alopecias.[65] In the early stages of disease, patients may present with hair breakage and thinning in the scalp vertex. As the disease progresses, hair loss becomes more severe, expands in an insidious centrifugal pattern, and ultimately results in permanent hair loss. The associated symptoms patients experience range from pruritus, tenderness, scale, papules, and pustules to no associated symptoms at all.[66] A diagnosis of CCCA often can be made through clinical examination; however, a scalp biopsy also can be performed to support the diagnosis.

Unlike other cicatricial alopecias where symptoms and inflammation are prominent and guide treatment duration, these are often is unclear in CCCA and requires patients to undergo lifelong treatment of this condition. First-line treatment options for CCCA include high-potency topical corticosteroids, often combined with intralesional corticosteroid injections in the scalp every 6 weeks to 12 weeks.[62] For those with signs of obvious inflammation, such as scalp erythema or follicular prominence, oral antibiotics, such as doxycycline, hydroxychloroquine, and mycophenolate mofetil, all have been useful when topical agents are unsuccessful.[67] Platelet-rich plasma injections and topical metformin also have shown some efficacy and may be beneficial as adjunct treatment in select patients.[45,68]

For women of African descent, nearly any discussion of treatment, regardless of alopecia subtype, should be accompanied by a discussion of hair styling practices. For many women, attempts to camouflage hair loss with extensions quickly can lead to end-stage traction alopecia, which is more difficult to camouflage than CCCA. Patients should be encouraged to avoid extensions if at all possible and, if they wish to resort to wigs, the use of satin-lined or velvet-lined wig caps to reduce friction along the hairline is recommended.

SUMMARY

An appropriate evaluation of hair disorders not only can address patient distress and quality of life but also can aid in the identification of underlying systemic processes. The ability to distinguish a nonscarring process with preservation of the hair follicle, as opposed to cicatricial hair loss resulting in permanent, progressive hair loss, is essential in developing a differential diagnosis and establishing prognosis for hair regrowth. Patients with significant disease involvement or signs and symptoms of a cicatricial process require prompt referral to a hair loss expert in dermatology for appropriate management.

CLINICS CARE POINTS

- Alopecia is the partial or complete loss of hair from 1 or more areas of the body, most commonly affecting the scalp. It can have an acute onset, such as with telogen effluvium and AA, or appear progressive in nature, such as with AGA or CCCA.

- For simplicity of distinction, alopecia can be categorized into 2 subtypes: nonscarring (noncicatricial) and scarring (cicatricial). AGA, AA, and traction alopecia are among several forms of nonscarring hair loss and do not necessarily require a punch biopsy of the scalp to make an accurate diagnosis. Treatment centers on restoration of hair growth. Contrarily, a punch biopsy often is useful for scarring alopecias, such as LPP, FFA, and CCCA, to identify subclinical inflammation, confirm the diagnosis, and estimate prognosis. Treatment of these conditions largely centers on limiting disease progression rather than hair regrowth.

- AGA is the most prevalent form of hair loss that affects primarily middle-aged men and women. Although the first-line treatment option is topical minoxidil, the use of finasteride in men and spironolactone in women also has proved efficacious. Patients with progressive disease resulting in extensive hair loss or balding mimicking end-stage fibrosis may benefit from hair transplantation.

- LPP and FFA are 2 forms of scarring alopecia that have become increasingly common in women. Treatment with superpotent and intralesional corticosteroids are useful for the prevention of disease progression. Hydroxycholoroqiune is an additional option for patients with extensive disease involvement or treatment-refractory disease.

- CCCA is a primary scarring alopecia with higher prevalence among women of African descent. It commonly presents as hair loss at the scalp vertex with evidence of fibrosis and loss of follicular ostia. Although treatment is targeted at reducing inflammation and preventing disease progression, therapies, such as topical metformin and platelet-rich plasma injections, offer the potential for regrowth of hair follicles that have not succumbed to complete destruction.

DISCLOSURE

Dr C. Aguh serves as consultant for L'oreal Inc, LEO Pharma, DevaConcepts, and UCB Pharma and receives royalties from UpToDate.

REFERENCES

1. Malkud S. A hospital-based study to determine causes of diffuse hair loss in women. J Clin Diagn Res 2015;9(8):WC01–4.
2. Koo JY, Shellow WV, Hallman CP, et al. Alopecia areata and increased prevalence of psychiatric disorders. Int J Dermatol 1994;33:849–50.
3. Ho CH, Sood T, Zito PM. Androgenetic alopecia. IStatPearls Publishing; 2020. Available at: https://www.ncbi.nlm.nih.gov/books/NBK430924.
4. Gan DC, Sinclair RD. Prevalence of male and female pattern hair loss in Maryborough. J Investig Dermatol Symp Proc 2005;10:184–9.
5. Sadick NS, Callender VD, Kircik LH, et al. New insight into the pathophysiology of hair loss trigger a paradigm shift in the treatment approach. J Drugs Dermatol 2017;16(11):s135–40.
6. Hamilton JB. Patterned hair loss in men: types and incidence. Ann NY Acad Sci 1951;53:708–14.
7. Olsen EA. Female pattern hair loss. J Am Acad Dermatol 2001;45:S70–80.

8. Futterweit W, Dunaif A, Yeh HC, et al. The prevalence of hyperandrogenism in 109 consecutive female patients with diffuse alopecia. J Am Acad Dermatol 1988; 19(5 Pt 1):831–6.

9. Tsuboi R, Itami S, Inui S, et al. Guidelines for the management of androgenetic alopecia (2010). J Dermatol 2012;39(2):113–20.

10. Messenger AG, Rundegren J. Minoxidil: mechanisms of action on hair growth. Br J Dermatol 2004;150(2):186–94.

11. Roberts JL. Androgenetic alopecia: treatment results with topical minoxidil. J Am Acad Dermatol 1987;16:705–10.

12. Olsen EA, Whiting D, Bergfeld W, et al. A multicenter, randomized, placebo-controlled, double-blind clinical trial of a novel formulation of 5% minoxidil topical foam versus placebo in the treatment of androgenetic alopecia in men. J Am Acad Dermatol 2007;57(5):767–74.

13. Okereke UR, Simmons A, Callender VD. Current and emerging treatment strategies for hair loss in women of color. Int J Women's Dermatol 2019;5:37–45.

14. Baas WR, Butcher MJ, Lwin A, et al. A review of the FAERS data on 5-alpha reductase inhibitors: implications for post finasteride syndrome. Urology 2018; 120:143–9.

15. Price VH, Roberts JL, Hordinsky M, et al. Lack of efficacy of finasteride in post-menopausal women with androgenetic alopecia. J Am Acad Dermatol 2000; 43(5 Pt 1):768–76.

16. Carmina E, Lobo RA. Treatment of hyperandrogenic alopecia in women. Fertil Steril 2003;79(1):91–5.

17. Burns LJ, De Souza B, Flynn E, et al. Spironolactone for treatment of female pattern hair loss. J Am Acad Dermatol 2020;83(1):276–8.

18. Sinclair RD. Female pattern hair loss: a pilot study investigating combination therapy with low-dose oral minoxidil and spironolactone. Int J Dermatol 2017;57(1): 104–9.

19. Camacho-Martínez FM. Hair loss in women. Semin Cutan Med Surg 2009;28(1): 19–32.

20. Dinh QQ, Sinclair R. Female pattern hair loss: current treatment concepts. Clin Interv Aging 2007;2(2):189–99.

21. Hughes EC, Saleh D. Telogen effluvium 2020. Available at: https://www.ncbi.nlm.nih.gov/books/NBK430848.

22. Harrison S, Sinclair R. Telogen effluvium. Clin Exp Dermatol 2002;27:389–95.

23. Barman JM, Astore I, Pecoraro V. The normal trichogram of the adult. J Invest Dermatol 1965;44:233–6.

24. Sinclair R. Diffuse hair loss. Int J Dermatol 1999;38:1–18.

25. Cline A, Kazemi A, Moy J, et al. A surge in the incidence of telogen effluvium in minority predominant communities heavily impacted by COVID-19. J Am Acad Dermatol 2020. https://doi.org/10.1016/j.jaad.2020.11.032.

26. Shapiro J, Wiseman M, Lui H. Practical management of hair loss. Can Fam Physician 2000;46:1469–77.

27. Malkud S. Telogen effluvium: a review. J Clin Diagn Res 2015;9(9):WE01–3.

28. Pratt CH, King LE Jr, Messenger AG, et al. Alopecia areata. Nat Rev Dis Primers 2017;3:17011.

29. Chu SY, Chen YJ, Tseng WC, et al. Comorbidity profiles among patients with alopecia areata: the importance of onset age, a nationwide population-based study. J Am Acad Dermatol 2011;65:949–56.

30. Alkhalifah A, Alsantali A, Wang E, et al. Alopecia areata update: part I. Clinical picture, histopathology, and pathogenesis. J Am Acad Dermatol 2010;62:177–88.

31. Islam N, Leung PS, Huntley AC, et al. The autoimmune basis of alopecia areata: a comprehensive review. Autoimmune Rev 2015;14(2):81–9.
32. Messenger AG, Slater DN, Bleehen SS. Alopecia areata: alterations in the hair growth cycle and correlation with the follicular pathology. Br J Dermatol 1986; 114(3):337–47.
33. Tosti A, Bellavista S, Iorizzo M. Alopecia areata: a long term follow-up study of 191 patients. J Am Acad Dermatol 2006;55(3):438–41.
34. Triyangkulsri K, Suchonwanit P. Role of janus kinase inhibitors in the treatment of alopecia areata. Drug Des Devel Ther 2018;12:2323–35.
35. Harel S, Higgins CA, Cerise JE, et al. Pharmacologic inhibition of JAK-STAT signaling promotes hair growth. Sci Adv 2015;1(9):e1500973.
36. Kennedy Crispin M, Ko JM, Craiglow BG, et al. Safety and efficacy of the JAK inhibitor tofacitinib citrate in patients with alopecia areata. JCI Insight 2016;1(15): e89776.
37. Liu LY, Craiglow BG, Dai F, et al. Tofacitinib for the treatment of severe alopecia areata and variants: a study of 90 patients. J Am Acad Dermatol 2017;76:22–8.
38. Alexis AF, Sergay AB, Taylor SC. Common dermatologic disorders in skin of color: a comparative practice survey. Cutis 2007;80(5):387–94.
39. Khumalo NP, Jessop S, Gumedze F, et al. Determinants of marginal traction alopecia in African girls and women. J Am Acad Dermatol 2008;59(3):432–8.
40. Khumalo NP, Jessop S, Gumedze F, et al. Hairdressing and the prevalence of scalp disease in African adults. Br J Dermatol 2007;157(5):981–8.
41. Samrao A, Price VH, Zedek D, et al. The "fringe sign" - a useful clinical finding in traction alopecia of the marginal hair line. Dermatol Online J 2011;17(11):1.
42. James J, Saladi RN, Fox JL. Traction alopecia in Sikh male patients. J Am Board Fam Med 2007;20(5):497–8.
43. Haskin A, Aguh C. All hairstyles are not created equal: what the dermatologist needs to know about black hairstyling practices and the risk of traction alopecia (TA). J Am Acad Dermatol 2016;75(3):606–11.
44. Somani N, Bergfeld WF. Cicatricial alopecia: classification and histopathology. Dermatol Ther 2008;21:221–37.
45. Dina Y, Aguh C. Use of platelet-rich plasma in cicatricial alopecia. Dermatol Surg 2019;45(7):979–81.
46. Chieregato C, Zini A, Barba A, et al. Lichen planopilaris: report of 30 cases and review of the literature. Int J Dermatol 2003;42(5):342–5.
47. Karnik P, Tekeste Z, McCormick TS, et al. Hair follicle stem cell-specific PPAR-gamma deletion causes scarring alopecia. J Invest Dermatol 2009;129(5): 1243–57.
48. Harries MJ, Meyer K, Chaudhry I, et al. Lichen planopilaris is characterized by immune privilege collapse of the hair follicle's epithelial stem cell niche. J Pathol 2013;231(2):236–47.
49. Poblet E, Jimenez F, Pascual A, et al. Frontal fibrosing alopecia versus lichen planopilaris: a clinicopathological study. Int J Dermatol 2006;45:375–80.
50. Sperling LC. Lichen planopilaris. An Atlas of hair Pathology with clinical correlations. New York: Parthenon Publishing Group; 2003. p. 101–6.
51. Lyakhovitsky A, Amichai B, Sizopoulou C, et al. A case series of 46 patients with lichen planopilaris: demographics, clinical evaluation, and treatment experience. J Dermatolog Treat 2015;26(3):275–9.
52. Dina Y, Okoye GA, Aguh C. The timing and distribution of non-scalp hair loss in patients with lichen planopilaris and frontal fibrosing alopecia: a survey-based study [published online ahead of print, 2018 Mar 17]. J Am Acad Dermatol 2018.

53. Assouly P, Reygagne P. Lichen planopilaris: update on diagnosis and treatment. Semin Cutan Med Surg 2009;28(1):3–10.
54. Callender VD, Reid SD, Obayan O, et al. Diagnostic clues to frontal fibrosing alopecia in patients of African descent. J Clin Aesthet Dermatol 2016;9(4):45–51.
55. Samrao A, Chew A-L, Price V. Frontal fibrosing alopecia: a clinical review of 36 patients. Br J Dermatol 2010;163(6):1296–300.
56. Bolduc C, Sperling LC, Shapiro J, et al. Primary cicatricial alopecia: lymphocytic primary cicatricial alopecias, including chronic cutaneous lupus erythematosus, lichen planopilaris, frontal fibrosing alopecia, and Graham–Little syndrome. J Am Acad Dermatol 2016;75:1081–99.
57. Debroy Kidambi A, Dobson K, Holmes S, et al. Frontal fibrosing alopecia in men: an association with facial moisturizers and sunscreens. Br J Dermatol 2017;177: 260–1.
58. Callander J, Frost J, Stone N. Ultraviolet filters in hair-care products: a possible link with frontal fibrosing alopecia and lichen planopilaris. Clin Exp Dermatol 2018;43:69–70.
59. Tosti A, Miteva M, Torres F. Lonely hair: a clue to the diagnosis of frontal fibrosing alopecia. Arch Dermatol 2011;147(10):1240.
60. Dlova NC, Salkey KS, Callender VD, et al. Central centrifugal cicatricial alopecia: new insights and a call for action. J Investig Dermatol Symp Proc 2017;18:S54–6.
61. Malki L, Sarig O, Romano MT, et al. Variant PADI3 in central centrifugal cicatricial alopecia. N Engl J Med 2019;380(9):833–41.
62. Aguh C, McMichael A. Central centrifugal cicatricial alopecia. JAMA Dermatol 2020;156(9):1036.
63. Dina Y, Okoye GA, Aguh C. Association of uterine leiomyomas with central centrifugal cicatricial alopecia. JAMA Dermatol 2018;154(2):213–4.
64. Coogan PF, Bethea TN, Cozier YC, et al. Association of type 2 diabetes with central-scalp hair loss in a large cohort study of African American women. Int J Women's Dermatol 2019;5(issue 4):261–6.
65. Olsen EA, Callender V, Sperling L, et al. Central scalp alopecia photographic scale in African American women. Dermatol Ther 2008;21(4):264–7.
66. Callender VD, Wright DR, Davis EC, et al. Hair breakage as a presenting sign of early or occult central centrifugal cicatricial alopecia: clinicopathologic findings in 9 patients. Arch Dermatol 2012;148:1047–52.
67. Ogunleye TA, McMichael A, Olsen EA. Central centrifugal cicatricial alopecia: what has been achieved, current clues for future research. Dermatol Clin 2014; 32:173–81.
68. Araoye EF, Thomas JAL, Aguh CU. Hair regrowth in 2 patients with recalcitrant central centrifugal cicatricial alopecia after use of topical metformin. JAAD Case Rep 2020;6(2):106–8.
69. Liyanage D, Sinclair R. Telogen effluvium. Cosmetics. 2016;3(2):13.

Diagnosis and Management of Dermatitis, Including Atopic, Contact, and Hand Eczemas

Cynthia X. Chan, BS[a],*, Kathryn A. Zug, MD[a,b]

KEYWORDS

- Eczema • Dermatitis • Atopic dermatitis • Irritant contact dermatitis
- Allergic contact dermatitis • Contact dermatitis • Asteatotic

KEY POINTS

- Most dermatitis is diagnosed based on clinical history and physical examination; patch testing is the gold standard for diagnosing allergic contact dermatitis.
- Common differential diagnoses for dermatitis include atopic dermatitis, contact dermatitis, asteatotic dermatitis, nummular dermatitis, seborrheic dermatitis, other dermatitis, psoriasis, tinea, scabies, and cutaneous T-cell lymphoma.
- The therapeutic ladder for dermatitis begins with frequent moisturization and minimization of allergens and irritants and progresses to topical corticosteroids and steroid-sparing agents, phototherapy, and finally systemic medications.

INTRODUCTION TO DERMATITIS DIAGNOSIS

The term "eczema" is derived from the Greek word "ekzein" meaning "to boil over." Dermatitis, a synonymous term, refers to conditions with spongiotic pathology. Acute eczematous dermatitis presents with severely pruritic erythematous, edematous, weeping plaques, vesicles, and/or bullae. Erythematous patches, juicy papules, and plaques with scale or crust are observed in subacute eczematous dermatitis, which lasts more than 1 week with variable pruritus. Chronic eczematous dermatitis results in moderate-to-intensely pruritic erythematous, dyspigmented, lichenified skin with scaling and excoriations, usually distributed on easily reached areas, intertriginous areas, eyelids, the posterior neck, ankles, and/or the anogenital region. Lesion borders are indistinct except in many cases of acute contact dermatitis. The primary symptom

[a] Geisel School of Medicine at Dartmouth, Hanover, NH, USA; [b] Department of Dermatology, Dartmouth-Hitchcock Medical Center, 18 Old Etna Road, Lebanon, NH 03766, USA
* Corresponding author.
E-mail address: Cynthia.X.Chan.med@dartmouth.edu

Med Clin N Am 105 (2021) 611–626
https://doi.org/10.1016/j.mcna.2021.04.003
0025-7125/21/© 2021 Elsevier Inc. All rights reserved.

medical.theclinics.com

is pruritus, which is often worse at bedtime and with certain triggers, but pain is sometimes prominent, such as in irritant contact dermatitis.

Although dermatitis is usually a clinical diagnosis, patch testing is the gold standard for diagnosing allergic contact dermatitis and is also indicated for recurrent or refractory dermatitis. Histology reveals spongiosis—fluid interspersed between keratinocytes—and is not diagnostic of a specific dermatitis but can help rule out other diagnoses. Patients frequently have multiple types of dermatitis.

INTRODUCTION TO DERMATITIS MANAGEMENT

The general management of dermatitis begins with minimizing exposure to irritants, allergens, and other triggers. The patient's topical regimen should be simplified accordingly. Best cleansing practices include using mild non–soap-based and non–detergent-based cleansers with neutral or physiologically acidic pH on the axilla, groin, face, soles, and scalp daily for 5 to 10 minutes in warm water.[1]

Patients are encouraged to moisturize as often as feasible daily to repair and protect their epidermis, even when there is no perceivable dermatitis. Moisturizing is recommended immediately after a wet activity and a few hours after applying topical corticosteroids.[1] Over-the-counter moisturizers free of common contact allergens are not more expensive than ones containing those allergens.[2] Moisturizers with special lipids formulations may have added benefits.[3–5]

As other topicals, moisturizers are available in different vehicles. Occlusive vehicles such as ointments and emollient creams contain higher lipid concentrations, lower water content, and fewer allergens and thus cause less stinging when applied to inflamed skin. Examples include petrolatum, vegetable shortening, and coconut oil. They are the most effective vehicles, especially for dry, lichenified, or exposed areas. However, greasiness may limit compliance. Nonocclusive vehicles such as lotions, foams, and liquids are appropriate for moist or occluded areas.[6]

Topical corticosteroids are a first-line therapy for decreasing inflammation and pruritus. They are safe for daily use for up to several weeks at a time and for long-term intermittent use.[7] Once cutaneous corticosteroid receptors are saturated, additional applications provide only an emollient effect. Thus, once a day dosing is preferred because, compared with multiple applications daily, it is nearly as effective, is cheaper and safer, and encourages better compliance.[8,9] In addition, when greater efficacy is desired, a higher potency corticosteroid is usually more appropriate than increasing the concentration of lower potency option. Groups I to III topical corticosteroids are appropriate for palms, soles, thick lesions, refractory lesions, and dermatitis flares but should be avoided for the face, intertriginous areas, and if younger than 1 year.

Less recommended routes of corticosteroid administration include intralesional and oral. Intralesional triamcinolone acetonide 2.5 to 5 mg/mL every 3 to 4 weeks as needed is typically reserved for lichenified or prurigo nodularis-like lesions. Short-term use of oral corticosteroid at a prednisone-equivalent dose of 0.5 to 1 mg/kg daily and then tapered over 2 to 3 weeks may be considered for severe or generalized dermatitis flares.

Steroid-sparing treatments include topical tacrolimus and pimecrolimus, crisaborole, tar, and phototherapy and systemic cyclosporin, azathioprine, methotrexate, mycophenolate mofetil, and injectable dupilumab.

There are no other well-proven antipruritics for dermatitis. Moisturizers with pramoxine 1% may be as antipruritic as hydrocortisone cream 1%.[10] Long-acting histamine H2-receptor antagonists may help decrease pruritus from environmental allergies. Cannabinoids are a promising antipruritic that lack randomized controlled trials.[11]

ATOPIC DERMATITIS
Clinics Care Points

- Essential features for the clinical diagnosis of atopic dermatitis include pruritus, eczema of typical morphology and distribution, and chronic or relapsing course.
- The differential diagnosis for atopic dermatitis differs slightly by age and includes contact dermatitis, seborrheic dermatitis, psoriasis, scabies, tinea, and cutaneous T-cell lymphoma (CTCL).
- The therapeutic ladder for atopic dermatitis is intended to control, not cure, the disease, and includes education, psychological support, epidermal barrier protection and repair, corticosteroids, calcineurin inhibitors, crisaborole, coal tar, phototherapy, and systemic medications including dupilumab.

Clinical Presentation

The clinical presentation of atopic dermatitis varies by stage. Several diagnostic criteria exist. The American Academy of Dermatology considers "essential features" necessary for diagnosis to be pruritus and eczema.[12] The latter should have a chronic or relapsing course or history, as well as typical morphology and distributions (eg, face, neck, and/or extensor surfaces in infants and children; flexural surfaces; sparing of the groin and axillae).[12] "Important features" with high sensitivity are early age of onset, xerosis, and immunoglobulin E reactivity or personal or family history of atopy (atopic dermatitis, allergic rhinitis, and/or asthma).[12] "Associated features" are atypical vascular responses (eg, facial pallor, white dermatographism, delayed blanch response); other filaggrin deficiency-associated conditions; perifollicular accentuation, lichenification, or prurigo lesions; and regional changes (eg, ocular, periorbital, perioral, periauricular, pityriasis alba).[12]

The infantile stage occurs between ages 2 months and 2 years. It begins as acute erythema and scaling on the bilateral cheeks that can extend symmetrically to the scalp, forehead, perioral area, neck, trunk, and extensor surfaces such as elbows and knees. Less commonly affected areas include the buttocks, anogenital region, central face, and intertriginous areas. Scratching, rubbing, and infection results in crusts, lichenification, and pustules, respectively.

The childhood stage occurs between ages 2 and 12 years. It presents subacutely as lichenified, indurated plaques and excoriated 2 to 4 mm papules distributed symmetrically (**Fig. 1**). It commonly affects the face, especially eyelids and ears, and flexural

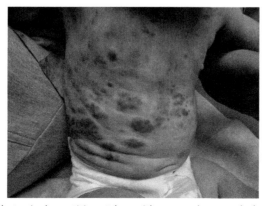

Fig. 1. Generalized atopic dermatitis patches with nummular morphology in a toddler.

surfaces, particularly antecubital and popliteal fossae, posterior neck, and flexor wrists and ankles, but can generalize.

The adolescent or adult stage presents after age 11 years with subacute and chronic lesions. Commonly affected areas in adolescents are flexural surfaces, forehead, and periorbital areas. Adults usually present with plaques that are erythematous, scaly, flat-topped, exudative, lichenified, or excoriated. In darker skin, lesions can be hyperpigmented with focal hypopigmentation corresponding to healed excoriations. Lesion distribution in adults is often localized, commonly to the hand, wrist, nipple, bilateral upper eyelids, or lips. However, it can generalize with flexural accentuation.

The differential diagnosis includes contact dermatitis, photodermatitis, seborrheic dermatitis, psoriasis, scabies, tinea, and ichthyosis vulgaris. In addition, Netherton syndrome, ectodermal dysplasia, Langerhans cell histiocytosis, certain primary immunodeficiency syndromes, and malnutrition may be considered in infants and children. Nummular dermatitis and pityriasis rosea are less likely in infants. CTCL is more likely in adults.

Management

The goal of treatment in atopic dermatitis is to control, not cure, the condition. Treatment plans should include both acute and maintenance therapies and regular long-term follow-up. Undertreatment can result in decreased provider-patient trust and prolonged patient suffering.

The therapeutic ladder for atopic dermatitis begins with education, psychological support, and epidermal barrier repair and protection for all patients. Education, including addressing corticosteroid phobia, and psychological support for patients and guardians reduces disease severity and improves quality of life.[13,14]

Epidermal barrier repair and protection is best achieved by minimizing triggers and increasing moisture. Common triggers include sweat, temperature extremes, low humidity, harsh cleansing practices, coarse fabrics, tight clothing, physical trauma, infections, allergens, and irritants. There is minimal evidence for bleach baths, which can decrease bacterial cutaneous colonization.[15] To increase epidermal moisture, refer to the moisturizer recommendations in the introduction; wet wraps are another option.[16] Wet wrap has many benefits—decreased flares, xerosis, pruritus, fissures, erythema, lichenification, and topical corticosteroid use—and may be sufficient monotherapy in mild cases.[17]

Topical corticosteroids are a first-line therapy. For moderate-to-severe cases or flares, apply once daily before bedtime for 1 to 4 weeks or for the duration of the flare, respectively.[1] For secondary prevention, apply a low-to-medium-potency corticosteroid once or twice weekly to areas that flare frequently.[18,19]

Topical tacrolimus and pimecrolimus decrease pruritus and corticosteroid use and are especially helpful for areas prone to steroid atrophy, including the face and intertriginous areas. They are approved by the Food and Drug Administration (FDA) as second-line therapies for ages 2 years and older, but pimecrolimus has demonstrated safety in ages as young as 3 months.[20] Pimecrolimus 1% cream is recommended for mild-to-moderate cases and has benefits similar to those of groups IV to VII corticosteroids.[21] Tacrolimus 0.03% or 0.1% ointment is recommended for moderate-to-severe cases and is more effective than pimecrolimus.[21–23]

Calcineurin inhibitors are safe for twice daily short-term use, such as during flares, or intermittent long-term use. For secondary prevention, apply on 2 consecutive days weekly to areas that flare frequently.[18,19] There is a black box warning of theoretic cancer risk that is based on data from mice studies and from oral calcineurin inhibitor use in humans.[24,25] Burning or stinging on application is common and usually decreases with usage. Adverse events of pimecrolimus include superimposed cutaneous infections.[26,27]

Topical crisaborole 2% ointment twice daily is another FDA-approved steroid-sparing second-line therapy for mild-to-moderate cases in ages 2 years and older but may be safe in as young as 3 months.[28] It has no adverse events but may burn or sting on initial applications.

Crude coal tar 1% to 5% or liquor carbonis detergens 5% to 20% are third-line options. They may be helpful for chronic, lichenified, or refractory lesions, especially those on the palms or soles, in adults with mild-to-moderate cases, particularly when used in conjunction with phototherapy.[29,30] They are well tolerated and cost-effective but have an odor and may cause staining, folliculitis, and contact dermatitis.[31]

Phototherapy is a third-line therapy that can improve nonscalp and nonintertriginous lesions and pruritus in moderate-to-severe cases refractory to topicals.[32] The preferred spectra are narrowband ultraviolet B (nbUVB), particularly for chronic moderate cases, or low-to-medium-dose ultraviolet A1, 2 to 5 times weekly for 3 to 12 weeks.[32] Psoralen and ultraviolet A (PUVA) has more adverse events, but oral PUVA may be considered for severe widespread chronic cases refractory to nbUVB and topical PUVA for lesions on the palms and soles.[31] Phototherapy requires patient compliance, as it often involves multiple outpatient visits over months.

Systemic medications are indicated for moderate-to-severe cases refractory to topicals and for severe flares. Dupilumab was the first option to gain FDA approval, for ages 6 years and older.[33] It is the most effective biologic, especially when used in conjunction with topical corticosteroids.[33,34] It is well tolerated, the main adverse event being keratoconjunctivitis.[33] If dupilumab is indicated but not an option, then other systemic medications may be considered.

Cyclosporine, 2.5 to 5 mg/kg daily, is usually the first nonbiological systemic medication to consider for severe chronic cases in ages 2 years and older.[35] It is more effective than phototherapy and oral corticosteroids, may be more effective during the first 4 months of treatment than methotrexate or azathioprine, and may be the most effective systemic option for children.[35–37] Because of its risk of adverse events including immunosuppression and dermatitis relapse, cyclosporine is safest as a short-term bridge for up to several months, with monitoring for hypertension and nephrotoxicity.[35] However, it can also be used intermittently, as well as continuously for up to 2 years.[35]

Azathioprine may be considered off-label for refractory severe cases mostly in adults. It achieves maximum benefits by 1 to 3 months.[31] The maintenance dose is usually 1.5 to 3.5 mg/kg daily but should be decreased to 0.5 to 1 mg/kg if the activity of thiopurine methyltransferase measured before initiation is low.[38] Adverse events include gastrointestinal upset, certain nonmelanoma skin cancers, possible increased risk of non-Hodgkin lymphoma with long-term use, and rare acute hypersensitivity syndrome. Use during pregnancy should be carefully considered. Live vaccines are contraindicated while on azathioprine. Complete blood count (CBC) and comprehensive metabolic panel (CMP) should be monitored.[35]

Methotrexate may be considered off-label for refractory severe cases.[31] It has similar efficacy to cyclosporine and azathioprine[35] and reaches maximum efficacy after 2 to 3 months.[31] Careful monitoring is required due to its many adverse events, including hepatoxicity and teratogenicity; patients with childbearing potential must use contraception concurrently.[34]

Mycophenolate mofetil may be considered off-label for severe cases refractory to the aforementioned medications, based on 1 controlled trial.[34,39] The recommended dose is 1 to 3 g daily for adults and 20 to 50 mg/kg daily for children.[31] Adverse effects include gastrointestinal upset, leukopenia, thrombocytopenia, hepatotoxicity, and teratogenicity; CBC and CMP should be monitored.[35]

Oral corticosteroid may be considered for severe flares while another treatment is being initiated.[40]

There are many therapeutic options in phase II and III trials. For example, Janus kinase inhibitors have decreased Eczema Area and Severity Index (EASI) and pruritus in mild-to-moderate cases in multiple trials.[41]

CONTACT DERMATITIS
Clinics Care Points

- Patch testing is the gold standard for diagnosing allergic contact dermatitis; irritant contact dermatitis is often a diagnosis of exclusion.
- Treatment of allergic contact dermatitis includes allergen identification and avoidance; moisturizers; corticosteroids; tacrolimus; UVB and PUVA; and for refractory cases, many of the systemic medications described for atopic dermatitis.

Clinical Presentation

Irritant contact dermatitis is the most common type of contact dermatitis. It usually presents as subacute or chronic eczematous dermatitis (**Fig. 2**). However, a strong irritant can result in lesions localized to areas of maximum contact within a few hours of exposure. These acute eruptions usually seem as edematous and erythematous vesicles, bullae, or ulcers with sharp borders. Irritant contact dermatitis is most common

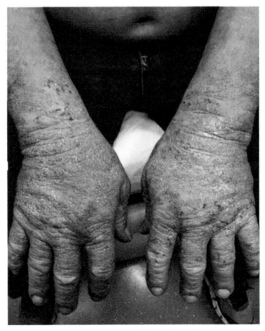

Fig. 2. Chronic lichenified eczematous dermatitis of the hands and wrists of a machinist caused by irritants and contact allergens.

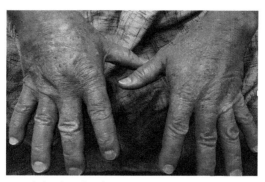

Fig. 3. Contact allergy of the hands of a surgeon to accelerators in gloves identified by patch testing as seen in **Fig. 5**.

on the face and hands. The primary symptom is burning pain that is worse than pruritus.

Allergic contact dermatitis presents after contact with an allergen within 8 to 120 hours in sensitized patients or 12 to 21 days in unsensitized patients. The lesions may be acute, lasting several weeks and localized to areas of contact, or chronic with a broader distribution. The face, forearms, and hands are the most commonly affected areas, followed by the trunk and groin (see **Fig. 2**; **Figs. 3** and **4**). There are some distinct presentations, including urushiol dermatitis and systemic contact dermatitis. Urushiol dermatitis, such as from poison ivy, appears within 48 hours of exposure and results in linear lesions and sometimes black spots that represent dried and oxidized urushiol and lasts 10 to 21 days without treatment. Systemic contact dermatitis results from systemic exposure to a contact allergen and can present as a generalized morbilliform or eczematous eruption or with other morphologic patterns such as symmetric drug-related intertriginous and flexural exanthema.

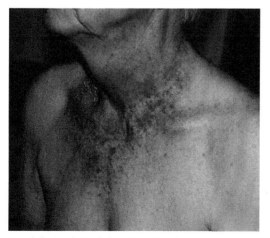

Fig. 4. Contact allergy of the neck and chest to propylene glycol contained in the patient's moisturizer and topical corticosteroid.

Diagnosis

Patch testing is the gold standard for diagnosing allergic contact dermatitis; results must be assessed for clinical relevance. Similarly, clinical data are insufficient, as dermatologists suspect the true allergens in only 50% of cases.[42]

For patch testing, only known materials in accepted concentrations should be used, and there are hundreds of allergens to choose from. The manual method involves placing allergens in a vehicle, usually petrolatum, into individual aluminum wells affixed to paper tape. The FDA-approved TRUE Test contains 35 screening allergens already affixed to paper tape. Patches are removed at 48 hours. Normal skin of the upper back is the preferred site for testing, but the upper lateral arm is also appropriate if testing only a few allergens (**Fig. 5**). Patients should avoid wetting and disturbing the test site such as with sweat or heavy lifting.

Because the test detects delayed-type hypersensitivity reactions, results should be read at 48 and 96 hours or 120 hours after application and sometimes at day 7 or later for greater accuracy (**Fig. 6**).[43,44] The TRUE Test detects 62% to 74% of the most common allergens; an expanded allergen series will often be positive in cases where TRUE test is negative but clinical suspicion for allergic contact dermatitis is high.[45]

Repeated open application test is indicated for negative patch testing with strong clinical suspicion for allergic contact dermatitis.[46] The patient's topical product is applied to the same test site twice to thrice daily for 1 to 2 weeks. Any dermatitis reaction is considered positive.

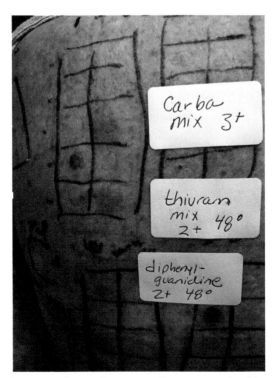

Fig. 5. Positive patch test reactions to 3 common allergens contained in synthetic nitrile and natural rubber latex gloves causing the dermatitis seen in **Fig. 3**.

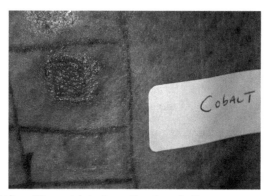

Fig. 6. A strong (3+) positive patch test reaction to cobalt.

Irritant contact dermatitis is often a diagnosis of exclusion. The differential diagnosis for contact dermatitis includes atopic dermatitis, nummular dermatitis, neurodermatitis, seborrheic dermatitis, photodermatosis, pigmented purpuric dermatoses, stasis dermatitis, recurrent vesicular dermatitis, fungal or bacterial cutaneous infection, connective tissue disease, CTCL, and drug eruptions.

Management

The cornerstone of irritant contact dermatitis management is avoidance of irritants including friction and wet-dry cycles, such as by using gloves and moisturizers.[47] Acute treatment often depends on the irritant, and topical corticosteroids are occasionally helpful.[47]

There are more options for allergic contact dermatitis, which can be treated empirically. The most important is avoidance of allergens and cross-reactive agents. Patient should receive oral and written education regarding their allergens, how to assess for product ingredients, and how to find product substitutes such as through the American Contact Dermatitis Society's Contact Allergen Management Program. Along with allergen avoidance, the patient's topical regimen should be simplified, for example to only moisturizer and topical corticosteroid twice daily for 1 to 3 weeks.[47]

In addition to topical corticosteroids and tacrolimus, there are several adjunctive therapies for allergic contact dermatitis.[48–52] Phototherapy may be considered for refractory, airborne, and hand cases, with UVB preferred over PUVA.[53,54] Only for severe acute or generalized cases should oral corticosteroids be considered. Many of the systemic medications described for atopic dermatitis may be considered for refractory cases.

HAND DERMATITIS
Clinics Care Points

- The most common subtypes of hand dermatitis are contact, atopic, recurrent vesicular, and hyperkeratotic.
- Treatments for hand dermatitis include irritant and allergen avoidance, frequent moisturizer use, corticosteroid ointments, phototherapy, botulinum toxin, and retinoids.

Clinical Presentation and Diagnosis

Hand dermatitis is a clinical diagnosis that often requires patch testing.[55] Many cases are a mixture of subtypes.[55] The most common subtype is irritant contact dermatitis, which presents with erythema, xerosis, and burning pain.[56] The next 2 most common subtypes are atopic dermatitis and allergic contact dermatitis.[55,56] Atopic dermatitis presents with erythema, scaling, and pruritus typically localized to the base of the fingers, dorsal hands, and volar wrists, as well as palmar hyperlinearity.[56] Allergic contact dermatitis presents with pruritic edema and vesicles on the fingertips and sometimes dorsal hands (see **Figs. 2** and **3**).[56] Patch testing is recommended for all chronic hand dermatitis, defined as lasting more than 3 months or recurring more than once within 12 months (see **Fig. 5**).[56–58]

Subtypes based on morphology include recurrent vesicular hand dermatitis, often referred to as dyshidrotic eczema or pompholyx, and hyperkeratotic hand dermatitis. The former is most prevalent in women in their 20s and men in their mid-40s.[55,56] It presents with monomorphic, deep-seated, clear ("tapioca-like") 1 to 5 mm pruritic vesicles without surrounding erythema that last 1 to 3 weeks; healing occurs as rings of thick scale, and peeling reveals a red cracked base with brown spots.[55,56] Chronic features include scaling, fissures, hyperkeratosis, and dystrophic nails.[56] Lesions are distributed symmetrically on the hands, especially palms and sides of fingers, in almost all cases and on the plantar feet in a minority of cases.[56] Hyperkeratotic hand dermatitis presents with discrete hyperkeratosis, fissures, and erythema on the palms and sometimes volar fingers and plantar feet of older adults.[55,56]

The differential diagnosis includes autoeczematization, tinea manuum, scabies, palmoplantar psoriasis, dyshidrosiform bullous pemphigoid, CTCL, and porphyria cutanea tarda.[55,56]

Management

There are 4 main guidelines for the management of hand dermatitis.[59] Patients should avoid irritants and allergens and use moisturizers in occlusive vehicles daily, as described in the introduction.[59] Palmar xerosis may benefit further from emollient under plastic or vinyl occlusion, whereas hyperkeratotic hand dermatitis benefits from keratolytic-rich and lipid-rich moisturizer ointments containing up to 20% salicylic acid or 10% to 20% urea.[56]

Topical corticosteroid applied before bedtime is a first-line therapy.[60] In general, groups II to IV ointment are used intermittently for flares until clear and for maintenance. Severe, weeping, or refractory cases may require short-term use of groups I to II ointment or creams under occlusion.

There are several other nonsystemic options. Tacrolimus and pimecrolimus are steroid sparing.[60] UVA or nbUVB may be considered for severe, chronic, or refractory cases, especially nonhyperkeratotic cases.[60,61] Intradermal botulinum toxin A 100 to 160 IU can improve palmar dermatitis, especially when palmar hyperhidrosis is present.[62–64] A solution of 1 part vinegar to 6 parts water sprayed on the skin and left to dry twice daily may help restore the acidic skin barrier.

Retinoids can improve chronic refractory cases, especially hyperkeratotic cases. Options include bexarotene gel; oral acitretin; and oral alitretinoin, which is approved for hand dermatitis in Europe and Canada.[60,65–67]

For cases that are severe, chronic, or refractory to the aforementioned treatments, consider cyclosporine, azathioprine, methotrexate, dupilumab, or oral corticosteroids.[63,64]

ASTEATOTIC DERMATITIS
Clinics Care Points

- The appearance of asteatotic dermatitis progresses from pruritic erythematous patches with fine scales to a "cracked porcelain" appearance followed by a painful "dried riverbed" appearance.

- First-line treatments for asteatotic dermatitis include frequent moisturization and judicious use of medium-potency corticosteroid ointments and creams.

Clinical Presentation

Asteatotic dermatitis is a chronic, low-grade dermatitis most prevalent in ages older than 55 years. It presents with erythematous patches with fine, flakey, powdery scales on a background of widespread xerosis. It resembles fine cracked porcelain early on and then develops erythematous fissures to resemble a dried riverbed when advanced. Lesions develop most commonly and initially on the pretibial area and may also involve the extensor arms, trunk, and axillae. The primary symptom is pruritis, although fissures are painful.

The differential diagnosis includes stasis dermatitis, contact dermatitis, adult atopic dermatitis, nummular dermatitis, cellulitis, and scabies.

Management

The key to asteatotic dermatitis management is minimizing transepidermal water loss, including through humidification and following the cleansing and moisturizer recommendations described in the introduction. Medium-potency corticosteroid ointments or creams can clear early inflammation within a few days but should be continued for 2 to 3 weeks. Corticosteroid application can be preceded by soak and smear or wet wrap only while lesions are weeping, indurated, and crusted. Pimecrolimus cream 1% may decrease EASI and pruritus in 2 to 4 weeks.[68] Flares require close follow-up because they can generalize.

NUMMULAR OR DISCOID DERMATITIS
Clinics Care Points

- Nummular dermatitis presents with pruritic, erythematous, edematous, coin-shaped 1 to 4 cm patches or plaques with scale and crust on the extensor legs and forearms and dorsal hands.
- First-line treatments for nummular dermatitis include sensitive skin care, moisturizers, medium-to-high-potency corticosteroid ointments and creams, tacrolimus, pimecrolimus, and crisaborole.

Clinical Presentation

Nummular dermatitis is most prevalent in ages 55 to 65 years. It begins as a solitary lesion and then quickly develops into discrete, round, coin-shaped, exudative, erythematous, edematous 1 to 10 cm patches or plaques with scale and crust that expand via papules or vesicles at the peripheral margin. These lesions are often lichenified, hyperkeratotic, and on a background of xerosis. The first few plaques are usually distributed symmetrically on the extensor lower legs in men and extensor forearms and dorsal hands in women, and subsequent lesions scatter inferior to the neck. Papules and weeping juicy vesicles are prominent during flares.

The differential diagnosis includes psoriasis, tinea corporis or autoeczematization, CTCL, contact dermatitis, atopic dermatitis, and pigmented purpura. More than 30% of cases that are patch tested are positive.[69]

Management

Nummular dermatitis can be very refractory to treatment. Management involves proper cleansing practices, simple topical regimens, humidification, and frequent moisturization as described in the introduction. Groups I to III corticosteroid ointment or cream applied once to twice daily for 3 to 4 weeks after hydration is a first-line therapy, but patients should eventually transition to tacrolimus, pimecrolimus, or crisaborole. nbUVB may be considered for cases refractory to topicals. Dupilumab resulted in improvement lasting at least 120 days in 1 case series.[70]

SUMMARY

Eczematous dermatitis has a significant chronic impact on quality of life. This comprehensive evidence-based review aids health care professionals in diagnosing specific types of dermatitis using clinical data and patch testing. The treatment approaches discussed should allow for best practice management.

DISCLOSURE

The authors have nothing to disclose.

REFERENCES

1. Eichenfield LF, Tom WL, Berger TG, et al. Guidelines of care for the management of atopic dermatitis: section 2. Management and treatment of atopic dermatitis with topical therapies. J Am Acad Dermatol 2014;71:116–32.
2. Xu S, Kwa M, Lohman ME, et al. Consumer preferences, product characteristics, and potentially allergenic ingredients in best-selling moisturizers. JAMA Dermatol 2017;153(11):1099–105.
3. Yang Q, Liu M, Li X, et al. The benefit of a ceramide-linoleic acid-containing moisturizer as an adjunctive therapy for a set of xerotic dermatoses. Dermatol Ther 2019;32(4):e13017.
4. Angelova-Fischer I, Rippke F, Richter D, et al. Stand-alone emollient treatment reduces flares after discontinuation of topical steroid treatment in atopic dermatitis: a double-blind, randomized, vehicle-controlled, left-right comparison study. Acta Derm Venereol 2018;98(5):517–23.
5. Koppes SA, Charles F, Lammers L, et al. Efficacy of a cream containing ceramides and magnesium in the treatment of mild to moderate atopic dermatitis: a randomized, double-blind, emollient- and hydrocortisone-controlled trial. Acta Derm Venereol 2016;96(7):948–53.
6. Buhse L, Kolinski R, Westenberger B, et al. Topical drug classification. Int J Pharm 2005;295(1–2):101–12.
7. Callen J, Chamlin S, Eichenfield LF, et al. A systematic review of the safety of topical therapies for atopic dermatitis. Br J Dermatol 2007;156:203–21.
8. National Institute for Health. Frequency of application of topical corticosteroids for atopic eczema. In: National Institute for Clinical Excellence Guidance. 2014. Available at: https://www.nice.org.uk/guidance/ta81. Accessed January, 18, 2021.
9. Green C, Colquitt JL, Kirby J, et al. Clinical and cost-effectiveness of once-daily versus more frequent use of same potency topical corticosteroids for atopic eczema: a systematic review and economic evaluation. Health Technol Assess 2004;8(47):iii–120.
10. Zirwas MJ, Barkovic S. Anti-pruritic efficacy of itch relief lotion and cream in patients with atopic history: comparison with hydrocortisone cream. J Drugs Dermatol 2017;16(3):243–7.
11. Avila C, Massick S, Kaffenberger BH, et al. Cannabinoids for the treatment of chronic pruritus: A review. J Am Acad Dermatol 2020;82(5):1205–12.

12. Eichenfield LF, Tom WL, Chamlin SL, et al. Guidelines of care for the management of atopic dermatitis: section 1. Diagnosis and assessment of atopic dermatitis. J Am Acad Dermatol 2014;70(2):338–51.
13. Langan SM, Irvine AD, Weidinger S. Atopic dermatitis. Lancet 2020;396(10247): 345–60 [Correction appears in 2020;396(10253):758].
14. Ersser SJ, Cowdell F, Latter S, et al. Psychological and educational interventions for atopic eczema in children. Cochrane Database Syst Rev 2014;2014(1): CD004054.
15. George SM, Karanovic S, Harrison DA, et al. Interventions to reduce Staphylococcus aureus in the management of eczema. Cochrane Database Syst Rev 2019;2019(10):CD003871.
16. Lee JH, Lee SJ, Kim D, et al. The effect of wet-wrap dressing on epidermal barrier in patients with atopic dermatitis. J Eur Acad Dermatol Venereol 2007;21(10): 1360–8.
17. van Zuuren EJ, Fedorowicz Z, Christensen R, et al. Emollients and moisturisers for eczema. Cochrane Database Syst Rev 2017;2(2):CD012119.
18. Sidbury R, Tom WL, Bergman JN, et al. Guidelines of care for the management of atopic dermatitis: Section 4. Prevention of disease flares and use of adjunctive therapies and approaches. J Am Acad Dermatol 2014;71(6):1218–33.
19. Schmitt J, von Kobyletzki L, Svensson A, et al. Efficacy and tolerability of proactive treatment with topical corticosteroids and calcineurin inhibitors for atopic eczema: systematic review and meta-analysis of randomized controlled trials. Br J Dermatol 2011;164:415–28.
20. Luger T, Augustin M, Lambert J, et al. Unmet medical needs in the treatment of atopic dermatitis in infants: An Expert consensus on safety and efficacy of pimecrolimus. Pediatr Allergy Immunol 2020. https://doi.org/10.1111/pai.13422.
21. Ashcroft DM, Dimmock P, Garside R, et al. Efficacy and tolerability of topical pimecrolimus and tacrolimus in the treatment of atopic dermatitis: meta-analysis of randomised controlled trials. BMJ 2005;330:516.
22. Cury Martins J, Martins C, Aoki V, et al. Topical tacrolimus for atopic dermatitis. Cochrane Database Syst Rev 2015;2015(7):CD009864.
23. Chapman MS, Schachner LA, Breneman D, et al. Tacrolimus ointment 0.03% shows efficacy and safety in pediatric and adult patients with mild to moderate atopic dermatitis. J Am Acad Dermatol 2005;53(2 Suppl 2):S177–85.
24. Paller AS, Fölster-Holst R, Chen SC, et al. No evidence of increased cancer incidence in children using topical tacrolimus for atopic dermatitis. J Am Acad Dermatol 2020;83(2):375–81.
25. Castellsague J, Kuiper JG, Pottegård A, et al. A cohort study on the risk of lymphoma and skin cancer in users of topical tacrolimus, pimecrolimus, and corticosteroids (Joint European Longitudinal Lymphoma and Skin Cancer Evaluation - JOELLE study). Clin Epidemiol 2018;10:299–310.
26. Leung DY, Hanifin JM, Pariser DM, et al. Effects of pimecrolimus cream 1% in the treatment of patients with atopic dermatitis who demonstrate a clinical insensitivity to topical corticosteroids: a randomized, multicentre vehicle-controlled trial. Br J Dermatol 2009;161(2):435–43.
27. Eichenfield LF, Lucky AW, Boguniewicz M, et al. Safety and efficacy of pimecrolimus (ASM 981) cream 1% in the treatment of mild and moderate atopic dermatitis in children and adolescents. J Am Acad Dermatol 2002;46:495–504.
28. Schlessinger J, Shepard JS, Gower R, et al. Safety, Effectiveness, and Pharmacokinetics of Crisaborole in Infants Aged 3 to < 24 Months with Mild-to-Moderate Atopic

Dermatitis: A Phase IV Open-Label Study (CrisADe CARE 1). Am J Clin Dermatol 2020;21(2):275–84.

29. van der Valk PG, Snater E, Verbeek-Gijsbers W, et al. Out-patient treatment of atopic dermatitis with crude coal tar. Dermatology 1996;193(1):41–4.
30. Munkvad M. A comparative trial of Clinitar versus hydrocortisone cream in the treatment of atopic eczema. Br J Dermatol 1989;121(6):763–6.
31. Wollenberg A, Christen-Zäch S, Taieb A, et al. ETFAD/EADV Eczema task force 2020 position paper on diagnosis and treatment of atopic dermatitis in adults and children. J Eur Acad Dermatol Venereol 2020;34(12):2717–44.
32. Garritsen FM, Brouwer MW, Limpens J, et al. Photo(chemo)therapy in the management of atopic dermatitis: an updated systematic review with implications for practice and research. Br J Dermatol 2014;170:501–13.
33. Blauvelt A, de Bruin-Weller M, Thaçi D, et al. Dupilumab with concomitant topical corticosteroid treatment in adults with atopic dermatitis with an inadequate response or intolerance to ciclosporin A or when this treatment is medically inadvisable: a placebo controlled, randomized phase III clinical trial (LIBERTY AD CAFÉ). Br J Dermatol 2018;178:1083–101.
34. Sawangjit R, Dilokthornsakul P, Lloyd-Lavery A, et al. Systemic treatments for eczema: a network meta-analysis. Cochrane Database Syst Rev 2020;2020(9): CD013206.
35. Wollenberg A, Barbarot S, Bieber T, et al. Consensus-based European guidelines for treatment of atopic eczema (atopic dermatitis) in adults and children: part II. J Eur Acad Dermatol Venereol 2018;32:850–78.
36. Drucker AM, Ellis AG, Bohdanowicz M, et al. Systemic immunomodulatory treatments for patients with atopic dermatitis. A systemic review and network meta-analysis. JAMA Dermatol 2020;156:1–10.
37. Seger EW, Wechter T, Strowd L, et al. Relative efficacy of systemic treatments for atopic dermatitis. J Am Acad Dermatol 2019;80:411–6.e4.
38. Meggitt SJ, Gray JC, Reynolds NJ. Azathioprine dosed by thiopurine methyltransferase activity for moderate-to-severe atopic eczema: a double-blind, randomised controlled trial. Lancet 2006;367:839–46.
39. Haeck IM, Knol MJ, Ten Berge O, et al. Enteric-coated mycophenolate sodium versus cyclosporin A as long-term treatment in adult patients with severe atopic dermatitis: a randomized controlled trial. J Am Acad Dermatol 2011;64(6): 1074–84.
40. Schmitt J, Schäkel K, Fölster-Holst R, et al. Prednisolone vs. ciclosporin for severe adult eczema. An investigator-initiated double-blind placebo-controlled multicentre trial. Br J Dermatol 2010;162:661–8.
41. Singh R, Heron CE, Ghamrawi RI, et al. Emerging role of janus kinase inhibitors for the treatment of atopic dermatitis. Immunotargets Ther 2020;9:255–72.
42. Podmore P, Burrows D, Bingham EA. Prediction of patch test results. Contact Dermatitis 1984;11(5):283–4.
43. van Amerongen CCA, Ofenloch R, Dittmar D, et al. New positive patch test reactions on day 7-The additional value of the day 7 patch test reading. Contact Dermatitis 2019;81(4):280–7.
44. Chaudhry HM, Drage LA, El-Azhary RA, et al. Delayed patch-test reading after 5 days: an update from the mayo clinic contact dermatitis group. Dermatitis 2017;28(4):253–60.
45. DeKoven JG, Warshaw EM, Zug KA, et al. North American contact dermatitis group patch test results: 2015-2016. Dermatitis 2018;29(6):297–309.

46. Nakada T, Hostynek JJ, Maibach HI. Use tests: ROAT (repeated open application test)/PUT (provocative use test): an overview. Contact Dermatitis 2000;43(1):1–3.
47. Saary J, Qureshi R, Palda V, et al. A systematic review of contact dermatitis treatment and prevention. J Am Acad Dermatol 2005;53(5):845.
48. Han JS, Won KH, Chang SE, et al. Tacrolimus 0.1% ointment in the treatment of allergic contact dermatitis: a new approach. Int J Dermatol 2014;53(10):e470–1.
49. Katsarou A, Armenaka M, Vosynioti V, et al. Tacrolimus ointment 0.1% in the treatment of allergic contact eyelid dermatitis. J Eur Acad Dermatol Venereol 2009; 23(4):382–7.
50. Pacor ML, Di Lorenzo G, Martinelli N, et al. Tacrolimus ointment in nickel sulphate-induced steroid-resistant allergic contact dermatitis. Allergy Asthma Proc 2006; 27(6):527–31.
51. Belsito D, Wilson DC, Warshaw E, et al. A prospective randomized clinical trial of 0.1% tacrolimus ointment in a model of chronic allergic contact dermatitis. J Am Acad Dermatol 2006;55(1):40–6.
52. Saripalli YV, Gadzia JE, Belsito DV. Tacrolimus ointment 0.1% in the treatment of nickel-induced allergic contact dermatitis. J Am Acad Dermatol 2003;49(3): 477–82.
53. Dogra S, Parsad D, Handa S. Narrowband ultraviolet B in airborne contact dermatitis: a ray of hope! Br J Dermatol 2004;150(2):373–4.
54. Cohen DE, Heidary N. Treatment of irritant and allergic contact dermatitis. Dermatol Ther 2004;17(4):334–40.
55. Agner T, Elsner P. Hand eczema: epidemiology, prognosis and prevention. J Eur Acad Dermatol Venereol 2020;34(Suppl 1):4–12.
56. Coenraads PJ. Hand eczema. N Engl J Med 2012;367(19):1829–37.
57. Diepgen TL, Andersen KE, Brandao FM, et al. Hand eczema classification: a cross-sectional, multicentre study of the aetiology and morphology of hand eczema. Br J Dermatol 2009;160:353–8.
58. Boonstra MB, Christoffers WA, Coenraads PJ, et al. Patch test results of hand eczema patients: relation to clinical types. J Eur Acad Dermatol Venereol 2015; 29(5):940–7.
59. Elsner P, Agner T. Hand eczema: treatment. J Eur Acad Dermatol Venereol 2020; 34(Suppl 1):13–21.
60. Christoffers WA, Coenraads PJ, Svensson Å, et al. Interventions for hand eczema. Cochrane Database Syst Rev 2019;4(4):CD004055.
61. Brass D, Fouweather T, Stocken DD, et al. An observer-blinded randomized controlled pilot trial comparing localized immersion psoralen-ultraviolet A with localized narrowband ultraviolet B for the treatment of palmar hand eczema. Br J Dermatol 2018;179(1):63–71.
62. Ismail A, El-Kholy S, Farid C. Botulinum toxin type A in chronic non-dyshidrotic palmar eczema: A side-by-side comparative study. J Dermatol 2020;47(6):601–8.
63. Swartling C, Naver H, Lindberg M, et al. Treatment of dyshidrotic hand dermatitis with intradermal botulinum toxin. J Am Acad Dermatol 2002;47(5):667–71.
64. Wollina U, Karamfilov T. Adjuvant botulinum toxin A in dyshidrotic hand eczema: a controlled prospective pilot study with left-right comparison. J Eur Acad Dermatol Venereol 2002;16:40–2.
65. Hanifin JM, Stevens V, Sheth P, et al. Novel treatment of chronic severe hand dermatitis with bexarotene gel. Br J Dermatol 2004;150(3):545–53.
66. Song M, Lee HJ, Lee WK, et al. Acitretin as a Therapeutic Option for Chronic Hand Eczema. Ann Dermatol 2017;29(3):385–7.

67. Luchsinger I, Vogler T, Schwieger-Briel A, et al. Safe and effective use of alitretinoin in children with recalcitrant hand eczema and other dermatoses - a retrospective analysis. J Eur Acad Dermatol Venereol 2020;34(5):1037–42.
68. Schulz P, Bunselmeyer B, Bräutigam M, et al. Pimecrolimus cream 1% is effective in asteatotic eczema: results of a randomized, double-blind, vehicle-controlled study in 40 patients. J Eur Acad Dermatol Venereol 2007;21(1):90–4.
69. Bonamonte D, Foti C, Vestita M, et al. Nummular eczema and contact allergy: a retrospective study. Dermatitis 2012;23(4):153–7.
70. Choi S, Zhu GA, Lewis MA, et al. Dupilumab treatment of nummular dermatitis: A retrospective cohort study. J Am Acad Dermatol 2020;82(5):1252–5.

Newer Therapies in Psoriasis

Justin W. Marson, MD[a],*, Margaret L. Snyder, MD[b],
Mark G. Lebwohl, MD[b]

KEYWORDS

- Psoriasis • Therapy • Biologics • Tumor necrosis factor-alpha • Interleukins
- Janus kinase inhibitor • Tyrosine kinase inhibitor
- Aryl hydrocarbon receptor modulator

KEY POINTS

- Mediators of inflammation in psoriasis pathogenesis include tumor necrosis factor-alpha, interleukin (IL)-17, IL-23, IL-36, as well as receptors that transduce and propagate these signals (Janus kinase, tyrosine receptor kinase).
- Newer targeted therapies, including biologics, oral agents, and topical agents, can maximize cutaneous and rheumatologic therapeutic benefit while minimizing adverse effects.
- Understanding nuances of therapeutic classes (eg, pharmacodynamics, route of administration, US Food and Drug Administration–approved usages) can maximize physicians' ability to provide the optimal care for patients.

INTRODUCTION

Psoriasis is a systemic inflammatory condition that negatively affects the quality of life and medical health of 125 million individuals globally.[1] Although psoriasis has historically been viewed as a skin-limited disease and managed with topical agents (eg, coal tar, corticosteroids, and vitamin D analogues),[2] the recontextualization of psoriasis as a systemic condition involving multiple organ systems has prompted the development of numerous immunomodulating, systemic agents with more targeted mechanisms of action.[3,4] This article briefly discusses the indications and nuances of new and developing therapeutic agents for psoriasis management (**Table 1**).

BACKGROUND OF PSORIASIS PATHOPHYSIOLOGY

Both the innate and adaptive immune systems contribute to the inflammatory pathways in psoriasis.[4] Damaged keratinocytes are thought to secrete antimicrobial peptides that interact with released cellular material, thereby locally activating dendritic cells, which in

Funding sources: None.
[a] National Society for Cutaneous Medicine, New York, NY, USA; [b] Department of Dermatology, Icahn School of Medicine at Mount Sinai, 5 East 98th Street, 5th Floor, New York, NY 10029, USA
* Corresponding author. 35 East 35th Street #208, New York, NY 10016.
E-mail address: justin.w.marson@gmail.com

Table 1
Summary of newer therapies for chronic plaque psoriasis and psoriatic arthritis

Class	Name	RoA	FDA-Approved Dosing: PsO	FDA-Approved Dosing: PsA	Regimen Adjustments[a]	Latest Findings
TNF-α	Certolizumab pegol	SubQ	400 mg QOW	400 mg on weeks 0, 2, 4 then c/w 200 mg QOW	PsO: <90 kg 400 mg on weeks 0, 2, 4 then c/w 200 mg QOW	• Efficacy and safety up to 3 y
IL-17A	Secukinumab	SubQ	300 mg on weeks 0,1,2,3, 4 then Q4W	Loading dose: 150 mg on weeks 0, 1, 2, 3, 4 then 150 mg Q4W, can increase to 300 mg Q4W. No loading dose: 150 mg Q4W, can increase to 300 mg Q4W	PsO: ≥90 kg, 300 mg Q2W[b] Pediatric (6–17 yo) dosing (high dose/low dose): <25 kg: 75 mg Q4W[b] 25–50 kg: 150/75 mg Q4W[b] >50 kg: 300/150 mg Q4W[b]	• Onset within 12 wk • Comparable with adalimumab for PsA • Potential efficacy and safety for pediatric PsO
IL-17A	Ixekizumab	SubQ	160 mg for 1 dose followed by 80 mg Q2W for 6 doses then 80 mg Q4W Pediatric (6–17 yo) dosing: <25 kg: 40 mg once then 20 mg Q4W 25–50 kg: 80 mg once then 40 mg Q4W >50 kg: 160 mg (2 separate 80 mg injections) then 80 mg Q2W for 6 doses then 80 mg Q4W	160 mg once, then 80 mg Q4W	PsA: can use in conjunction with other DMARDs	• Onset within 12 wk

Class	Drug	Route	Dosing	Dosing		Comments
IL-17A and IL-17F	Bimekizumab	SubQ	160 mg Q4W[b] 320-mg loading dose then 160 mg Q4W[b] 320 mg Q8W[c]	160 mg Q4W[b] 320-mg loading dose then 160 mg Q4W[b] 320 mg Q8W[c]	—	• Efficacious for PsO • Potential benefits for PsA
IL-23p19	Guselkumab	SubQ	100 mg on weeks 0, 4 then then Q8W	100 mg on weeks 0,4 then Q8W	PsA: can use in conjunction with other DMARDs	• Benefits for PsA • Increased durability vs IL-17
IL-23p19	Tildrakizumab	SubQ	100 mg on weeks 0, 4 then Q12W	20 mg Q12W[b] 100 mg Q12W[b] 200 mg Q12W[b] 200 mg Q4W[b]	—	• Potential benefits for PsA • Efficacy for up to 4 y; retreatment after lapsed dose; despite long-standing/previously treated PsO • Increased durability vs IL-17
IL-23p19	Risankizumab	SubQ	150 mg (2 consecutive 75-mg doses) on weeks 0, 4 then Q12W	—	—	• Preliminary data: efficacy up to 136 wk; increased efficacy vs adalimumab and ustekinumab
IL-23p19	Mirikizumab	SubQ	Induction: 250 mg Q4W[b] 30 mg Q8W[b] 100 mg Q8W[b] 300 mg Q8W[b] Maintenance: 125 mg Q8W[b] 250 mg Q8W[b] 300 mg Q8W[b]	—	250 mg Q4W for 16 weeks then 250 mg Q8W 250 mg Q4W for 16 weeks then 125 mg Q8W	• Preliminary data: efficacy for PsO; increased durability vs IL-17

(continued on next page)

Table 1
(continued)

Class	Name	RoA	FDA-Approved Dosing: PsO	FDA-Approved Dosing: PsA	Regimen Adjustments[a]	Latest Findings
IL-36	Spesolimab	Parenteral	One dose 10 mg/kg[b]	—	—	• Preliminary data: efficacy and safety up to week 20 after 1 dose; efficacy for pustular PsO
JAK1/2	Baricitinib[b]	Oral	2 mg QD[b] 4 mg QD[b] 8 mg QD[b] 10 mg QD[b]	—	Avoid in severe hepatic/renal (eGFR<15–30 mL/min/1.73 m²) impairment	—
TyK	BMS-986165 (deucravacitinib)	Oral	3 mg QOD[b] 3 mg QD[b] 3 mg BID[b] 6 mg BID[b] 12 mg QD[b]	—	—	• Efficacious for PsO
PDE-4 inhibitor	Roflumilast	Topical	0.15% QD 0.3% QD	—	—	• Efficacious for mild-moderate PsO
Aryl hydrocarbon receptor modulator	Tapinarof	Topical	0.5% QD[b] 0.5% BID[b] 1.0% QD[b] 1.0% BID[b]	—	—	• Efficacious for mild-moderate PsO

Abbreviations: BID, twice a day; *c/w*, continue with; DMARDs, disease-modifying antirheumatic drugs; eGFR, estimated glomerular filtration rate; FDA, United States Food and Drug Administration; IL, interleukin; JAK, Janus kinase; PDE-4, phosphodiesterase 4; PsA, psoriatic arthritis; PsO, plaque psoriasis; Q12W, every 12 weeks; Q4W, every 4 weeks; Q8W, every 8 weeks; QD, daily; QOD, every other day; QOW, every other week; RoA, route of administration; SubQ, subcutaneous injection; TNF-α, tumor necrosis factor-alpha; TyK, tyrosine receptor kinase; yo, years old.

[a] No studies detailing necessary dose adjustment for renal or hepatic adjustments (unless otherwise noted).

[b] Reported dosages in clinical trial.

[c] Recent studies suggest equivalent efficacy with 320 mg Q8W dosing regimen compared to 320 mg Q4W.

turn locally and distally activate various T-cell lineages (most notably T-helper [Th] 1 and Th17 subsets) by secreting cytokines, including tumor necrosis factor alpha (TNF-α), interleukin (IL)-12, and IL-23.[4] Upregulation of IL-23 drives increases in Th17 lymphocyte activity and expression of IL-17, a dimeric cytokine wherein 2 of the 6 known isoforms (A and F) are clinically relevant to psoriasis pathogenesis.[4] Transmission of these extracellular signals requires transmembrane signaling receptors, notably Janus kinase (JAK) and tyrosine receptors kinases (TyKs).[4] When activated, JAKs and TyKs selectively phosphorylate intracellular proteins, leading to signal transduction, subsequent alteration of gene expression, and, ultimately, protein synthesis involved in propagating inflammation. Additional cytokines, such as IL-36 released by keratinocytes and modified by neutrophils, are also thought to be contributory.[4]

TUMOR NECROSIS FACTOR-α INHIBITORS
Certolizumab Pegol

TNF-α inhibitors have been used for psoriasis for more than a decade. Certolizumab pegol is a combination of a human monoclonal antibody and a polyethylene glycol moiety capable of binding free and soluble TNF-α that has been US Food and Drug Administration (FDA) approved since 2018 for the treatment of plaque psoriasis, psoriatic arthritis, and other inflammatory arthropathies.[5] Data from phase II trials have shown efficacy for certolizumab pegol for up to 48 weeks. 68.2% of patients receiving 200 mg doses every other week saw at least a 75% improvement in their psoriasis area and severity index (PASI 75) score, while 49.1% achieved at least PASI 90 compared to 9.9% and 2.5% for patients on placebo. Additionally, 81.6% and 60.1% of patients on certolizumab pegol 400 mg every other week achieved PASI75/90.[6] More recent data from the CIMPASI-1 and CIMPASI-2 trials have shown efficacy for up to 3 years (144 weeks) with 70.6% and 48.7% of patients on the 200-mg dose and 72.9% and 42.7% of patients on the 400-mg regimen reaching PASI 75/90, respectively.[7] The same trial also pooled data on safety for the 200-mg and 400-mg dosing regimens and found treatment-emergent adverse effects (TEAEs) were transiently higher during the first 16 weeks of treatment, were similar between treatment groups across adverse events (AEs) by week 48, remained stable through week 144, and that less than 9% of patients discontinued treatment as a result of AEs.[8] Out of nearly 1000 participants over 3 years, there were 2 study-related deaths (1 myocardial infarction and another a complication of hemorrhagic pancreatic necrosis, both with significant comorbidities), 3 study-related opportunistic infections (legionella pneumonia, fungal esophagitis, and tuberculosis in a patient from an endemic area with initially negative prestudy screen), 11 malignancies, 5 nonmelanoma skin cancers, 9 major adverse cardiovascular events, and 2 demyelinating events (although 1 patient had reported symptoms before the study). The most common TEAE was mild to moderate infection, with 41 infections reported (including upper and lower respiratory infections, skin and soft tissue infection, and endophthalmitis).[8] These data show the durability of certolizumab efficacy as well as its relative safety.

INTERLEUKIN-17 INHIBITORS
Secukinumab

Secukinumab is an anti–IL-17A agent that has been FDA approved for psoriasis, psoriatic arthritis, and other inflammatory arthropathies since 2015. Real-world studies have shown efficacy with PASI 75/90/100 of 83.8%/70%/46.3% at week 16 and drug survival of up to 74.5% at 2 years.[9] In a study of 10,416 patients with psoriasis and 3866 patients with psoriatic arthritis, the respective incidence per

100 patient-years of serious infections was 1.4 and 1.9; candidal infections were 2.2 and 1.5; and major adverse cardiac events were 0.3 and 0.4.[10] There were no cases of tuberculosis reactivation.[10]

New data from several comparator trials have shown clinical nuances for secukinumab. The phase III, double-blinded, randomized ECLIPSE trial showed differences in time to clinical efficacy, wherein, at week 12, a larger percentage of patients on secukinumab 300 mg weekly for 5 doses then every 4 weeks (76.2%) reached PASI90 than those receiving guselkumab 100 mg every 4 weeks for 2 doses then every 8 weeks (69.1%); however, by week 16 to 20, similar proportions of both arms (~80%) reached PASI90.[11] Another comparator trial for psoriatic arthritis (EXCEED) found that, within 52 weeks, 67% of participants on secukinumab attained 20% improvement per American College of Rheumatology response criteria (ACR20) versus 62% on adalimumab (odds ratio [OR], 1.3; 95% confidence interval, 0.98–1.72). Interestingly, there were similar TEAEs compared with prior studies, with 1% of the adalimumab group and 2% of the secukinumab group developing serious infections. Furthermore although 24% of participants on adalimumab discontinued prematurely, only 14% on secukinumab did not reach week 52.[12]

Additional studies have also shown secukinumab's efficacy for additional populations. For patients weighing more than 90 kg, preliminary studies have found more frequent dosing may better control disease burden. For example, 73.2% of patients with a mean body weight of 111.5 kg ($\pm$17.5 kg) on 300 mg every 2 weeks achieved PASI90 versus 55.5% of patients with a mean body weight of 110.7 kg ($\pm$18.5 kg) on 300 mg every 4 weeks ($P<.0003$).[13]

New data from phase III, double-blind trials also suggests weight-based dosing of secukinumab may have potential benefits for the adolescent population with plaque psoriasis.[14] In 1 study, participants aged 6 to 17 years were stratified by weight (<25 kg, 25–50 kg, >50 kg) and then randomized into either high-dose or low-dose groups. By week 12, significantly more participants in both the high-dose and low-dose secukinumab groups reached PASI75/90 (80%/73%, 78%/68%, respectively) than placebo (15%/2%) ($P<.0001$).[14] Interestingly, significantly more ($P<.05$) participants also reached PASI90 compared with etanercept (29%). By week 52, safety data showed similar rates of injection-site reactions and candidal infections across treatment arms; however, there were increased rates of hypersensitivity reactions in the high-dose group.[14] Although further studies are needed to fully elucidate TEAE, efficacy has been shown in patients previously on biologics or with long-standing psoriasis.

These findings suggest utility for secukinumab for quick-onset management of adult and pediatric plaque psoriasis as well as psoriatic arthritis.

Ixekizumab

Ixekizumab, an IL-17A antagonist, has also shown efficacy for both plaque psoriasis and psoriatic arthritis. Similarly to the ECLIPSE trial, the IXORA-R study showed early superiority of IL-17 compared with IL-23 blockade. In this trial, 1027 patients were randomized 1:1 to receive standard dosages of either ixekizumab or guselkumab.[15] IL-17 inhibition showed faster onset of skin clearance and greater efficacy, with 28% of patients on ixekizumab achieving a PASI50 response at week 1, versus 9% for guselkumab. This effect continued to be apparent throughout the studied time period, with 41% in the ixekizumab group achieving PASI100 at week 12, compared with only 25% receiving guselkumab.[15] Long-term data are needed in order to evaluate the relative maintenance of this clinical response over time.

Ixekizumab has also been shown to be effective in pediatric patients with plaque psoriasis. By week 12 in the IXORA-PEDS study, 89% of pediatric patients treated with ixekizumab achieved a PASI75 response, compared with 25% in the placebo group.[16] Similarly, 81% and 11% achieved an static physician's global assessment (sPGA) of 0 out of 1 in ixekizumab and placebo groups, respectively. Ixekizumab was also superior in important secondary end points such as improvement in skin itch and quality of life. Clinical response was maintained through 48 weeks of treatment, and safety profiles were similar among drug-treated and placebo-treated groups aside from injection-site reactions and inflammatory bowel disease, which were seen more frequently with ixekizumab.

Ixekizumab has likewise shown to be a promising treatment of patients with joint manifestations. One randomized, open-label, 24-week clinical trial comparing ixekizumab with adalimumab in 500 patients found ixekizumab to be noninferior to adalimumab in improving joint disease as determined by ACR50 response. Furthermore, ixekizumab was superior in the clearance of skin lesions (PASI 100 of 60% vs 47%, respectively).[17] The current evidence suggests ixekizumab is a well-tolerated therapeutic option for both adult and pediatric patients with plaque psoriasis and/or psoriatic arthritis, and may be superior in rate of onset of clinical response compared with agents that inhibit IL-23, an important factor to consider when counseling patients.

Bimekizumab

Bimekizumab is the first bispecific antibody capable of targeting 2 isoforms of IL-17, IL-17A and IL-17F, both of which have been shown to have a pathogenic role in psoriasis and psoriatic arthritis.[18] In the BE ACTIVE study, a multiple-site, randomized, double-blind, controlled phase IIb trial, 206 adult participants with psoriatic arthritis were randomized to 1 of 4 doses of bimekizumab (16 mg, 160 mg, 160 mg after a 1-time 320-mg loading dose, or 320 mg) every 4 weeks or placebo over 12 weeks.[19] At 12 weeks, participants treated with bimekizumab had a significantly higher OR ACR50, with OR increasing in a dose-dependent manner, versus placebo. Furthermore, AEs were predominately mild to moderate in severity and had similar rates across placebo and treatment arms.[19] Preliminary data from phase III of the BE ACTIVE study at 48 weeks show similar continued efficacy.

In a multiarmed, double-blind, randomized, placebo-controlled phase IIb study (BE ABLE 1), participants showed a dose-dependent response to bimekizumab by week 12 with PASI 90/100 scores of 46.2% to 79.1% and 27.9% to 60% compared with the placebo group (0%).[20] TEAEs were reported in 61% of the bimekizumab group versus 36% in the placebo group, including mild to moderate viral and fungal infections that resolved, and only 4.8% of TEAEs led to discontinuation.[20] Continuation of this study in the BE ABLE 2 trial showed both lasting efficacy of bimekizumab for skin lesions in plaque psoriasis as well as efficacy in other clinical domains of psoriasis.[21] At week 60, participants continued to have high efficacy, with 80% to 100% maintaining PASI90.[21] The most common AEs observed were oral/esophageal candidiasis (13.4%) and nasopharyngitis (12.9%), with only 6.9% of participants reporting serious TEAEs.[21]

A phase III, randomized, double-blinded, placebo-controlled study (BE READY)[22] and a comparator-controlled study versus ustekinumab (BE VIVID)[23] are currently underway with promising results in terms of longevity of efficacy between dosages (up to 8 weeks without loss of efficacy). Preliminary data show notable skin clearance by week 16, which is sustained through week 52, despite participants' prior use of systemics (~80% of patients) and/or biologics (~40% of patients).[22,23] Further studies will be needed to fully elucidate bimekizumab's safety profile with respect to inflammatory bowel disease, (candida) infection risk, as well as efficacy for inflammatory arthropathies. Overall, these studies show the efficacy and safety of a novel agent capable of blocking a broader range of IL-17 isoforms in the management of psoriasis and psoriatic arthritis.

INTERLEUKIN-23 INHIBITORS
Guselkumab

Guselkumab is an FDA-approved (since June 2017) human monoclonal immunoglobulin (Ig) G antibody that inhibits IL-23 at its p19 subunit. Previous phase III clinical trials (eg, VOYAGE 2) have shown guselkumab's efficacy for plaque psoriasis, and new data suggest its utility in managing psoriatic arthritis.[3,24] In the multisite, double-blind, randomized-controlled phase III trial, DISCOVER 1, guselkumab achieved ACR20 by week 24 in 59% of patients on 100 mg every 4 weeks and 52% of patients receiving 100 mg every 8 weeks (after administration of 100 mg on weeks 0 and 4) compared with only 22% of patients on placebo. In addition, preliminary data from DISCOVER-2 suggest that guselkumab 100 mg every 4 weeks may have advantages compared with both placebo and every-8-weeks dosing in preventing radiographic progression of psoriatic joint disease.[25]

Additional findings from the ECLIPSE trial found that, although guselkumab had lower PASI90scores than secukinumab at week 12, by week 48, guselkumab's PASI90 was ~84.5% compared with 70% for secukinumab.[11] These differences in pharmacokinetics likely reflect the mechanism of action of these agents and are being further studied in additional head-to-head trials.[15] Clinically, these differences add a dimension to patient counseling of goals regarding response time versus durability of response.

Tildrakizumab

FDA approved since 2018, tildrakizumab is a humanized monoclonal IgG antibody that antagonizes IL-23 via the p19 subunit.[3] Although already approved for moderate to severe chronic plaque psoriasis,[3] data from a phase IIb study suggest future utility for psoriatic arthritis.[26] ACR20/50/70 for patients with active psoriatic arthritis that received at least 1 dose of tildrakizumab were significantly greater than (71.4%–79.5%/39.7%–52.6%/16.7%–29.1%), and increased in a dose-dependent manner compared with placebo (50.6%/24.1%/10.1%) by week 24.[26] Preliminary data are also promising for crossover participants (either crossing from placebo to drug or increasing to a higher dose of tildrakizumab) by week 52.

In terms of chronic plaque psoriasis, efficacy data for tildrakizumab are now available for up to 4 years. Data from the original reSURFACE 1 trial now show that tildrakizumab 100 mg and 200 mg had similar and durable PASI 75/90/100 (82%/56%/28%) at 144 weeks.[27] The reSURFACE 1 trial also showed durability of tildrakizumab for patients that may miss a dose with a median of 20/25 weeks (tildrakizumab 100/200 mg respectively) before losing PASI75.[28,29] After lapses in treatment, no rebound was observed and, following retreatment for at least 12 weeks, 85.7%/83.3% (100/200 mg respectively) were able to recapture PASI75.

Another consideration is that tildrakizumab seems to have similar efficacy despite the chronicity that patients have had psoriasis. For example, 72.6% and 48.2% of patients who have had long-standing moderate-severe psoriasis achieved PASI75/90 on tildrakizumab 100 mg compared with only 54.4% and 26.9% PASI75/90 on etanercept.[30]

Risankizumab

Risankizumab is a subcutaneously administered anti–IL-23 blocker at the p19 subunit that was FDA approved in 2019 for moderate to severe plaque psoriasis.[31] Initial results from 2 phase 3 randomized, double-blind, head-to-head trials (UltIMMA and IMMvent) showed efficacy compared with ustekinumab (UltIMMa-1/UltMMA-2) and adalimumab (IMMvent). Specifically, 74.8% to 75.3% of patients on risankizumab achieved PASI90 by week 16 without incurring unexpected AEs, compared with 2.0% to 4.6% on placebo and 42.0% to 47.5% on ustekinumab.[32] Similar results were found in the IMMvent trial, with 72% of participants on risankizumab 150 mg achieving PASI90 by week 16 versus 47% on adalimumab 40 mg. Furthermore, 66% of adalimumab-intermediate responders who were switched to risankizumab achieved PASI90.[33] Preliminary data from LIMMitless, the open-label extension of the UltIMMA/IMMvent trials, have shown lasting efficacy of risankizumab for up to 136 weeks, with PASI90/100 up to 87%/61%, respectively, and similar PASI90/100 for patients who transitioned from adalimumab to risankizumab.[34,35]

Mirikizumab

Mirikizumab (LY3074828) is a humanized antibody against the p19 subunit of IL-23 that is currently undergoing randomized, placebo-controlled trials to determine its efficacy for chronic plaque psoriasis. In initial phase 2, 4-armed, parallel trials, mirikizumab showed PASI90 in 67% of participants on 300 mg every 8 weeks, 59% on 100 mg every 8 weeks, 29% on 30 mg every 8 weeks and in 0% in those on placebo with similar serious AEs in participants on mirikizumab (1%) and placebo (2%).[36] Preliminary data out to 52 weeks showed additional efficacy of mirikizumab 300 mg every 8 weeks for participants who had not reached PASI90 (on other doses/placebo). Sixty-eight percent of participants previously on placebo and 69%/60%/57% of participants previously on mirikizumab 30/100/300 mg every 8 weeks until week 16 achieved PASI90 by week 52. These results suggest mirikizumab may have similar delayed-onset pharmacodynamics to other IL-23p19 inhibitors.[37]

At present, the phase 3, randomized, double-blind, placebo-controlled, head-to-head trial comparing mirikizumab with secukinumab (OASIS-2) is underway.[38] Preliminary data suggest mirikizumab 250 mg every 4 weeks is noninferior to secukinumab 300 mg in attaining PASI90/100 at week 16 and that both the 125-mg and 250-mg every 8 weeks dosing patterns may have significantly greater efficacy by week 52.[38]

Interleukin-36 Inhibitors

Recent studies have found that IL-36, driven by IL-17, may play a role in epidermal hyperplasia and the clinical and histologic development of scale and parakeratosis, respectively.[39] To that end, a new biologic, BI 655130 (spesolimab), has entered phase 1 trials to determine efficacy and safety for use in generalized pustular psoriasis.[40] Thus far, preliminary data show that blockade of IL-36 achieved a physician global assessment score of 0 out of 1 for 4 out of 4 patients beginning at week 4 of treatment, without serious drug-related AEs or AEs leading to discontinuation up to week 20.[40] Imsidolimab, another anti–IL-36 antibody that inhibits the function of the IL-36 receptor, is also being investigated for pustular psoriasis.

ORAL THERAPIES
Baricitinib

Baricitinib is an oral JAK1/2 inhibitor that has been studied for treatment of moderate to severe psoriasis.[41] In the 2016 phase 2 study, 271 patients were randomized to baricitinib 2 mg, 4 mg, 8 mg, 10 mg, or placebo once daily and assessed for PASI75 response over 12 weeks. By 12 weeks, 42.9% of participants on 8 mg ($P<.05$) and 54% on 10 mg ($P<.001$) achieved PASI75, compared with only 17% in the placebo group. Statistically significant results were observable by week 8 in the 8-mg and

10-mg groups versus placebo (P<.01).[41] More than 81% of patients maintained PASI75 response through 24 weeks. Over the course of the study, the most common TEAEs were infections, predominantly nasopharyngitis, in 21.1% of all participants on baricitinib and 26.5% on placebo. No opportunistic infections were observed.[41] However, mild dose-associated increases in creatine kinase, high-density lipoprotein, and low-density lipoprotein levels, and decreases in hemoglobin level and neutrophil count, were reported.[41]

Tyrosine Receptor Kinase Inhibitor

BMS-986165, also called deucravacitinib, is a selective TYK2 inhibitor that is currently undergoing phase 3 trials for the treatment of moderate to severe plaque psoriasis. Results from the phase 2 trials, wherein 267 patients were randomized to 1 of 6 interventions (placebo, 3 mg every other day, 3 mg daily, 3 mg twice daily, 6 mg twice daily, 12 mg daily), have shown that, by 12 weeks, PASI 75/90 was attained by 39%/16% of participants on 3 mg daily (P<.001, P<.05), 69%/44% on 3 mg twice daily, 67%/44% on 6 mg twice daily, and 75%/43% on 12 mg daily (all P<.0001) compared with only 7%/2% of those on placebo.[42] Similar results were found for achieving PASI 100 (or completely lesion-free skin) with 18% of participants on 6 mg twice daily (P<.01) and 25% of participants on 12 mg daily (P<.001), compared with 0% on placebo.[42] The most common AEs were upper respiratory infections and nasopharyngitis.[42] Of note, there were no deaths or serious AEs recorded in either the 6 mg twice daily or 12 mg daily groups.[42]

TOPICAL THERAPIES
Roflumilast

Phosphodiesterase-4 inhibitors are a novel class of medications first FDA approved in 2014.[43] Although originally only available orally (as apremilast),[43] a new topical formulation, ARQ-151 (roflumilast) has recently completed phase 2b double-blind, placebo-controlled trials. Of participants randomized to either 0.3% or 0.15% roflumilast cream daily for 12 weeks, 28% (P<.001) and 23% (P<.004) achieved investigator's global assessment (IGA) of clear or nearly clear by 6 weeks, compared with only 8% on vehicle.[44] Furthermore, participants had at least a 2-grade improvement in intertriginous psoriasis in 73%/44% of the 0.3%/0.15% groups, respectively, versus 29% on placebo.[44] Phase 3 trials for ARQ-151 are ongoing to determine long-term safety and efficacy.

Tapinarof

Tapinarof, an aryl hydrocarbon receptor modulator, has shown significant efficacy in clearing plaque psoriasis lesions in phase 2 clinical trials. In a double-blind, randomized, vehicle-controlled study, treatment success, defined as both achievement of a PGA of 0/1 and a 2-grade overall improvement, was significantly higher in patients receiving tapinarof than in those on placebo after only 8 weeks of treatment. This effect was increased by week 12, with treatment success achieved in 36% to 65% of patients in tapinarof arms versus 5% to 11% receiving placebo (P<.05).[45] Likewise, PASI75 response was significantly higher in the tapinarof groups at these time points. Statistically significant improvement was witnessed with both once-daily and twice-daily application and with both 1% and 0.5% formulations, and treatment success persisted throughout the 16-week study. Therefore, tapinarof represents a promising nonsteroidal option for patients with limited involvement who are suitable for topical therapy, and phase 3 trials are ongoing to determine long-term safety and efficacy.

SUMMARY

Although the most conspicuous symptoms are often cutaneous, psoriasis is a systemic, inflammatory condition. To that end, newer therapies have been developed to target key mediators in the psoriatic-inflammatory cascade. Although preliminary data are promising for various therapeutic options in the treatment of both psoriasis and psoriatic arthritis, there are nuances between agents that should be taken into account when counseling patients. Although data suggest IL-17 inhibitors may have superior efficacy earlier in the treatment course than IL-23 inhibitors, the latter may prove more efficacious in the long term. Furthermore, secukinumab may have efficacy for managing psoriasis in pediatric patients and patients weighing more than 90 kg. For patients averse to injections, oral JAK and TyK inhibitors may provide suitable alternatives. In addition, newer topical, nonsteroidal agents using both known and novel pathways are being implemented to control mild to moderate plaque psoriasis. As the scope of understanding of psoriasis pathogenesis improves, so too will the efficacy and safety of the agents in the armament.

CLINICS CARE POINTS

- Current data suggest IL-17 inhibitors may have quicker onset than IL-23 inhibitors; however, longitudinal data suggest IL-23 inhibitors may have more sustained efficacy.

- JAK and selective TyK inhibitors provide targeted oral therapeutic options for patients who are not amenable to infusion or subcutaneous biologic therapies.

- New targeted topical therapies (tapinarof, roflumilast) may provide efficacious nonsteroidal options for limited chronic plaque psoriasis.

- The most common adverse effects of targeted, systemic immunomodulating therapies are upper respiratory infections, nasopharyngitis, and mild to moderate candida infections. However, prescribers should still be diligent about conducting screening laboratory assessments before initiating therapy.

CONFLICTS OF INTEREST

Drs J.W. Marson and M.L. Snyder have no relevant disclosures. M.G. Lebwohl is an employee of Mount Sinai and receives research funds from Abbvie, Amgen, Arcutis, Boehringer Ingelheim, Dermavant, Eli Lilly, Incyte, Janssen Research & Development, Leo Pharmaceuticals, Ortho Dermatologics, Pfizer, and UCB, and is a consultant for Aditum Bio, Allergan, Almirall, Arcutis, Avotres Therapeutics, BirchBioMed, BMD skincare, Boehringer-Ingelheim, Bristol-Myers Squibb, Cara Therapeutics, Castle Biosciences, Corrona, Dermavant Sciences, Evelo, Facilitate International Dermatologic Education, Foundation for Research and Education in Dermatology, Inozyme Pharma, Kyowa Kirin, LEO Pharma, Meiji Seika Pharma, Menlo, Mitsubishi, Neuroderm, Pfizer, Promius/Dr Reddy's Laboratories, Serono, Theravance, and Verrica.

REFERENCES

1. Armstrong AW, Read C. Pathophysiology, Clinical Presentation, and Treatment of Psoriasis: A Review. JAMA 2020;323(19):1945–60.

2. Elmets CA, Korman NJ, Prater EF, et al. Joint AAD-NPF Guidelines of care for the management and treatment of psoriasis with topical therapy and alternative medicine modalities for psoriasis severity measures. J Am Acad Dermatol 2020. https://doi.org/10.1016/j.jaad.2020.07.087.

3. Menter A, Strober BE, Kaplan DH, et al. Joint AAD-NPF guidelines of care for the management and treatment of psoriasis with biologics. J Am Acad Dermatol 2019. https://doi.org/10.1016/j.jaad.2018.11.057.

4. Rendon A, Schäkel K. Psoriasis Pathogenesis and Treatment. Int J Mol Sci 2019. https://doi.org/10.3390/ijms20061475.

5. Highlights of Prescribing Information. Available at: https://www.accessdata.fda.gov/drugsatfda_docs/label/2019/125160s237lbl.pdf. Accessed September 22, 2020.

6. Gottlieb AB, Blauvelt A, Thaçi D, et al. Certolizumab pegol for the treatment of chronic plaque psoriasis: Results through 48 weeks from 2 phase 3, multicenter, randomized, double-blinded, placebo-controlled studies (CIMPASI-1 and CIMPASI-2). J Am Acad Dermatol 2018;79(2):302–14.e6.

7. Gordon KB, Warren RB, Gottlieb AB, et al. Long-term efficacy of certolizumab pegol for the treatment of plaque psoriasis: 3-year results from two randomized phase III trials (CIMPASI-1 and CIMPASI-2). Br J Dermatol 2020. https://doi.org/10.1111/bjd.19393.

8. Blauvelt A, Paul C, Van De Kerkhof P, et al. Long-Term Safety of Certolizumab Pegol in Plaque Psoriasis: Pooled Analysis over 3 Years from Three Phase 3, Randomised, Placebo-Controlled Studies. Br J Dermatol 2020. https://doi.org/10.1111/bjd.19314.

9. Rompoti N, Katsimbri P, Kokkalis G, et al. Real world data from the use of secukinumab in the treatment of moderate-to-severe psoriasis, including scalp and palmoplantar psoriasis: A 104-week clinical study. Dermatol Ther 2019;32(5):e13006.

10. Deodhar A, Mease PJ, McInnes IB, et al. Long-term safety of secukinumab in patients with moderate-to-severe plaque psoriasis, psoriatic arthritis, and ankylosing spondylitis: integrated pooled clinical trial and post-marketing surveillance data. Arthritis Res Ther 2019;21(1):111.

11. Reich K, Armstrong AW, Langley RG, et al. Guselkumab versus secukinumab for the treatment of moderate-to-severe psoriasis (ECLIPSE): results from a phase 3, randomised controlled trial. Lancet 2019;394(10201):831–9.

12. McInnes IB, Behrens F, Mease PJ, et al, EXCEED Study Group. Secukinumab versus adalimumab for treatment of active psoriatic arthritis (EXCEED): a double-blind, parallel-group, randomised, active-controlled, phase 3b trial. Lancet 2020;395(10235):1496–505 [Erratum in: Lancet. 2020;395(10238):1694].

13. Augustin M., Patekar M., Yamauchi P., Pinter A., Bagel J., Xia S., Charef P., Keefe D. Secukinumab dosing every two weeks demonstrated superior efficacy compared to dosing every four weeks in psoriasis patients weighing 90 kg or more. 29th European Academy of Dermatology and Venereology (EADV) Congress: Posters P1391. Virtually Presented October 29–31, 2020.

14. Bodemer C, et al. Secukinumab demonstrated high efficacy and a favorable safety profile in pediatric patients with severe chronic plaque psoriasis: One-year results. FC02.08, EADV Virtual Congress, October 29–31, 2020.

15. Blauvelt A, Papp K, Gottlieb A, et al. A head-to-head comparison of ixekizumab vs. guselkumab in patients with moderate-to-severe plaque psoriasis: 12-week efficacy, safety and speed of response from a randomized, double-blinded trial. Br J Dermatol 2020;182(6):1348–58.

16. Paller AS, Seyger MMB, Magarinos GA, et al. Efficacy and safety of ixekizumab in a phase III, randomized, double-blind, placebo-controlled study in paediatric patients with moderate-to-severe plaque psoriasis (IXORA-PEDS). Br J Dermatol 2020;183(2):231–41.

17. Mease PJ, Smolen JS, Behrens F, et al. A head-to-head comparison of the efficacy and safety of ixekizumab and adalimumab in biological-naïve patients with active psoriatic arthritis: 24-week results of a randomised, open-label, blinded-assessor trial. Ann Rheum Dis 2020;79(1):123–31.

18. Reis J, Vender R, Torres T. Bimekizumab: the first dual inhibitor of interleukin (IL)-17A and IL-17F for the treatment of psoriatic disease and ankylosing spondylitis. BioDrugs 2019;33(4):391–9.

19. Ritchlin CT, Kavanaugh A, Merola JF, et al. Bimekizumab in patients with active psoriatic arthritis: results from a 48-week, randomised, double-blind, placebo-controlled, dose-ranging phase 2b trial. Lancet 2020;395(10222):427–40.

20. Papp KA, Merola JF, Gottlieb AB, et al. Dual neutralization of both interleukin 17A and interleukin 17F with bimekizumab in patients with psoriasis: Results from BE ABLE 1, a 12-week randomized, double-blinded, placebo-controlled phase 2b trial. J Am Acad Dermatol 2018;79(2):277–86.e10.

21. Blauvelt A, Papp KA, Merola JF, et al. Bimekizumab for patients with moderate to severe plaque psoriasis: 60-week results from BE ABLE 2, a randomized, double-blinded, placebo-controlled, phase 2b extension study. J Am Acad Dermatol 2020. https://doi.org/10.1016/j.jaad.2020.05.105. S0190-9622(20)30980-4.

22. Gordon, K., Foley, P., Krueger, J., Pinter, A., Reich, K., Vender, R., Vanvoorden, V., Madden, C., Peterson, L., Blauvelt, A. Efficacy and safety of bimekizumab in patients with moderate-to-severe plaque psoriasis: results from BE READY, a 56-week Phase 3, randomized, double-blinded, placebo-controlled study with randomized withdrawal. Poster presented at: AAD 2020, March 22–24, 2020; Denver, CO.

23. Reich, K., Papp, K.A., Blauvelt, A., Langley, R., Armstrong, A., Warren, R.B., Gordon, K., Merola, J.F., Madden, C., Wang, M., Vanvoorden, V., Lebwohl, M. Efficacy and safety of bimekizumab in patients with moderate-to-severe plaque psoriasis: results from BE VIVID, a 52-week Phase 3, randomized, double-blinded, ustekinumab- and placebo-controlled study. Poster presented at: AAD 2020, March 22–24, 2020; Denver, CO.

24. Deodhar A, Helliwell PS, Boehncke WH, et al, DISCOVER-1 Study Group. Guselkumab in patients with active psoriatic arthritis who were biologic-naive or had previously received TNFα inhibitor treatment (DISCOVER-1): a double-blind, randomised, placebo-controlled phase 3 trial. Lancet 2020;395(10230):1115–25 [Erratum in: Lancet. 2020;395(10230):1114].

25. Mease PJ, Rahman P, Gottlieb AB, et al. ACR 2019. ePoster: L13. qq. Available at: https://acrabstracts.org/abstract/guselkumab-an-anti-interleukin-23p19-monoclonal-antibody-in-biologic-naive-patients-with-active-psoriatic-arthritis-week-24-results-of-the-phase-3-randomized-double-blind-placebo-controlled-stud/. Accessed December 3, 2020.

26. Mease P, Chohan S, Fructuoso F, et al. Efficacy and Safety of Tildrakizumab, a High-Affinity Anti-Interleukin-23P19 Monoclonal Antibody, In Patients with Active Psoriatic Arthritis in a Randomized, Double-Blind, Placebo-Controlled, Multiple-Dose, Phase 2B Study. Abstract, EULAR 2020; Presented June 5, 2020. Available at: http://scientific.sparx-ip.net/archiveeular/index.cfm?. Accessed December 2, 2020.

27. Crowley, J, Korman, N, Spelman, L, Igarashi, A, Ohtsuki, M, Gupta, A, Mendelsohn, A, Rozzo, S, Guenthner, S. Efficacy and Safety of Long-Term Tildrakizumab

for Plaque Psoriasis: 4-Year Results from reSURFACE 1. 28th European Academy of Dermatology and Venereology (EADV) Congress: Posters P1646. Presented October 9, 2019.

28. Reich K, Papp KA, Blauvelt A, et al. Tildrakizumab versus placebo or etanercept for chronic plaque psoriasis (reSURFACE 1 and reSURFACE 2): results from two randomised controlled, phase 3 trials. Lancet 2017. https://doi.org/10.1016/s0140-6736(17)31279-5.

29. Reich, K et al. Time to relapse in patients with moderate-to-severe psoriasis who were tildrakizumab responders at week 28: post-hoc analysis through 64 weeks from reSURFACE 1 trial. 28th European Academy of Dermatology and Venereology (EADV) Congress: Posters P1697. Presented October 9, 2019.

30. Thaci, D et al. Efficacy of tildrakizumab in patients with moderate-to-severe psoriasis according to disease duration: pooled analysis from reSURFACE 1 and reSURFACE 2 phase 3 trials at week 28. 28th European Academy of Dermatology and Venereology (EADV) Congress: Posters P1754. Presented October 9, 2019.

31. Highlights of Prescribing Information. Available at: https://www.accessdata.fda.gov/drugsatfda_docs/label/2019/761105s000lbl.pdf. Accessed November 22, 2020.

32. Gordon KB, Strober B, Lebwohl M, et al. Efficacy and safety of risankizumab in moderate-to-severe plaque psoriasis (UltIMMa-1 and UltIMMa-2): results from two double-blind, randomised, placebo-controlled and ustekinumab-controlled phase 3 trials. Lancet 2018;392(10148):650–61.

33. Reich K, Gooderham M, Thaçi D, et al. Risankizumab compared with adalimumab in patients with moderate-to-severe plaque psoriasis (IMMvent): a randomised, double-blind, active-comparator-controlled phase 3 trial. Lancet 2019; 394(10198):576–86 [Erratum in: Lancet. 2019].

34. Papp, K, Lebwohl, M, Ohtsuki, M, Puig, L, Zeng, J, Rubant, S, Valdes, J, Leonardi, C. Long-term Efficacy and Safety of Continuous Q12W Risankizumab: Results from the Open-Label Extension LIMMitless. 28th European Academy of Dermatology and Venereology (EADV) Congress: Posters FC01.01. Presented October 9, 2019.

35. Reich, K et al. Long-term Efficacy and Safety of Switching from Adalimumab to Risankizumab: Results from the Open-Label Extension LIMMitless. 28th European Academy of Dermatology and Venereology (EADV) Congress: Posters P1713. Presented October 9, 2019.

36. Reich K, Rich P, Maari C, et al. Efficacy and safety of mirikizumab (LY 3074828) in the treatment of moderate-to-severe plaque psoriasis: results from a randomized phase II study. Br J Dermatol 2019;181:88–95.

37. Rich P, Igarashi A, Patel D, et al. Impact of mirikizumab treatment on psoriasis disease activity at week 52 based upon prior treatment with biologic therapy. J Eur Acad Dermatol Venereol 2019;33:25. Discussed E-Poster Presentations.

38. ClinicalTrials.gov Identifier: NCT03535194. A Study to Assess if Mirikizumab is Effective and Safe Compared to Secukinumab and Placebo in Moderate to Severe Plaque Psoriasis (OASIS-2). Available at: https://clinicaltrials.gov/ct2/show/NCT03535194. Accessed December 6, 2020.

39. Hawkes JE, Yan BY, Chan TC, et al. Discovery of the IL-23/IL-17 Signaling Pathway and the Treatment of Psoriasis. J Immunol 2018;201:1605–13.

40. Balachez, H. et al. Efficacy and safety of BI 655130, an anti-interleukin-36 receptor antibody, in patients with acute generalized pustular psoriasis. 27th European Academy of Dermatology and Venereology (EADV) Congress: Posters D3T01.1E. Presented September 15, 2018.

41. Papp KA, Menter MA, Raman M, et al. A randomized phase 2b trial of baricitinib, an oral Janus kinase (JAK) 1/JAK2 inhibitor, in patients with moderate-to-severe psoriasis. Br J Dermatol 2016;174(6):1266–76.
42. Papp K, Gordon K, Thaçi D, et al. Phase 2 Trial of Selective Tyrosine Kinase 2 Inhibition in Psoriasis. N Engl J Med 2018;379(14):1313–21.
43. Menter A, Gelfand JM, Connor C, et al. Joint American Academy of Dermatology–National Psoriasis Foundation guidelines of care for the management of psoriasis with systemic nonbiologic therapies. J Am Acad Dermatol 2020;82:1445–86.
44. Lebwohl MG, Papp KA, Stein Gold L, et al. ARQ-151 201 Study Investigators. Trial of Roflumilast Cream for Chronic Plaque Psoriasis. N Engl J Med 2020; 383(3):229–39.
45. Robbins K, Bissonnette R, Maeda-Chubachi T, et al. Phase 2, randomized dose-finding study of tapinarof (GSK2894512 cream) for the treatment of plaque psoriasis. J Am Acad Dermatol 2019;80(3):714–21.

Recognition, Staging, and Management of Melanoma

Sarem Rashid[a,b], Hensin Tsao, MD, PhD[a],*

KEYWORDS

- Melanoma • Staging • Management • Treatment • Heterogeneity

KEY POINTS

- Over the past 50 years, melanoma has been one of the fastest-growing cancers in the United States.
- The major pathologic subtypes for melanoma include superficial spreading melanoma, nodular melanoma, acral lentiginous melanoma, and lentigo maligna melanoma.
- Histopathologic features such as thickness, mitoses, and ulceration are currently incorporated into the eighth edition of the tumor, node, metastasis melanoma staging system.
- BRAF and NRAS, the most common gene mutations in cutaneous melanoma, are widely studied for their therapeutic potential.

INTRODUCTION

Melanoma originates from melanin-producing melanocytes of the skin (basal epidermis and hair follicles), eye (choroid layer), leptomeninges, brain, and heart, among other tissues, which suggests that melanoma is a clinically heterogenous disease.[1] Melanin is an endogenous pigment that fulfills a variety of biological functions, such as protection from ultraviolet (UV) genotoxicity and pigmentation of the skin and eye.[2] In later stages, the migratory nature of the neural crest stem cell origin of melanocytes may contribute to the invasiveness of melanoma cells into the skin and its metastatic potential to other organs, such as the brain and lungs.[3]

Melanoma is stratified into 1 of 3 categories depending on the tissue type of the primary tumor: cutaneous melanoma, mucosal melanoma, and ocular melanoma. Cutaneous melanoma is the most prevalent out of the 3, and is the focus of this article.

EPIDEMIOLOGY

According to the National Cancer Institute, there were more than 100,000 new cases of melanoma and 6850 deaths nationwide in 2020.[4,5] The risk of melanoma

[a] Department of Dermatology, Wellman Center for Photomedicine, Massachusetts General Hospital, Boston, MA 02466, USA; [b] Boston University School of Medicine, Boston, MA, USA
* Corresponding author. Massachusetts General Hospital, Edwards 211, 50 Blossom Street, Boston, MA 02114.
E-mail address: htsao@mgh.harvard.edu

Med Clin N Am 105 (2021) 643–661
https://doi.org/10.1016/j.mcna.2021.04.005
0025-7125/21/© 2021 Elsevier Inc. All rights reserved.

increases with age, with mean age of onset at 65 years.[4] Notably, melanoma is one of the most common cancers in young adults less than 30 years old, particularly in women.[4–7] Surveillance, Epidemiology, and End Results (SEER) data from 2012 to 2016 suggest that the age-adjusted rate of melanoma increased 1.8% per year on average for men and 2.5% per year on average for women.[8] One explanation is the widespread use of indoor tanning in the young female demographic, which is associated with a dose-dependent risk for many skin cancers.[9] Individuals with decreased tanning ability, particularly light-skinned individuals, have an increased propensity to use tanning beds, suggesting a behavioral association to increased melanoma susceptibility.[9,10]

Melanoma incidence varies significantly based on ethnicity and race.[4,5,7] More than 95% of cases are diagnosed in lightly pigmented populations; white individuals are 5 to 25 times more likely to be diagnosed than nonwhite races, such as black, Hispanic, American Indian, and Pacific Islander.[5] From 2006 to 2015, SEER analysis revealed that black patients had thicker and more ulcerated melanomas compared with non-Hispanic white people, with significantly decreased survival in stages I ($P = .004$) and III ($P = .005$).[11] Although a biological explanation is not yet established, the nature of melanomas in skin of color (ie, non–sun-exposed sites) and health care access may both contribute to discrepancies in morbidity and mortality for these patients.

In 1975, Dr Thomas Fitzpatrick at Harvard University created a skin phototype (SPT) scheme to predict overall risk for skin cancer. Lower SPT (I–III) is associated with fairer skin and an increased propensity to burn, whereas higher SPT (IV–VI) is associated with darker skin and a decreased propensity to burn.[12] Variations in melanoma incidence are probably related to decreased photoprotection from reduced melanin, leading to increased susceptibility for both UVA and UVB penetration through the skin.[1,13] The melanocortin 1 receptor (MC1R), a 7-transmembrane G protein–coupled receptor that increases intracellular cyclic AMP level, is frequently implicated in ethnic skin differences through the modulation of eumelanin and pheomelanin. When MC1R is mutated, eumelanin production is compromised to prioritize pheomelanin production. Pheomelanin is frequently implicated in melanoma pathogenesis through decreased photostability and increased susceptibility to reactive oxygen species.[14]

UV light exposure remains the most widely recognized environmental risk factor for melanoma; the pattern and duration of exposure have been suggested to influence presentation.[1,6,15] Within the UV spectrum, UVB (290–320 nm) and UVA (320–400 nm) are frequently implicated in mutagenesis. A history of intense and intermittent sun exposure, characteristic in individuals with prior sunburn history, is associated with higher melanoma risk compared with those with chronic sun exposure at moderate intensity.[16] Geographically, melanoma incidence has been observed to increase with altitude and decrease with geographic latitude (toward the equator), supporting the causal role of sun exposure in similar races and ethnicities.[7,10,13]

Melanoma is often discovered incidentally during a routine skin examination. Although many lesions are asymptomatic, patients may report ongoing crusting, itching, or bleeding of a pigmented lesion.[17–19]

Early lesions of concern may be monitored by the patient or physician using visual recognition tools. The most widely used tools in a clinical setting include the ABCDE criteria, ugly duckling sign, and simple change in a preexisting lesion. For the ABCDE criteria, the following characteristics are described: A is for asymmetry, B is for border irregularity, C is for color heterogeneity, D is for diameter larger than 6 mm, and E is for evolution with regard to shape and size (or elevation). As an alternative, the ugly duckling sign approach screens for nevi that are atypical from other banal nevi on the patient's body.[15–17]

Routine complete skin examinations by a dermatologist are recommended for patients at increased risk for melanoma. Examples of high-risk features include personal history of skin cancer, family history of skin cancer, frequent sunburns, excessive tanning bed use, a history of familial atypical multiple-mole melanoma (FAMMM) syndrome, and, very rarely, tumor syndromes such as xeroderma pigmentosum. However, there is no consensus regarding routine melanoma screening for patients without these risk factors in the United States.[17]

TYPES OF MELANOMA

Superficial spreading melanomas (SSMs) are the most common pathologic subtype, comprising more than 60% to 70% of melanoma diagnoses (**Fig. 2**A).[20–22] Lesions of this type are most likely to have mixed-color pigmentation and irregular borders with a notched appearance. Pathogenesis may occur de novo or in association with preexisting nevi (**Fig. 1**).[23] SSMs tend to occur head, neck, and truncal areas in men, and lower legs in women.[22,24] Unlike many epithelial tumors, these lesions are prevalent throughout adulthood, with peak incidence in the fifth decade.[25]

Nodular melanomas (NMs) comprise approximately 10% to 20% of diagnoses and are second most common after SSM (**Fig. 2**B).[20–22] These lesions tend to be smooth nodules with dark and homogeneous pigmentation. Like SSM lesions, NM is preferentially located in truncal locations. NM is typically thicker than SSM and is associated with predominant vertical growth phase (VGP). Therefore, this subtype is considered biologically aggressive and more likely to metastasize.[22,26] Features of this lesion are distinct from other cutaneous melanoma subtypes, and commonly do not meet ABCDE criteria.[27,28]

Acral lentiginous melanomas (ALMs) comprise approximately 2% to 5% of all melanomas; however, they comprise 35% to 65% of cutaneous melanomas in dark-skinned individuals (such as African American, Asian, or Hispanic people) (**Fig. 2**C).[10,29–31] Lesions typically present as darkly pigmented macules with irregular borders. Most ALM lesions arise in the palms, soles, subungual areas, and

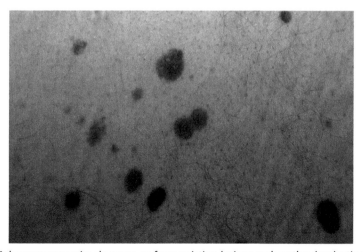

Fig. 1. Melanoma may arise de novo, or from existing lesions such as the dysplastic nevi represented here. Dysplastic nevi may present with mixed-color pigmentation, irregular borders, and an enlarged appearance.

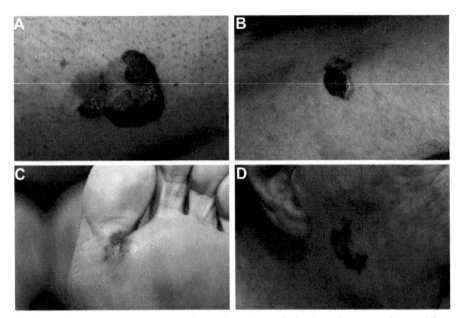

Fig. 2. (*A–D*) Representative images for each major pathologic melanoma subtype: (*A*) superficial spreading melanoma, (*B*) nodular melanoma, (*C*) acral lentiginous melanoma, (*D*) lentigo maligna melanoma.

occasionally in mucosal surfaces.[25] ALM is associated with advanced stage and poor prognosis, although it is controversial whether ALM is more aggressive than other subtypes.[32–34]

In addition, lentigo maligna melanomas (LMMs) comprise approximately 4% to 15% of all melanomas (**Fig. 2**D).[22,35] These lesions result from chronic sun radiation to bare skin, thus often appear in the head and neck area of elderly individuals. Incidence increases with age and peaks in the seventh or eighth decade of life.[35,36] LMMs can arise from a slow-growing patch of discolored skin called lentigo maligna, often referred to as Hutchinson melanotic freckle or circumscribed precancerous melanosis of Dubreuilh.

STAGING
Staging Overview

After melanoma is diagnosed, staging of the melanoma is important to inform prognostic assessment and clinical decision making. The American Joint Commission for Cancer (AJCC) is a tumor-node-metastasis (TNM)–based classification scheme that includes histopathologic features, including thickness and ulceration. Pathologic staging requires assessment of the primary tumor biopsy in addition to examination of surrounding lymph nodes. More than 80% of patients diagnosed with cutaneous melanoma are classified as either stage I or stage II[25] (**Table 1**).

If a biopsy contains multiple samples, AJCC staging integrates the summative worst features.[37] For example, if significantly increased mitotic rate is detected in a subsequent biopsy specimen, it is recommended for the pathologist to include the later recorded value. Furthermore, the single highest-stage group applies for patients with several primary cutaneous melanomas. In addition to the parameters required for AJCC staging, the Melanoma Expert Panel strongly recommends collection of

Table 1
Description of pathological stages in the 8th edition AJCC

Stage Group	Thickness Cutoff (mm)	T-Category	N-Category	M-Category
0	-	Tis	N0	M0
IA	<0.8	T1a	N0	M0
IB	0.8–1.0 or ≤1.0[a]/1.1–2.0	T1b/T2a	N0	M0
IIA	1.1–2.0[a]/2.1–4.0	T2b/T3a	N0	M0
IIB	2.1–4.0[a]/>4.0	T3b/T4a	N0	M0
IIC	>4.0[a]	T4b	N0	M0
IIIA	<0.8/0.8–1.0 or ≤1.07[a]/1.1–2.0	T1a-T2a	N1a/N2a	M0
IIIB	-	T0	N1b/N1c	M0
IIIB	0.8/0.8–1.0 or ≤1.0[a]/1.1–2.0	T1a-T2a	N1b/N1c/N2b	M0
IIIB	1.1–2.0[a]/2.1–4.0	T2b/T3a	N1a-N2b	
IIIC	<4.0	T1a-T3a	N2c/N3a/N3b/N3c	M0
IMC	2.1–4.0[a]/>4.0	T3b/T4a	At least N1	M0
IMC	>4.0[a]	T4b	N1a-N2c	M0
MID	>4.0[a]	T4b	N3a/N3bN3c	M0
IV	-	All T-Categories	All N-Categories	M1

[a] Presence of ulceration required for T-stage cut-off range.

other histopathologic features, such as Clark level, tumor regression, angioinvasion, neural/perineural invasion, and infiltrating lymphocytes for their noncanonical prognostic value.[38]

T Category of the American Joint Committee on Cancer Eighth Edition for Tumor-Node-Metastasis Staging

T-category domains include thickness and ulceration.[38] The Breslow microstaging method for thickness, which is like Clark level (although no longer considered by the AJCC), measures primary tumor depth of invasion in millimeters. Breslow thickness is measured from the granular layer of the epidermis to the bottom of the tumor using an ocular micrometer placed perpendicular to the skin. For ulcerated lesions, thickness is measured from the base of the ulceration.[39] T-category thresholds for melanoma thickness are defined at 1.0, 2.0, and 4.0 mm. Of note, nonulcerated tumors with thickness from 0.8 to 1.0 are classified in the T1b category. The AJCC eighth edition recommends thickness to be reported to the nearest 0.1 mm because measurement to the nearest 0.01 mm offers little prognostic advantage and is likely to be imprecise.[38] Microsatellites and other foci of neurotropism are excluded in the measurement of thickness.[37]

Mitotic rate, defined in terms of number of mitoses per square millimeter in the invasive tumor component, is measured by the so-called hot-spot approach. Univariate survival analysis for patients with node-negative stage I and II melanoma report mitotic rate to be a significant adverse prognostic factor for survival.[38,40] The AJCC eighth edition notably excludes mitotic rate as a staging criterion for several reasons. Gershenwald and colleagues[38] analyzed survival in 7568 patients with T1 N0 melanoma from the International Melanoma Database and Discovery Platform by thickness (<0.8 mm and 0.8mm−1.0 mm), ulceration (presence or absence), and mitoses (<1/mm^2 and ≥1/mm^2). Mitotic rate was not found to be a significant predictor of melanoma-specific survival in their final analysis. The establishment of mitotic rate as a staging parameter in the seventh edition is thought to have influenced fewer mitotically negative melanomas to be correctly identified. Nonetheless, there is consensus that mitotic rate, when applied as a range across all tumor thicknesses, is an important independent prognostic factor.[40] Despite exclusion as a staging parameter, the AJCC Melanoma Expert Panel continues to recommend assessment of mitotic rate for all primary cutaneous melanomas.[38]

Per the AJCC, ulceration is defined as the absence of intact epidermis overlying a major portion of the primary melanoma based on microscopic examination of the histologic sections.[41] Positive ulceration corresponds to the b subcategory for stage T1 to T4 melanomas. Similar to tumor thickness and mitotic rate, presence of ulceration is an adverse prognostic factor in primary melanoma.[42–44] For example, Balch and colleagues reported that 5-year survival rate decreased from 80% to 55% and 53% to 12% in the presence of ulceration for patients with stage I and II melanoma respectively (P<.001). A common pitfall for this feature is misclassification of epidermal loss caused by previous traumatic surgery (including past biopsy) or scratching by the patient. Therefore, correlation to clinical history is essential for accurate assessment. If there is doubt with regard to the cause of epidermal loss, then the tumor should be considered ulcerated.

N Category of the American Joint Committee on Cancer Eighth Edition for Tumor-Node-Metastasis Staging

The N category classifies metastatic spread to regional lymph nodes or satellite areas. Microscopic distance between the primary tumor and satellite area is used to further describe these nonnodal locoregional metastases. Microsatellite metastases are visualized directly adjacent to the primary tumor. In contrast, satellite and in-transit metastases are respectively located less than 2 cm or greater than or equal to 2 cm from the primary tumor. All 3 metastases are considered independent adverse prognosticators.[45–47] Univariate analysis of prognosis in patients with nonnodal locoregional metastases (microsatellite, satellite, or in-transit metastases) showed no significant differences in prognosis.[38] Therefore, all 3 types are combined into a single category in the eighth edition AJCC. The presence of nonnodal locoregional metastases further designates the c subcategory for stages N1 to N3.

Recent breakthroughs in lymphatic mapping and sentinel lymph node biopsy have tremendously improved staging protocols for patients with melanoma.[38,48] The National Comprehensive Cancer Network recommends consideration of sentinel lymph node biopsy for all melanomas that are T1b or greater.[49] For these patients, the eighth edition AJCC considers both the number of affected nodes and the degree of regional lymph node involvement. Microscopically identified regional node metastasis but clinically, radiographically, or ultrasonography-negative metastases are considered clinically occult (or microscopic). Patients with regional node metastasis with clinically, radiographically, or ultrasonography-positive assessment are clinically detected (or macroscopic).[38] Consistent with previous editions of the AJCC staging system, no threshold has yet been defined for designating a tumor-involved lymph node. Therefore, the presence of any metastatic tumor cells identified on hematoxylin-eosin–stained specimens should be recorded as positive. Five-year survival for patients with a single clinically occult or clinically detected tumor-involved lymph node was 71% and 50% respectively (P = .004).[50]

M Category of the American Joint Committee on Cancer Eighth Edition for Tumor-Node-Metastasis Staging

The presence and anatomic location of distant metastasis are classified by the M category.[38] New to the eighth edition AJCC is designation of 1 and 0 subcategories for

M1a-M1d melanomas. These labels correspond with increased serum lactate dehydrogenase (LDH) and nonincreased serum LDH respectively.

Future Directions for Tumor-Node-Metastasis Staging

A long-standing clinical goal in dermatology is to increase prognostic precision for existing classification schemes. The conventional AJCC melanoma staging system uses a limited set of parameters for all patients, irrespective of clinical context. Combination of existing staging schemes with computer-aided technologies and expanded variable lists from the patient record may greatly improve personalized prediction.[37] For example, univariate analyses detail the role of primary anatomic location, radial growth phase, VGP, gender, and age in determining survival.[51–54] Gene expression profiling for high-risk patients has also offered promising results, although further studies are recommended before routine clinical use.[55]

GENETIC RISK FACTORS

Melanoma has a tumor mutation burden of approximately 100/Mb, which is among the highest mutation frequencies reported alongside lung cancer.[56] More than 80% of these mutations are found to UVB signatures. An important feature in melanoma pathogenesis is the capacity for different passenger mutations to take driver roles to maintain cell viability in different physiologic contexts or treatments. For example, somatic *NRAS* mutations are commonly observed in resistance pathways against mutant-selective BRAF inhibitor regimens. Molecular genotyping has broadened the capacity for use of these genetic events as prognostic markers and therapeutic targets.[57]

Germline risk variants also dictate individual risk. Polymorphisms of the *MC1R* gene modulate several physiologic functions such as skin/hair pigmentation, UV cancer susceptibility, and DNA repair.[58,59] Loss-of-function *MC1R* mutations increase relative production of pheomelanin, which confers an increased risk of skin cancer.[60] This mutation is commonly observed in patients with red-yellow hair and lightly pigmented skin.[61]

Approximately 3% to 15% of all malignant melanomas are associated with family history.[62] Of these cases, nearly 40% of familial melanomas are found to contain germline mutations in *CDKN2A*.[63,64] FAMMM syndrome is a familial melanoma variant that is frequently associated with germline *CDK2NA* mutation. This condition is characterized by the presence of numerous clinically atypical (dysplastic) nevi, often exceeding 50 in number, and heightened risk of pancreatic cancer. Melanomas may arise de novo or from existing nevi as early as the second decade of life.[65] Thus, biannual skin examinations are recommended for affected patients starting at age 10 years and should be offered to first-degree and second-degree relatives. Endoscopic ultrasonography, computed tomography, and MRI are indicated for screening of pancreatic masses in adulthood, although exact guidelines may vary per institution.[65] Notably, *CD2KNA* mutations are also enriched in patients with sporadic multiple primary melanomas.[60]

TREATMENT
Surgery

Surgical removal and biopsy, usually by wide local excision (WLE), remains the primary treatment of all early-stage or localized melanomas. For WLE, margin size is varied according to thickness. According to the American Academy of Dermatology and National Comprehensive Cancer Network (NCCN) guidelines, melanoma in situ and primary melanomas with Breslow thickness less than or equal to 1.0, 1.01 to 2, 2.01

to 4, and greater than 4 mm are indicated to be excised with margins of 0.5 to 1, 1, 1 to 2, 2, and 2 cm, respectively (**Table 2**).[66–68]

Several biopsy techniques are used in clinic, including shave, punch, incisional, and excisional. Both the AJCC and NCCN strongly recommend excisional biopsy because it can be used to definitively establish T stage while reducing potential sampling errors caused by partial resection. Incisional and punch biopsies are recommended for sampling focally suspicious areas in larger lesions. Recommended use of shave biopsies remains controversial because of potential transection of the deep aspects of the tumor, although Zager and colleagues[69] found the technique to be accurate in 97% of patients.[41,67,69]

Mohs micrographic surgery is a tissue-sparing procedure that allows optimal clearance through complete evaluation of the peripheral and deep margins in house. Although highly effective in keratinocyte tumors, use of this procedure has not yet been established for routine use in invasive melanoma but is appropriate for in situ melanoma, LMM type.[68,70] One advantage of this procedure is for removal of larger melanomas, particularly those in cosmetically sensitive areas such as the eyelid, ears, or cheek. In these lesions, precise evaluation of the margins reduces the amount of removed skin and overall scar size. Furthermore, the preestablished margins for WLE may not be suitable for asymmetric peripheral growth pattern in certain melanoma types.[71]

There is some evidence that supports metastasectomy for melanomas of all stages. In a retrospective study using data from the Multicenter Selective Lymphadenectomy Trial (MSLT-1), combined surgical treatment of patients with stage IV melanoma was shown to improve clinical outcomes compared with systemic therapy alone. Four-year survival was 20.8% for patients who underwent combined surgical treatment and systemic medical treatment (SMT) compared with 7.0% for those with SMT alone for AJCC stages M1a to M1d ($P<.0001$). Metastatic melanoma to the skin, subcutaneous lymph nodes, or distant lymph nodes (M1a) was associated with the largest survival advantage (69% in patients who underwent surgery vs 0% for patients treated with SMT alone).[72,73] It is unclear whether the improved survival benefit associated with surgical treatment is caused by impediment of primary tumor metastasis versus decreased immunosuppression from metastasis, or both.

Chemotherapy

Traditional chemotherapy is rarely used now given the advent of highly efficacious molecular and immune-based therapies. However, it is indicated for combination therapy in certain cases of advanced melanoma and in palliative treatments.[74,75] These earlier treatments are reviewed here mostly for historical value.

Table 2
Recommended surgical excision margins for primary cutaneous melanoma by the National Comprehensive Cancer Network

Melanoma Thickness (mm)	Surgical Margin (cm)
In situ	0.5–1.0
≤1.0	1.0
1.0–2.0	1.0–2.0
>2.0	2.0

Intravenous dacarbazine (DTIC), an alkylating agent, is currently the only non-immune/targeted agent approved by the US Food and Drug Administration (FDA). DTIC was associated with a response rate of 7% to 12% and median overall survival of 5.6 to 7.8 months after initiation of treatment in phase III studies.[76–78] A prodrug of DTIC called temozolomide (TMZ) has also been used as an oral treatment alternative for advanced melanomas.[76] Biochemotherapy is the combined use of chemotherapy and immunotherapy (usually interleukin-2). The prognostic value of this combined regimen remains to be determined, although frequent use is uniformly discouraged because of high toxicity.[79]

Since the early 1990s, isolated limb infusion (ILI) has been used as a proxy for limb amputation in treatment of refractory or localized melanomas with in-transit metastasis.[29,80] Catheters are inserted into the axial vasculature of a tumor-bearing limb, while pressure is applied proximally to prevent leakage into systemic circulation. Combinations of chemotherapeutics and biologics (such as tumor necrosis factor and melphalan) are commonly used for ILI. Drawbacks to this procedure include significant functional sequelae (ie, redness, lymphoedema, or damage to vessels) caused by drug toxicity, although the limb may potentially be spared from amputation.

Immunotherapy

Since 2010, immunotherapy has emerged as an effective treatment in part because of melanoma's high immunogenicity resulting from UV mutagenesis. The tumor extracellular matrix poses a complex physiologic environment in which normal cell functions, such as immunosurveillance and cell growth, are compromised. Two pathways to immunosuppression that have been identified in T cells are downregulation of surface major histocompatibility complex-1, and upregulation of cell surface inhibitory proteins. Recent advances in immunotherapy involve blocking the activation of these inhibitory proteins to reinforce host immune responses.[81]

Cytotoxic T-lymphocyte-associated antigen-4 (CTLA4) is a T-cell surface protein that engages B7 on antigen-presenting cells during the priming phase of immune engagement. CTLA4 functions to scavenge CD80/CD86 ligands away from its costimulatory receptor, CD28. Both CTLA4 and CD28 on the cell surface compete to bind to CD80/CD86, either resulting in the propagation of stimulatory or inhibitory T-cell signals. In this regard, CTLA4 serves as a molecular brake to dampen proliferation of physiologic immune responses.[30] A CTLA4 antibody (ipilimumab), a human monoclonal IgG4 variant, was the first immune checkpoint inhibitor designated by the FDA for clinical use. Ipilimumab binds to the CTLA4 receptor, thereby sustaining a prolonged immune response against tumor cells. Response to CTLA4 therapy is associated with posttreatment increase in tumor-infiltrating lymphocytes.[82] A phase III clinical trial (**Table 3**) showed significantly increased 5-year survival in patients receiving ipilimumab compared with placebo ($P = .002$), with an associated plateau in survival benefit after 3 years.[31,83] Severe toxicity occurs in 70% to 89% of patients on ipilimumab and frequently requires reductions in either, or both, dose and duration of use.[84,85]

Programmed cell death 1 receptor (PD-1) is another widely studied immune checkpoint receptor found on T-cell surfaces and operates during the effector stage of tumor destruction. When bound to its tumor-based target, programmed death-ligand 1, PD-1 acts via phosphatase SHP2 to inhibit kinases associated with T-cell activation and autoimmune response. Expression of PD-1, in turn, is cyclically induced by T-cell activation. After an acute antigen encounter, PD-1 expression eventually declines, whereas, during chronic antigen exposure, expression remains increased. In prolonged antigen encounters, the increased expression of inhibitory receptors (such as PD-1 and CTLA4) and reduced capacity to secrete cytokines may develop into a

Table 3
Efficacy of combination immunotherapy regimens

Trial	Phase	Treatment Arms	OS (Median)	PFS (Median)	ORR (%)
CheckMate 067 (NCT01844505)	Phase III	Nivolumab and ipilimumab vs ipilimumab vs nivolumab vs	19.98 (nivolumab and ipilimumab)	11.50 (nivolumab and ipilimumab) vs 2.89 (ipilimumab monotherapy) vs 6.87 (nivolumab monotherapy)	57.6 (nivolumab and ipilimumab) vs 43.7 (ipilimumab monotherapy) vs 19.0 (nivolumab monotherapy)
CheckMate 069 (NCT01927419)	Phase II	Ipilimumab and nivolumab vs ipilimumab	22.30 (ipilimumab and nivolumab) vs (nivolumab monotherapy)	8.57 (ipilimumab and nivolumab) vs 3.73 (nivolumab monotherapy)	59 (ipilimumab and nivolumab) vs 11 (nivolumab monotherapy)
COMBI-i (NCT02967692)	Phase III	Spartalizumab, dabrafenib, and trametinib	Not reported	Not reported	75 (spartalizumab, dabrafenib, and trametinib)
Keynote-252/ECHO-301 (NCT02752074)	Phase III	Pembrolizumab and epacadostat vs pembrolizumab	87.2 (pembrolizumab and epacadostat) vs 84.1 (pembrolizumab monotherapy)	4.7 (pembrolizumab and epacadostat) vs 4.9 (pembrolizumab monotherapy)	34.2 (pembrolizumab and epacadostat) vs 31.5 (pembrolizumab monotherapy)
IMspire150	Phase III	Spartalizumab, vemurafenib, and cobimetinib versus vemurafenib and cobimetinib	28.8 (spartalizumab, vemurafenib, and cobimetinib) vs 25.1 (vemurafenib and cobimetinib)	15.1 (spartalizumab, vemurafenib, and cobimetinib) vs 10.6 (vemurafenib and cobimetinib)	66 (spartalizumab, vemurafenib, and cobimetinib) vs 65 (vemurafenib and cobimetinib)

characteristic phenotype described as T-cell exhaustion.[81,86] PD-1 inhibitors (nivolumab and pembrolizumab) are used additively with ipilimumab for cases of metastatic melanoma, although they have shown superior single-agent survival.[87,88] Furthermore, combination therapy with PD-1 and CTLA4 inhibitors is associated with improved survival compared with any single-agent regimen.

Targeted therapy

Approximately 70% of patients with cutaneous melanoma show mutations in key molecular signaling pathways.[89] Mutations in protein kinase B-raf (BRAF), a serine-threonine kinase that acts in the mitogen-activated protein kinase (MAPK) (or RAS-RAF-MEK-ERK) pathway, are found in nearly half of cutaneous melanomas.[90] More than 40 different mutations have been reported for this gene; however, the most common is the substitution of glutamate for valine at codon 600 (V600E) in exon 15. BRAF mutations have been associated with superficial spreading and nodular pathologic subtypes, with evidence to support the causal role of UVB.[91] Other histopathologic features associated with BRAF include the presence of mitoses, truncal location, and early age of onset (<50 years).[89] Less commonly reported BRAF mutations include V600K and V600G/R. NRAS mutations are the second most common in oncogenic lesions and are found in approximately 20% of cutaneous melanomas. Melanomas may harbor many different mutations in toto; however, at the cellular level, mutations in BRAF(V600) and NRAS(Q61) are described to be mutually exclusive.[54] Still, there are currently no effective targeted therapies for patients with wild-type BRAF.[3]

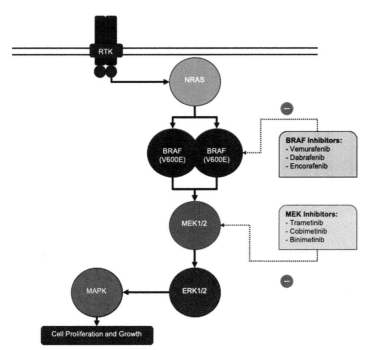

Fig. 3. The *MAPK* pathway is an important regulator of cell proliferation in melanocytes. Dysregulation of this pathway usually occurs because of activating *BRAF* or *NRAS* mutations, and may promote tumorigenic behavior.

Table 4
Efficacy of BRAF and MEK inhibitor combination trials

Trial	Phase	Treatment Arms	OS (Median)	PFS (Median)	ORR (%)
BRIM7 (NCT01271803)	Phase Ib	Vemurafenib and cobimetinib (BRAF-naive patient group) vs vemurafenib and cobimetinib (recently progressed patient group)	31.8 (BRAF-naive patient group) vs 8.5 (recently progressed patient group)	13.7 (BRAF-naive patient group) vs 2.8 (recently progressed patient group)	87 (BRAF-naive patient group) vs 15 (recently progressed patient group)
BRF113220 (NCT01072175)	Phase II	Dabrafenib and trametinib (150:2 dose) vs dabrafenib and trametinib (150:1 dose) vs dabrafenib	25.0 (150:2 dose) vs 18.7 (150:1 dose) vs 20.2 (dabrafenib monotherapy)	9.4 (150:2 dose) vs 9.2 (150:1 dose) vs 5.8 (dabrafenib monotherapy)	Not reported
coBRIM (NCT01689519)	Phase III	Vemurafenib and cobimetinib versus vemurafenib	22.5 (vemurafenib and cobimetinib) vs 17.4 (vemurafenib monotherapy)	12.6 (vemurafenib and cobimetinib) vs 7.2 (vemurafenib monotherapy)	68 (vemurafenib and cobimetinib) vs 45 (vemurafenib monotherapy)
COMBI-d (NCT01584648)	Phase III	Dabrafenib and trametinib vs dabrafenib	25.1 (dabrafenib and trametinib) vs 18.7 (dabrafenib monotherapy)	9.3 (dabrafenib and trametinib) vs 8.8 (dabrafenib monotherapy)	66 (dabrafenib and trametinib) vs 51 (dabrafenib monotherapy)
COMBI-v (NCT01597908)	Phase III	Dabrafenib and trametinib vs vemurafenib	17.2 (vemurafenib monotherapy)	11.4 (dabrafenib and trametinib) vs 7.3 (vemurafenib monotherapy)	64 (dabrafenib and trametinib) vs 51 (vemurafenib monotherapy)
COLOMBUS (NCT01909453)	Phase III	Encorafenib and binimetinib vs encorafenib vs vemurafenib	33.6 (encorafenib and binimetinib) vs 16.9 (vemurafenib monotherapy)	14.9 (encorafenib and binimetinib) vs 7.3 (vemurafenib monotherapy)	Not reported

Abbreviations: ORR, overall response rate; OS, overall survival; PFS, progression free survival.

PLX4032, or vemurafenib, is a potent and selective inhibitor of BRAF(V600E) that shows marked inhibition of the MAP pathway (**Fig. 3**). Cells that do not harbor the *BRAF* mutation are not affected. A phase II study showed at least a 50% response rate and median duration of response of 6.7 months.[92] In a phase III study comparing the effects of vemurafenib with dacarbazine, vemurafenib was associated with a relative reduction of 63% in the risk of death and 70% in the risk of tumor progression for BRAF(V600E) mutant melanomas.[78] Dabrafenib and encorafenib are additional BRAF mutant-selective inhibitors that have offered promising results in clinical trials.[74,93,94]

For treatment of melanomas bearing BRAF or NRAS mutations, selective MEK inhibitors can also impair activation of the MAPK cascade to inhibit cell growth and induce cell death[95] (**Table 4**). Compared with single-agent BRAF inhibitors, combination therapy with BRAF and MEK inhibitors is associated with improved overall survival and progression-free survival.[96] There are currently 3 combinations approved by the FDA for clinic use: (1) dabrafenib and trametinib, (2) encorafenib plus binimetinib, and (3) vemurafenib and cobimetinib. Addition of PD-1 antibodies to this regimen has been shown to decrease response rates but increase response duration.[96]

Acquired resistance continues to be a major therapeutic pitfall for BRAF mutant-selective inhibitors. Unregulated MAPK pathway activation may persist because of several physiologic mechanisms.[97] Common genetic causes include mutations in *NRAS*, *BRAF* (amplification), *MAP2K1/MAP2K2*, or other mutations in the phosphoinositide 3-kinase (PI3K) pathway. In a phenomenon known as the *BRAF* inhibitor paradox, MAPK signaling activation in nonmutant BRAF cells facilitates transactivation of the RAF protein in drug-free cells. Screening for RAF inhibitor resistance genes has been associated with improved clinical outcomes for patients receiving target therapy. Use of downstream RAF or MEK inhibitors in combination regimens has been shown to reduce MAPK-driven acquired resistance.[98,99]

SUMMARY

This article began by reflecting on the distinct epidemiology of melanoma in the United States. As one of the most prevalent and fastest-growing cancers in the United States, the disease has emerged as an important public health concern these past few decades. Notably, melanoma is a disease with highly varied incidence and severity. The functional diversity of melanin was explored in the context of race, gender, and geography. Discovery of the MC1R receptor in the mid-1990s has allowed clinicians to conceptualize the physiologic mechanisms underlying pigmentation control and set the foundation for understanding UV-induced melanoma pathogenesis. Histological staging has emerged as a useful classification scheme for predicting prognosis and treatment pattern by similar groupings. Although the scientific body of research surrounding melanoma continues to rapidly change, the impetus remains clear: the complexity of this disease will require further efforts to unravel the gap between gene alterations at the cellular level, and tumor histopathology.

CLINICS CARE POINTS

- Melanoma is the most lethal form of skin cancer in the United States. Incidence rates are rapidly increasing in adults, particularly in the female young adult demographic.
- Melanoma results from malignant proliferation of pigment-producing cells called melanocytes. Although classically located in the epidermis, these cells may also be tumorigenic in various organ tissues, including the eye and meninges.

- Pathogenesis is thought to occur through the interaction of environmental exposures (such as UV radiation) and genetic susceptibilities. Mutations in BRAF are widely investigated because of their high prevalence and therapeutic potential.
- The clinical landscape for melanoma treatment is quickly evolving. Adjuvant immunotherapy and targeted therapy have been shown to increase survival in advanced melanomas.
- Drug resistance is a major limitation to current targeted treatments and immunotherapy. Further research is required to gain a better understanding of these highly diverse mechanisms.

REFERENCES

1. Matthews NH, Li W-Q, Qureshi AA, et al. Epidemiology of melanoma. In: Ward WH, Farma JM, editors. Cutaneous melanoma: etiology and therapy. Brisbane, AU: Codon Publications; 2017. p. 1–2. Available at: http://www.ncbi.nlm.nih.gov/books/NBK481862/. Accessed November 30, 2020.
2. Schlessinger DI, Anoruo M, Schlessinger J. Biochemistry, melanin. In: StatPearls. Treasure Island, FL: StatPearls Publishing; 2020. p. 1–4. Available at: http://www.ncbi.nlm.nih.gov/books/NBK459156/. Accessed November 30, 2020.
3. Rebecca VW, Somasundaram R, Herlyn M. Pre-clinical modeling of cutaneous melanoma. Nat Commun 2020;11(1):2858.
4. Melanoma Skin Cancer | Understanding Melanoma. Available at: https://www.cancer.org/cancer/melanoma-skin-cancer.html. Accessed November 30, 2020.
5. SEER Cancer Statistics Review, 1975-2017. SEER. Available at: https://seer.cancer.gov/csr/1975_2017/index.html. Accessed November 30, 2020.
6. Erdei E, Torres SM. A new understanding in the epidemiology of melanoma. Expert Rev Anticancer Ther 2010;10(11):1811–23.
7. Houghton AN, Polsky D. Focus on melanoma. Cancer Cell 2002;2(4):275–8.
8. Melanoma Incidence and Mortality, United States–2012–2016 | CDC. 2020. Available at: https://www.cdc.gov/cancer/uscs/about/data-briefs/no9-melanoma-incidence-mortality-UnitedStates-2012-2016.htm. Accessed November 30, 2020.
9. Zhang M, Qureshi AA, Geller AC, et al. Use of tanning beds and incidence of skin cancer. J Clin Oncol 2012;30(14):1588–93.
10. Chang Y, Barrett JH, Bishop DT, et al. Sun exposure and melanoma risk at different latitudes: a pooled analysis of 5700 cases and 7216 controls. Int J Epidemiol 2009;38(3):814–30.
11. Huang K, Fan J, Misra S. Acral Lentiginous Melanoma: Incidence and Survival in the United States, 2006-2015, an Analysis of SEER Registry. Gen Surg 2020;251: 329–39.
12. Merrill SJ, Subramanian M, Godar DE. Worldwide cutaneous malignant melanoma incidences analyzed by sex, age, and skin type over time (1955–2007): Is HPV infection of androgenic hair follicular melanocytes a risk factor for developing melanoma exclusively in people of European-ancestry? Dermatoendocrinol 2016;8(1). https://doi.org/10.1080/19381980.2016.1215391.
13. Brenner M, Hearing VJ. The protective role of melanin against UV damage in human skin. Photochem Photobiol 2008;84(3):539–49.
14. Nasti TH, Timares L. Invited Review MC1R, Eumelanin and Pheomelanin: their role in determining the susceptibility to skin cancer. Photochem Photobiol 2015; 91(1):188–200.
15. Lin JY, Fisher DE. Melanocyte biology and skin pigmentation. Nature 2007; 445(7130):843–50.

16. Leonardi GC, Falzone L, Salemi R, et al. Cutaneous melanoma: From pathogenesis to therapy (Review). Int J Oncol 2018;52(4):1071–80.
17. Ward WH, Lambreton F, Goel N, et al. Clinical presentation and staging of melanoma. In: Ward WH, Farma JM, editors. Cutaneous melanoma: etiology and therapy. Brisbane, AU: Codon Publications; 2017. p. 1–10. Available at: http://www.ncbi.nlm.nih.gov/books/NBK481857/. Accessed January 17, 2021.
18. Gaudy-Marqueste C, Wazaefi Y, Bruneu Y, et al. Ugly duckling sign as a major factor of efficiency in melanoma detection. JAMA Dermatol 2017;153(4):279.
19. Grob JJ. The "ugly duckling" sign: identification of the common characteristics of nevi in an individual as a basis for melanoma screening. Arch Dermatol 1998;134(1):103–4.
20. Greenwald HS, Friedman EB, Osman I. Superficial spreading and nodular melanoma are distinct biological entities: a challenge to the linear progression model. Melanoma Res 2012;22(1):1–8.
21. Shaikh WR, Xiong M, Weinstock MA. The contribution of nodular subtype to melanoma mortality in the United States, 1978 to 2007. Arch Dermatol 2012;148(1):30–6.
22. Morton DL, Essner R, Kirkwood JM, et al. Clinical characteristics. Holl-frei cancer med 6th edition 2003. Available at: https://www.ncbi.nlm.nih.gov/books/NBK13375/. Accessed January 17, 2021.
23. Markovic SN, Erickson LA, Rao RD, et al. Malignant melanoma in the 21st century, part 1: epidemiology, risk factors, screening, prevention, and diagnosis. Mayo Clin Proc 2007;82(3):364–80.
24. Cutaneous Malignant Melanoma: A Primary Care Perspective - American Family Physician. Available at: https://www.aafp.org/afp/2012/0115/p161.html. Accessed January 17, 2021.
25. Cummins DL, Cummins JM, Pantle H, et al. Cutaneous Malignant Melanoma. Mayo Clin Proc 2006;81(4):500–7.
26. Faut M, Wevers KP, van Ginkel RJ, et al. Nodular histologic subtype and ulceration are tumor factors associated with high risk of recurrence in sentinel node-negative melanoma patients. Ann Surg Oncol 2017;24(1):142–9.
27. Kelly JW, Chamberlain AJ, Staples MP, et al. Nodular melanoma. No longer as simple as ABC. Aust Fam Physician 2003;32(9):706–9.
28. Bradford PT, Goldstein AM, McMaster ML, et al. Acral Lentiginous Melanoma: Incidence and Survival Patterns in the United States, 1986-2005. Arch Dermatol 2009;145(4). https://doi.org/10.1001/archdermatol.2008.609.
29. Giles MH, Coventry BJ. Isolated limb infusion chemotherapy for melanoma: an overview of early experience at the Adelaide Melanoma Unit. Cancer Manag Res 2013;5:243–9.
30. Alegre M-L, Frauwirth KA, Thompson CB. T-cell regulation by CD28 and CTLA-4. Nat Rev Immunol 2001;1(3):220–8.
31. Maio M, Grob J-J, Aamdal S, et al. Five-year survival rates for treatment-naive patients with advanced melanoma who received ipilimumab plus dacarbazine in a phase III trial. J Clin Oncol 2015;33(10):1191–6.
32. Howard MD, Xie C, Wee E, et al. Acral lentiginous melanoma: differences in survival compared with other subtypes. Br J Dermatol 2020;182(4):1056–7.
33. Han B, Hur K, Ohn J, et al. Acral lentiginous melanoma in situ: dermoscopic features and management strategy. Sci Rep 2020;10(1):20503.
34. Saida T, Koga H, Uhara H. Key points in dermoscopic differentiation between early acral melanoma and acral nevus. J Dermatol 2011;38(1):25–34.

35. McKenna JK, Florell SR, Goldman GD, et al. Lentigo maligna/lentigo maligna melanoma: current state of diagnosis and treatment. Dermatol Surg 2006;32(4): 493–504.
36. Smalberger GJ, Siegel DM, Khachemoune A. Lentigo maligna. Dermatol Ther 2008;21(6):439–46.
37. Scolyer RA, Rawson RV, Gershenwald JE, et al. Melanoma pathology reporting and staging. Mod Pathol 2020;33(1):15–24.
38. Gershenwald JE, Scolyer RA, Hess KR, et al. Melanoma Staging: Evidence-Based Changes in the American Joint Committee on Cancer Eighth Edition Cancer Staging Manual. CA Cancer J Clin 2017;67(6):472–92.
39. Trinidad CM, Torres-Cabala CA, Curry JL, et al. Update on eighth edition American Joint Committee on Cancer classification for cutaneous melanoma and overview of potential pitfalls in histological examination of staging parameters. J Clin Pathol 2019;72(4):265–70.
40. Thompson JF, Soong S-J, Balch CM, et al. Prognostic significance of mitotic rate in localized primary cutaneous melanoma: an analysis of patients in the multi-institutional American Joint Committee on Cancer melanoma staging database. J Clin Oncol 2011;29(16):2199–205.
41. Balch CM, Gershenwald JE, Soong S, et al. Final Version of 2009 AJCC Melanoma Staging and Classification. J Clin Oncol 2009;27(36):6199–206.
42. Balch CM, Wilkerson JA, Murad TM, et al. The prognostic significance of ulceration of cutaneous melanoma. Cancer 1980;45(12):3012–7.
43. Bønnelykke-Behrndtz ML, Steiniche T. Ulcerated melanoma: aspects and prognostic impact. In: Ward WH, Farma JM, editors. Cutaneous melanoma: etiology and therapy. Brisbane, AU: Codon Publications; 2017. p. 1–10. Available at: http://www.ncbi.nlm.nih.gov/books/NBK481861/. Accessed December 27, 2020.
44. Jewell R, Elliott F, Laye J, et al. The clinico-pathological and gene expression patterns associated with ulceration of primary melanoma. Pigment Cell Melanoma Res 2015;28(1):94–104.
45. Rao UNM, Ibrahim J, Flaherty LE, et al. Implications of microscopic satellites of the primary and extracapsular lymph node spread in patients with high-risk melanoma: pathologic corollary of Eastern Cooperative Oncology Group Trial E1690. J Clin Oncol 2002;20(8):2053–7.
46. Read RL, Haydu L, Saw RPM, et al. In-transit melanoma metastases: incidence, prognosis, and the role of lymphadenectomy. Ann Surg Oncol 2015;22(2): 475–81.
47. Harrist TJ, Rigel DS, Day CL, et al. Microscopic satellites" are more highly associated with regional lymph node metastases than is primary melanoma thickness. Cancer 1984;53(10):2183–7.
48. Morton DL, Wen DR, Wong JH, et al. Technical details of intraoperative lymphatic mapping for early stage melanoma. Arch Surg 1992;127(4):392–9.
49. Egger ME, Stevenson M, Bhutiani N, et al. Should sentinel lymph node biopsy be performed for All T1b Melanomas in the New 8th Edition American Joint Committee on Cancer Staging System? J Am Coll Surg 2019;228(4):466–72.
50. Balch CM, Gershenwald JE, Soong S, et al. Multivariate analysis of prognostic factors among 2,313 patients with stage III melanoma: comparison of nodal micrometastases versus macrometastases. J Clin Oncol 2010;28(14):2452–9.
51. Crowson AN, Magro CM, Mihm MC. Prognosticators of melanoma, the melanoma report, and the sentinel lymph node. Mod Pathol 2006;19(2):S71–87.

52. Betti R, Agape E, Vergani R, et al. An observational study regarding the rate of growth in vertical and radial growth phase superficial spreading melanomas. Oncol Lett 2016;12(3):2099–102.
53. Bellenghi M, Puglisi R, Pontecorvi G, et al. Sex and Gender Disparities in Melanoma. Cancers 2020;12(7). https://doi.org/10.3390/cancers12071819.
54. Gupta S, Artomov M, Goggins W, et al. Gender Disparity and Mutation Burden in Metastatic Melanoma. JNCI J Natl Cancer Inst 2015;107(11). https://doi.org/10.1093/jnci/djv221.
55. Gerami P, Cook RW, Russell MC, et al. Gene expression profiling for molecular staging of cutaneous melanoma in patients undergoing sentinel lymph node biopsy. J Am Acad Dermatol 2015;72(5):780–5.e3.
56. Lawrence MS, Stojanov P, Polak P, et al. Mutational heterogeneity in cancer and the search for new cancer-associated genes. Nature 2013;499(7457):214–8.
57. Glitza IC, Davies MA. Genotyping of cutaneous melanoma. Chin Clin Oncol 2014; 3(3):27.
58. Wolf Horrell EM, Boulanger MC, D'Orazio JA. Melanocortin 1 receptor: structure, function, and regulation. Front Genet 2016;7. https://doi.org/10.3389/fgene.2016.00095.
59. Chen S, Han C, Miao X, et al. Targeting MC1R depalmitoylation to prevent melanomagenesis in redheads. Nat Commun 2019;10(1):877.
60. Potrony M, Badenas C, Aguilera P, et al. Update in genetic susceptibility in melanoma. Ann Transl Med 2015;3(15). https://doi.org/10.3978/j.issn.2305-5839.2015.08.11.
61. Beaumont KA, Shekar SN, Cook AL, et al. Red hair is the null phenotype of MC1R. Hum Mutat 2008;29(8):E88–94.
62. Dębniak T. Familial malignant melanoma - overview. Hered Cancer Clin Pract 2004;2(3):123–9.
63. Goldstein AM, Chan M, Harland M, et al. High-risk melanoma susceptibility genes and pancreatic cancer, neural system tumors, and uveal melanoma across GenoMEL. Cancer Res 2006;66(20):9818–28.
64. Soura E, Eliades P, Shannon K, et al. Hereditary Melanoma: Update on Syndromes and Management - Genetics of familial atypical multiple mole melanoma syndrome. J Am Acad Dermatol 2016;74(3):395–407.
65. Eckerle Mize D, Bishop M, Resse E, et al. Familial atypical multiple mole melanoma syndrome. In: Riegert-Johnson DL, Boardman LA, Hefferon T, et al, editors. Cancer syndromes. Bethesda, MD: National Center for Biotechnology Information (US); 2009. p. 12-3. Available at: http://www.ncbi.nlm.nih.gov/books/NBK7030/. Accessed January 18, 2021.
66. Gupta S, Tsao H. Epidemiology of Melanoma. In: Loda M, Mucci L, Mittelstadt M, et al, editors. Pathology and Epidemiology of Cancer. Cham: Springer; 2017. https://doi.org/10.1007/978-3-319-35153-7_31.
67. Niknam Leilabadi S, Chen A, Tsai S, et al. Update and review on the surgical management of primary cutaneous melanoma. Healthcare 2014;2(2):234–49.
68. Swetter SM, Tsao H, Bichakjian CK, et al. Guidelines of care for the management of primary cutaneous melanoma. J Am Acad Dermatol 2019;80(1):208–50.
69. Zager JS, Hochwald SN, Marzban SS, et al. Shave Biopsy Is a Safe and Accurate Method for the Initial Evaluation of Melanoma. J Am Coll Surg 2011;212(4):454–62.
70. Hoc Task Force Ad, Connolly SM, Baker DR, et al. AAD/ACMS/ASDSA/ASMS 2012 appropriate use criteria for Mohs micrographic surgery: a report of the American Academy of Dermatology, American College of Mohs Surgery,

American Society for Dermatologic Surgery Association, and the American Society for Mohs Surgery. J Am Acad Dermatol 2012;67(4):531–50.

71. Beaulieu D, Fathi R, Srivastava D, et al. Current perspectives on Mohs micrographic surgery for melanoma. Clin Cosmet Investig Dermatol 2018;11:309–20.

72. Howard JH, Thompson JF, Mozzillo N, et al. Metastasectomy for distant metastatic melanoma: Analysis of data from the first Multicenter Selective Lymphadenectomy Trial (MSLT-I). Ann Surg Oncol 2012;19(8):2547–55.

73. Tyrell R, Antia C, Stanley S, et al. Surgical resection of metastatic melanoma in the era of immunotherapy and targeted therapy. Melanoma Manag 2017;4(1):61–8.

74. Domingues B, Lopes JM, Soares P, et al. Melanoma treatment in review. Immunotargets Ther 2018;7:35–49.

75. Wilson MA, Schuchter LM. Chemotherapy for Melanoma. Cancer Treat Res 2016; 167:209–29.

76. Middleton MR, Grob JJ, Aaronson N, et al. Randomized phase III study of temozolomide versus dacarbazine in the treatment of patients with advanced metastatic malignant melanoma. J Clin Oncol 2000;18(1):158–66.

77. Chapman PB, Einhorn LH, Meyers ML, et al. Phase III multicenter randomized trial of the Dartmouth regimen versus dacarbazine in patients with metastatic melanoma. J Clin Oncol 1999;17(9):2745–51.

78. Chapman PB, Hauschild A, Robert C, et al. Improved Survival with Vemurafenib in Melanoma with BRAF V600E Mutation. N Engl J Med 2011;364(26):2507–16.

79. Verma S, Petrella T, Hamm C, et al. Biochemotherapy for the treatment of metastatic malignant melanoma: a clinical practice guideline. Curr Oncol 2008; 15(2):85–9.

80. Hannay J, Davis JJ, Yu D, et al. Isolated limb perfusion: a novel delivery system for wild-type p53 and fiber-modified oncolytic adenoviruses to extremity sarcoma. Gene Ther 2007;14(8):671–81.

81. Pardoll DM. The blockade of immune checkpoints in cancer immunotherapy. Nat Rev Cancer 2012;12(4):252–64.

82. Murciano-Goroff YR, Warner AB, Wolchok JD. The future of cancer immunotherapy: microenvironment-targeting combinations. Cell Res 2020;30(6):507–19.

83. Linck RDM, Costa RL de P, Garicochea B. Cancer immunology and melanoma immunotherapy. An Bras Dermatol 2017;92(6):830–5.

84. O'Day SJ, Maio M, Chiarion-Sileni V, et al. Efficacy and safety of ipilimumab monotherapy in patients with pretreated advanced melanoma: a multicenter single-arm phase II study. Ann Oncol 2010;21(8):1712–7.

85. Hodi FS, O'Day SJ, McDermott DF, et al. Improved survival with ipilimumab in patients with metastatic melanoma. N Engl J Med 2010. https://doi.org/10.1056/NEJMoa1003466.

86. Blank CU, Haining WN, Held W, et al. Defining 'T cell exhaustion. Nat Rev Immunol 2019;19(11):665–74.

87. Weiss SA, Wolchok JD, Sznol M. Immunotherapy of Melanoma: Facts and Hopes. Clin Cancer Res 2019;25(17):5191–201.

88. Wolchok JD, Chiarion-Sileni V, Gonzalez R, et al. Overall Survival with Combined Nivolumab and Ipilimumab in Advanced Melanoma. N Engl J Med 2017;377(14): 1345–56.

89. Davies H, Bignell GR, Cox C, et al. Mutations of the BRAF gene in human cancer. Nature 2002;417(6892):949–54.

90. Khattak M, Fisher R, Turajlic S, et al. Targeted therapy and immunotherapy in advanced melanoma: an evolving paradigm. Ther Adv Med Oncol 2013;5(2): 105–18.

91. Hocker T, Tsao H. Ultraviolet radiation and melanoma: a systematic review and analysis of reported sequence variants. Hum Mutat 2007;28(6):578–88.
92. BRIM-2: An open-label, multicenter phase II study of vemurafenib in previously treated patients with BRAF V600E mutation-positive metastatic melanoma. | Journal of Clinical Oncology. Available at: https://ascopubs.org/doi/abs/10.1200/jco.2011.29.15_suppl.8509. Accessed January 14, 2021.
93. Hauschild A, Grob J-J, Demidov LV, et al. Dabrafenib in BRAF-mutated metastatic melanoma: a multicentre, open-label, phase 3 randomised controlled trial. Lancet 2012;380(9839):358–65.
94. Dummer R, Ascierto PA, Gogas HJ, et al. Overall survival in patients with BRAF-mutant melanoma receiving encorafenib plus binimetinib versus vemurafenib or encorafenib (COLUMBUS): a multicentre, open-label, randomised, phase 3 trial. Lancet Oncol 2018;19(10):1315–27.
95. Grimaldi AM, Simeone E, Festino L, et al. MEK inhibitors in the treatment of metastatic melanoma and solid tumors. Am J Clin Dermatol 2017;18(6):745–54.
96. Ribas A, Lawrence D, Atkinson V, et al. Combined BRAF and MEK inhibition with PD-1 blockade immunotherapy in BRAF -mutant melanoma. Nat Med 2019;25(6):936–40.
97. Kakadia S, Yarlagadda N, Awad R, et al. Mechanisms of resistance to BRAF and MEK inhibitors and clinical update of US Food and Drug Administration-approved targeted therapy in advanced melanoma. Oncotargets Ther 2018;11:7095–107.
98. Patel H, Yacoub N, Mishra R, et al. Current Advances in the Treatment of BRAF-Mutant Melanoma. Cancers 2020;12(2). https://doi.org/10.3390/cancers12020482.
99. Eroglu Z, Ribas A. Combination therapy with BRAF and MEK inhibitors for melanoma: latest evidence and place in therapy. Ther Adv Med Oncol 2016;8(1):48–56. https://doi.org/10.1177/1758834015616934.

Lower Extremity Ulcers

Caralin Schneider, BA, Scott Stratman, BS, Robert S. Kirsner, MD, PhD*

KEYWORDS

- Leg ulcer • Venous ulcer • Venous insufficiency • Arterial ulcer
- Peripheral artery disease • Diabetic ulcer • Diabetic neuropathy • Wound care

KEY POINTS

- Lower extremity ulcers affect more than 6.5 million Americans each year causing significant morbidity and cost to health care systems both in the United States and globally.
- Venous leg ulcers are the most common ulcers found on the legs (80%–90%) and diabetic foot ulcers are the most common ulcers found on the feet (80%).
- Atypical ulcers make up 10% of lower extremity ulcers and arterial disease may complicate up to one-third of lower extremity ulcers.
- Lower extremity ulcers often require a multidisciplinary approach with referral to a wound care center when wound healing stalls.

INTRODUCTION

Lower extremity ulcerations affect up to 49 million people annually worldwide with a cumulative lifetime risk of 1.0% to 1.8%, causing significant morbidity, mortality, and cost to health care systems globally. In the United States alone, the treatment of chronic wounds, or wounds that do not progress through healing in a timely manner, conservatively costs an estimated $25 billion annually.[1] Multidisciplinary care by the primary care practitioners, internists, dermatologists, vascular, general and plastic surgeons, podiatrists, and wound care providers is often required in the management of these wounds.

Lower extremity ulcers can be divided into leg and foot ulcers. The predominate ulceration found on the leg is a venous leg ulcer (VLU) comprising up to 80% to 90% of leg ulcers or ulcers located between the knee and the ankle. Diabetic foot ulcers (DFU) caused by neuropathy, vascular disease, or a combination of the two are the most common cause of foot ulcers. Arterial ulcers, pressure ulcers, and atypical ulcers all contribute to lower extremity ulcer prevalence and are discussed throughout this article.

Dr. Phillip Frost Department of Dermatology & Cutaneous Surgery, University of Miami Miller School of Medicine, 1600 N.W. 10th Avenue, RMSB, Room 2023-A, USA
* Corresponding author.
E-mail address: Rkirsner@med.miami.edu

Med Clin N Am 105 (2021) 663–679
https://doi.org/10.1016/j.mcna.2021.04.006
0025-7125/21/© 2021 Elsevier Inc. All rights reserved.

medical.theclinics.com

PATHOPHYSIOLOGY
Venous Leg Ulcers

VLUs are the most common leg ulcers, comprising up to 80% to 90% of lower extremity ulcers. The primary underlying mechanism for VLU formation is due to failure of the calf muscle pump to appropriately return blood to the heart from the legs. Veins, their working valves, and the muscles of the leg and feet make up the calf muscle pump. Most commonly, venous reflux occurs, which causes sustained elevated venous pressures that, under normal conditions, decrease with ambulation. This sustained elevation in venous pressure during ambulation owing to calf muscle pump failure most commonly results from incompetent valves or obstruction in the superficial and/or deep venous systems. Other possible causes include calf muscle failure owing to muscle disease or decreased ankle range of motion. Blood subsequently pools in the lower extremities, leading to increased local pressures, endothelial cell separation, and extravasation of fluid, cells, and macromolecules. This leads to the signs and symptoms patients with chronic venous insufficiency present with including edema, dermatitis, dyspigmentation, atrophie blanche, lipodermatosclerosis, and eventually ulceration.

The pathophysiology of a patient's first VLU is not understood fully, and multiple hypotheses have been suggested. One hypothesis suggests fibrin leakage secondary to increased intraluminal pressure in the capillaries, causing deposition of pericapillary fibrin cuffs.[2–4] This process consequently causes impairment in oxygen and nutrient diffusion, leading to inhibition in healing and potentially ulcer formation. Another hypothesis concerns the accumulation and activation of white blood cells around the dermal capillaries secondary to sustained elevated venous pressures (venous hypertension). These white blood cells subsequently release free radicals and destructive enzymes that may cause skin damage, resulting in ulceration.[5] Finally, a third hypothesis posits that the fibrin cuffs generated from leakage of dermal capillaries work to trap growth factors and matrix material.[6] This trapping of material precludes effective wound healing and maintenance of tissue integrity, causing its breakdown and eventual ulceration. More recently, the presence of excessive iron and hemosiderin deposited in tissues leads to prolongation of inflammation owing to dysregulation of macrophage influx and efflux. All of these mechanisms likely occur and contribute to disease development. Although the pathophysiologic mechanisms leading to venous insufficiency have been thoughtfully considered, the cause for development of first VLU is still under debate.

Arterial Ulcers

Arterial ulcerations result from arterial insufficiency leading to inadequate oxygen and nutrient delivery and tissue ischemia and breakdown. The most common etiology of arterial ulcers is peripheral arterial disease (PAD) caused by atherosclerosis and stenosis of the arterial lumen. PAD-induced tissue ischemia is often exacerbated by prolonged cutaneous pressure against a hard surface, such as a bone. This entity is often considered large vessel arterial disease. Smaller vessels may also be affected and, therefore, other causes of arterial ulcers often indicate an atypical etiology, such as thromboangiitis obliterans, arteriovenous malformation, Raynaud's phenomenon, microthrombotic disease, coagulopathies, cryoprecipitable diseases (cryoglobulinemia and cryofibrinogenemia), vasculitis, sickle cell disease, and polycythemia vera, among others.[7] Arterial disease may also complicate venous insufficiency and up to 25% to 33%% of patients with chronic venous insufficiency may have concomitant arterial disease, which may alter therapeutic approaches, such as debridement and compression.

Diabetic Foot Ulcers

In patients with diabetes mellitus, DFUs often result from neuropathy, particularly sensory neuropathy, and the subsequent loss of protective sensation in the foot. This condition leads to undetected prolonged pressure and repetitive traumatic tissue injury of the foot. Diabetic neuropathy develops secondary to hyperglycemia and hyperlipidemia induced hypermetabolic state of nerve cell bodies leading to reactive oxygen species and resulting distal to proximal axonal damage.[8] Sensory neurons including those for pain and temperature as well as vibration and proprioception are most susceptible to this metabolic damage; however, larger motor neurons are also susceptible. This neuropathy leads to muscle atrophy and anatomic bony abnormalities and deformities including Charcot foot, and this combination leads to an increased propensity for undetected pressure and trauma.[9,10] Repetitive trauma and friction may result in hyperkeratosis of high-pressure areas, leading to impaired cutaneous blood flow. Furthermore, diabetes mellitus leads to endothelial cell dysfunction as well as advanced glycation end products. Patients with diabetes mellitus have a higher incidence of peripheral vascular disease contributing to the pathogenesis and chronicity of ulcers.[11]

Atypical Ulcers

Atypical ulcers encompass ulcers that do not fit into the categories of VLUs, DFUs, arterial ulcers owing to large vessel disease, or pressure ulcers and represent up to 10% of ulcers on the leg.[7] Several thousand causes of atypical ulcers exist with etiologies including but not limited to inflammatory processes (ie, pyoderma gangrenosum, vasculitis, immunobullous disease), infection, vasculopathy, malignancy, metabolic disorders (ie, calciphylaxis), vasculitis, vasculopathy, sickle cell disease, drugs, or an externally induced mechanism. Suspicion should be raised for an atypical etiology when a leg ulcer presents in an uncommon anatomic location, has an unusual appearance or presentation, or is refractory to standard of care treatment.

CLINICAL PRESENTATION
Venous Leg Ulcers

VLUs are the most common leg ulcer, affecting 1% of the adult population and up to 3.6% of people older than 65 years. VLUs are also among the most common medical conditions in the Western world. VLUs have significant socioeconomic impact and millions of health care dollars are spent each year in their treatment and management. Risk factors for VLUs include both nonmodifiable factors such as age, female sex, White race, hypertension, a family history of VLUs, a history of superficial or deep venous thrombosis, reflux of the superficial, perforating, and/or deep venous systems; and modifiable risk factors such as type 2 diabetes and a high body mass index with physical inactivity (**Table 1**).[12]

History taking for diagnosis of VLUs should revolve around underlying conditions and the location of the ulceration. A history of varicose veins, multiparity, obesity, and prior venous thrombosis all help to support the clinical diagnosis of VLU. Patients with venous disease and venous ulcers may have a propensity of thromboembolism. In the setting of a patient with VLUs with recurrent thrombosis, miscarriages, or platelet disorders, an investigation into coagulation disorders is warranted. On physical examination, VLUs are commonly located near the medial malleolus, also called the gaiter region because it to corresponds with this location on certain styles of boots. This location is the medial aspect of the lower leg between the lower calf and the medial malleolus (**Fig. 1**). Lateral malleoli located VLUs also occur, and 1 in 20 patients

Table 1
Diagnosis and management of the most commonly encountered lower extremity ulcers

	VLU	Arterial Ulcer	DFU
History	Prior venous thrombosis Obesity Female sex Multiparity Physical inactivity Family history of VLU	Claudication symptoms Rest pain Cardiovascular risk factors Age >40 Smoking Male sex Hypertension Hyperlipidemia Diabetes Hyperhomocysteinemia Family history of PAD	Diabetes Prior DFU Neuropathy Insensate feet
Examination			
Location	Medial or lateral lower leg; gaiter region 1/20 on dorsal or lateral feet	Bony prominences Anteriorly Pressure sites Heel, malleoli, shin, distal toes	Foot below the ankle Pressure sites or sites of repetitive trauma
Appearance	Superficial with sloping flat borders Edema Pigment deposition Varicose veins Venous dermatitis Atrophie blanche Lipodermatosclerosis	"Punched out" sharply demarcated borders Necrotic Weak/absent distal pulses Pale skin Capillary refill >3 seconds Positive Beurger's test	Surrounding callous Peripheral neuropathy Vibration, monofilament, reflexes, gait

Imaging investigations	Duplex ultrasound examination Plethysmography Venous volume Venous filling index Ejection fraction Residual volume fraction	ABI TBI PVR Arterial duplex ultrasound examination Transcutaneous oximetry Contrast angiography	
Treatment		Risk factor reduction Wound care Infection management	
	ABI >0.9 Compression ABI 0.50–0.8 Light compression with close monitoring ABI <0.5 No compression Caution with debridement Consider venous surgery and arterial revascularization	Augment arterial flow including revascularization Avoid debridement until after revascularization	Mechanical offloading Debridement
Adjunctive therapies	Pentoxifylline Aspirin Statins Cell and tissue–based therapies	Consider after revascularization, if needed	Hyperbaric oxygen therapy NPWT PDGF Cell and tissue–based products

Abbreviations: ABI, ankle-brachial index; NPWT, negative pressure wound therapy; PDGF, platelet-derived growth factor; PVR, pulse volume readings; TBI, toe-brachial index.

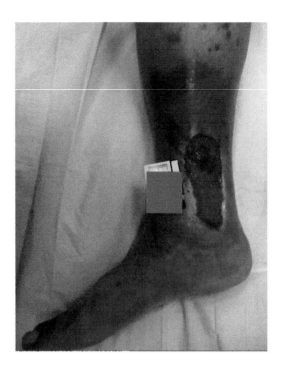

Fig. 1. VLU.

with VLU may have an ulcer on the dorsum or lateral aspects of the feet. VLUs may be painful in up to three-quarters of patients, but typically the pain is either dull or burning pain and relieved by leg elevation. VLUs are typically associated with edema, pigment deposition (from hemosiderin and melanin), venous dermatitis, atrophie blanche (white, porcelain scars), and lipodermatosclerosis (induration and fibrosis of the dermis and subcutaneous tissue). Because of concomitant sustained high ambulatory venous pressures, so-called venous hypertension, in these patients, moderate to heavy exudate may occur. The quality of the exudate, whether serous or purulent, may be a clinical clue to wound infection. Typically, VLUs are relatively superficial or shallow with sloping flat borders. Punched out ulcers, ulcers deep to tendon or bone, and ulcers with eschar are typically not due (at least solely) to venous disease. More commonly, VLUs have a variable degree of granulation and devitalized tissue (slough).

Arterial Leg Ulcers

Arterial ulcers most often occur in people with large vessel PAD with risk factors similar to coronary artery disease including older age, male sex, smoking, hypertension, diabetes, hyperlipidemia, hyperhomocysteinemia, a family history of PAD, and low socioeconomic status. The American College of Cardiology/American Heart Association guidelines recommend screening for PAD in patients more than 70 year old, 50 to 69 years old with a history of smoking or diabetes, and 40 to 49 years old with diabetes and at least 1 other atherosclerotic risk factor.[13] Arterial ulcers, therefore, typically present after the age of 40 when the effects of atherosclerosis begin to manifest. On history, patients may also report intermittent claudication or pain in the legs exacerbated by exercise or leg elevation, and relieved by rest and gravity such as dangling the leg from the edge of the bed or light walking.

On physical examination, arterial ulcers seem to be "punched-out" with sharply demarcated borders, often distally over a bony prominence, anteriorly on the leg where reduplication of vascular supply is less likely or sites of pressure (heel, malleoli, shin, and distal toes) (**Fig. 2**). The wound base may seem to be necrotic, and is often painful, unlike most venous ulcerations. The surrounding skin may seem to be pale and demonstrate decreased capillary refill time (>3 seconds). The Beurger's test or elevation of the leg to 45° for 1 minute may be positive for pallor. The absence of peripheral pulses, including the dorsalis pedis and posterior tibial, are highly sensitive for PAD; however, their presence does not exclude PAD. In fact, up to 80% of patients with arterial ulcers have palpable peripheral pulses.[14]

Diabetic Foot Ulcers

DFUs burden up to 25% of people with diabetes in their lifetime leading to morbidity, mortality, and health care costs of $6.2 to $18.7 billion annually in the United States alone.[15] With diabetes mellitus increasing globally, DFUs and their complications are and will become increasingly prevalent. Therefore, DFU prevention, diagnosis, and treatment are paramount. The most important risk factor for DFU is peripheral neuropathy with a 7-fold increased risk compared with patients with diabetes without peripheral neuropathy. Other important risk factors include duration of diabetes, age, severity of hyperglycemia, co-occurring peripheral artery disease, and renal disease. A thorough history of the wound course, the history of diabetes history and its management, smoking history, claudication history, previous ulcerations, vascular interventions, and amputations provide important insight.

DFUs occur below the level of the ankle, most commonly on the forefoot owing to orthopedic deformities such as neuropathic (Charcot) arthropathy and resulting motor impairments. Insensate areas of the foot exposed to prolonged pressure are susceptible to tissue injury and DFU formation (**Figs. 3** and **4**). On physical examination of patients with diabetes mellitus presenting with a foot ulcer, neurologic, peripheral vascular, and dermatologic assessments provide valuable clinical information of the etiology and treatment targets. For example, the presence of impaired vibration, monofilament sensation, reflexes, and gait suggest neuropathy. The absence of distal pulses implies concurrent PAD, but all patients with DFU (and all leg ulcers for that

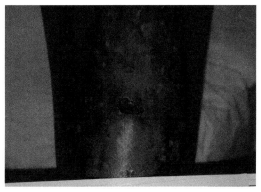

Fig. 2. Arterial ulcer on the anterior shin.

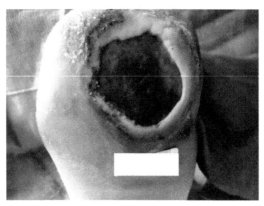

Fig. 3. DFU of the plantar heel.

matter) should have arterial vascular evaluation performed. Hyperkeratosis or callous formation clues to high pressure point areas of the foot at risk for ulceration.

DFUs may be deep to the tendon or bone and the use of a sterile, blunt probe may aid in the identification of possible bone or undermined borders. Probing to the bone increases the likelihood of having osteomyelitis. Skin, soft tissue, and bone infection in patients with DFU have the potential for significant consequence and diagnosis is often delayed. The presence of multiple cardinal signs of inflammation (redness, warmth, pain, and swelling), which may be blunted in diabetic patients, may suggest infection. Empiric treatment is needed, and culture results often help to direct antibiotic therapy if the infection persists. If an infection is suspected or the presence of bone is noted, imaging and laboratory tests may assist with identifying underlying osteomyelitis.

DIAGNOSTIC WORKUP FOR LEG ULCERS
Laboratory Tests

Although laboratory tests are not required for every patient with leg wounds, those with slow or nonhealing wounds should have an assessment to ensure there are no comorbid conditions that might delay healing. For example, anemia, renal

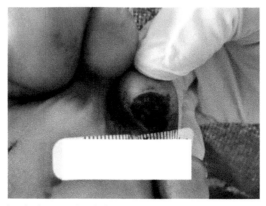

Fig. 4. DFU of the third plantar, distal digit.

insufficiency, and hypoalbuminemia can all deter healing. Additionally, further focused laboratory evaluation may be helpful in those with unknown or atypical etiologies. For example, an elevated An erythrocyte sedimentation rate of more than 60 mm/hr or a C-reactive protein of more than 7.9 mg/dL not otherwise explained suggests osteomyelitis in DFU patients.[16]

Vascular Studies

Venous studies

Two commonly implemented venous studies used to evaluate the severity of venous disease include the duplex ultrasound examination and plethysmography (**Figs. 5** and **6**). Through duplex ultrasound examination, one can directly visualize the veins in the lower extremities. By direct visualization, venous flow and the presence of venous thrombosis can be evaluated. The identification of obstruction or incompetent valves via duplex ultrasound examination can be later used in the treatment of patients with chronic venous insufficiency, by way of venous intervention, which was recently proved effective in speeding healing of VLU. Plethysmography is another commonly used venous study that can be used to measure the venous volume, venous filling index, ejection fraction, and residual volume fraction. The venous filling index is a good predictor of venous reflux and clinical severity of disease.[17] Other options for venous studies include contrast venography, foot volumetry, and phlebography.

Arterial studies

To detect large vessel disease, measurement of the ankle-brachial index (ABI) is the most sensitive form of testing.[18] The ABI has a predictive value in detecting coronary artery (CAD) with an increased risk of CAD in those with ABI less than 0.9. Patients with

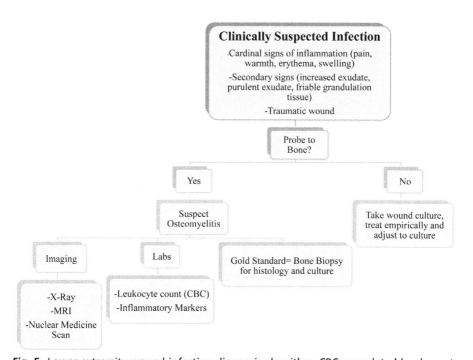

Fig. 5. Lower extremity wound infection diagnosis algorithm. CBC, complete blood count.

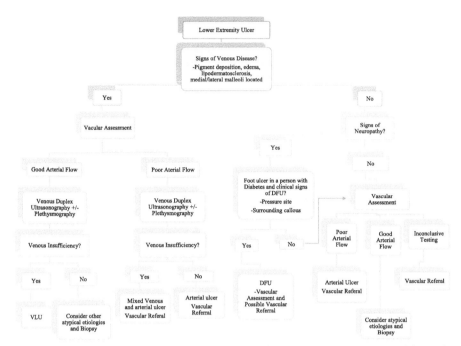

Fig. 6. Systematic approach to the lower extremity ulcer. (Note: partially adapted from Abbade et al.[42])

moderate to severe large vessel disease will have an ABI of less than 0.7, compatible with PAD. Lower ABIs correlate with more severe arterial disease. Arterial insufficiency can be further corroborated via Doppler flowmeter, especially if peripheral pulses are not palpable. Patients with a decreased ABI and/or weak peripheral pulses should be further evaluated with arterial duplex ultrasound examination, to measure the extent of arterial disease. Although contrast angiography is the gold standard in the diagnosis of arterial insufficiency, it is invasive and thus carries some risk. Other noninvasive studies that can be used to measure the extent of arterial insufficiency include the toe-brachial index, pulse volume recordings, and transcutaneous oximetry measurements. Adequate blood flow is necessary for the healing of all wounds, so study-guided evaluation of arterial disease is paramount before treatment implementation, whether it is less (ie, compression therapy or debridement) or more (ie, vascular intervention including, bypass surgery) invasive.

Biopsy

Although not necessary for all chronic wounds, biopsy can be a useful diagnostic tool when the ulcer etiology remains unclear, and an atypical cause of an ulcer is suspected. Wound biopsies are sent for histology and for tissue culture to identify atypical causes of infection including mycobacterial infection and subcutaneous fungal infections. Biopsies should be taken from the wound edge (including ulcer and adjacent edge) with either a punch biopsy encompassing subcutaneous tissue or wedge biopsy. Although, in the case of pyoderma gangrenosum, a risk of pathergy is present, overall the research suggests that a biopsy does not hinder the healing of chronic wounds.[19,20]

A biopsy may also be considered in a chronic wound with transformation when malignancy is clinically suspected.[20] Although the incidence of malignant transformation of chronic wounds has been studied, a consensus has not been reached. One prospective study of 154 VLUs with and without arterial insufficiency that failed healing after 3 months, however, showed a 10% prevalence of skin cancer in the chronic ulcers.[20] Therefore, if malignancy is suspected clinically, a biopsy should be performed without fear of exacerbating the ulcer. In these cases of suspected malignancy, a second biopsy for histology should be taken for the ulcer center as well as from the ulcer edge.

Biopsies of bone can be useful, as well, to help diagnose osteomyelitis. The gold standard for the diagnosis of osteomyelitis is a positive histology and tissue culture of the bone, which has the added benefit of identifying a causative organism.

Radiographic Studies

Imaging studies can offer clinicians invaluable information about a wound, including its depth, surrounding blood flow, and presence of inflammation and/or infection. The significance of ultrasound imaging has already been discussed in the management of wounds, but radiographs, computed tomography scans, and MRI also have usefulness in wound management. Osteomyelitis, an infection of the surrounding bone, can potentially be diagnosed through radiographic studies, but these have low sensitivity and specificity for diagnosing osteomyelitis.[21] Although MRI is the most sensitive imaging study in diagnosing osteomyelitis, computed tomography scans are also useful in many clinical contexts; the drawback of computed tomography scanning, however, is its use of ionizing radiation, thereby making it more invasive.

GENERAL WOUND TREATMENT
Debridement

Wound debridement consists of removing necrotic tissue, slough, and bacterial biofilms from the wound bed, as well as hyperkeratotic tissue from the wound edges to allow for optimal healing.[22] Debridement should be limited in arterial ulcers owing to inadequate blood supply, as well as in suspected and untreated pyoderma gangrenosum owing to the possibility of pathergy, or wound worsening. Five different types of debridement (autolytic, enzymatic, mechanical, surgical, and biologic) exist with their associated advantages (**Table 2**). Clinicians most often use surgical debridement either with a scalpel or sharp curette, but autolytic, enzymatic, and biologic forms of debridement are often less painful and can be incorporated into selective debridement that may occur in subsequent visits.

Infection Management

Even though most, if not all, chronic leg ulcerations are colonized with bacteria, this does imply an infected wound. Systemic antibiotic therapy should only be implemented if there is clinical suspicion for infection (eg, host response with increased pain or tenderness, warmth, redness, or swelling). Finding increasing or purulent drainage or abnormal granulation tissue suggests a high local bioburden and may be treated with topical antimicrobials. When infection is suspected, cultures can be used to identify the specific infectious micro-organism that could be either colonizing or infecting a wound and subsequently help guide antibiotic therapy, should empiric antibiotics based on algorithms fail to resolve infection (**Fig. 5**).

Of note, systemic antibiotic therapy seems neither to decrease biofilm formation nor does it increase healing rates in noninfected wounds. Topical antimicrobials have also

Table 2 Debridement methods		
Method	Description	Examples
Surgical	Sharp removal of the wound base and edge with pain control needed (local or general anesthesia)	
Mechanical	Moisten wound environment to allow for removal of adherent slough	Wet saline gauze High-pressure irrigation Pulsed lavage Hydrotherapy
Autolytic	Maintenance of a moist wound environment to allow for the body's own enzymes (metalloproteases) to breakdown necrotic tissue	Occlusive dressings
Enzymatic	Added enzymes to the wound base to allow breakdown of tissue Will breakdown normal tissue and can lead to wound enlargement if not carefully placed only in the wound	Collagenase Papain–urea preparations
Biological	Sterile maggots placed directly on the wound bed to consume necrotic tissue while preserving normal tissue	Larvae (sterile maggots of *Lucilia sericata*)

been explored in various systematic reviews; clinically uninfected wounds that are healing do not require topical antibiotics.[23] Newer nontoxic, antiseptics (eg, slow release cadexomer iodine or silver dressings) have now become preferable to other antiseptics that can damage healthy granulation tissue.

Dressings

When dressing lower extremity wounds, the type of wound, wound moisture, and vascular supply of the lower extremity should be taken into consideration. A moist wound environment should be maintained to allow for autolytic debridement, alteration of the wound microbiome, and promotion of an electrical gradient to promote keratinocyte migration for healing. Dressings that help to moisturize wounds include occlusive dressings such as hydrocolloids or hydrogels. Although a desiccated wound should be avoided, so should a macerated wound. Absorptive wound dressings for exudative wounds include foams and alginates. The periwound skin should also be protected from excessive moisture by protective barrier creams and dryness by moisturizing lotions.

In addition to moisture retention, dressings may be impregnated with therapeutic treatments including silver as an antimicrobial or collagen, which incorporates into the wound bed and may accelerate healing by attracting growth factors, decreasing reactive oxygen species, and hastening granulation tissue formation.[24]

Management of Venous Leg Ulcers

When it comes to the treatment of VLUs, compression therapy is the cornerstone of treatment. By increasing the local hydrostatic pressure and, thereby, decreasing the superficial venous pressure, compression decreases the leakage of fluid into the interstitial space, thus decreasing edema and swelling. Improving venous return, stimulating fibrinolysis and decreasing wound bioburden are additional benefits of compression therapy. This decrease in edema ultimately improves healing; several clinical trials and systematic reviews have identified the usefulness of compression in the healing of VLUs and decreasing recurrences.[25,26] However, close follow-up is required in patients with arterial disease (eg, an ABI of 0.5–0.8), because compression can impede arterial blood flow and risk ischemia. In severe cases (an ABI of <0.5), compression should not be used. An alternative, albeit more invasive, therapy for venous reflux aside from compression is venous intervention, including surgery.

Through venous interventions such as phlebectomy, sclerotherapy, laser or other ablation techniques, endoscopic procedures, or ligation and stripping, venous reflux can be treated, thus improving healing outcomes in those with VLUs. More recently, laser or radiofrequency ablation are favored owing to less invasive aspects, decreasing the risk associated with other surgical interventions. Additionally, patients can actively participate in their care—regular leg elevation, especially at night, can help to ameliorate the edema and swelling that normally impede effective wound healing in patients with VLUs.

Healing outcomes in patients with VLUs can be further optimized through medical management. The efficacy of pentoxifylline, a substituted xanthine derivative, in the treatment of VLUs has been investigated and results summarized in a systematic review.[27] Pentoxifylline was found to be a useful adjunct to compression therapy in the treatment of VLUs; pentoxifylline and compression were more effective than placebo and compression (relative risk, 1.30; 95% confidence interval, 1.10–1.54). Aspirin, considering its inhibition of inflammation and platelet activity, has also been implicated in the healing of VLUs. Although prior randomized controlled trials suggested that full-dose aspirin (300 mg/d) improved healing outcomes in patients with VLUs, these trials were limited in quality because of the potential for selection bias and their small sizes.[28] More recently, a single-center randomized controlled trial suggested that statins might result in improved healing.

Management of Arterial Ulcerations

Arterial ulcer treatment centers on improving arterial blood flow, including revascularization and pain control. Patients with arterial ulcers who need intervention, where medical management fails, should be referred to a vascular surgeon or interventional radiologist for the evaluation for percutaneous balloon angioplasty with or without stenting or surgical revascularization. Amputation may be necessary in the event of progressive gangrene or severe rest pain. In the circumstance that the patient is not a candidate for revascularization, the ulcer may be managed conservatively with wound care and reduction and treatment of PAD risk factors.[29] Debridement should be limited until adequate blood supply to the wound has been established by a revascularization procedure.[30]

All patients with arterial ulcers should be encouraged to exercise to incite collateral circulation. Additionally, all reversible risk factors for PAD should be corrected and hypercholesterolemia, hyperlipidemia, and diabetes should be treated to target levels. Protection of the lower extremities from further trauma and infection to avoid worsening of the existing ulcer, amputation, or new ulcerations is crucial.[31]

Management of Diabetic Foot Ulcers

The hallmarks of DFU treatment are diabetes management, mechanical offloading, debridement, and wound care. Debridement of any surrounding hyperkeratosis removes genotypically and phenotypically abnormal cells and aids in offloading of new border epithelium. Debridement of adherent slough at the wound base increases growth factors important for infection prevention and healing. Adjunctive therapies shown to aid in DFU healing include hyperbaric oxygen therapy, cell and tissue–based products, negative pressure wound therapy (NPWT), and platelet-derived growth factor (using various formulations), with others in development.[32] After wound closure, continued diabetes management, offloading, and vigilance cannot be underestimated owing to high recurrence rates. Up to 40% of DFUs recur after 1 year, 66% recur in 3 years, 75% in 5 years; and close to 100% at 10 years; therefore, prevention and monitoring are paramount.[33]

Adjunctive Therapies

When the standard of care for the wound stalls, referral to a wound care center, if not already made, and adjunctive therapies should be considered.

Autologous skin grafts

Split or partial thickness skin grafts may be used to treat large or refractory ulcers. These procedures include taking epidermis and only part of the dermis from a donor site and transferring it to the wound bed. Split thickness skin grafts have associated donor site morbidity, but typically the donor site heals relatively quickly. A newer technique of epidermal skin grafting allows the harvesting of epidermal grafts without the need for anesthesia or a trained surgeon, making it more cost effective. Epidermal wounds heal quickly without scarring, and thus have limited donor site morbidity.[34] Epidermal skin grafting may also be advantageous in patients who have a disease process that exhibits pathergy, such as pyoderma gangrenosum.

Cell and tissue–based products

Numerous cell and tissue–based products are available commercially for the treatment of chronic wounds and are categorized into a few different groups based on the presence of cells (cellular vs acellular), source (allogenic, xenogeneic, and autologous), conformation (single layer, bilayered, trilayered, and spray), and anatomic structure (epidermal, dermal, and composite).[35]

An example of a cellular product currently available and approved by the US Food and Drug Administration for the treatment of VLUs is a bilayered product composed of human growth-arrested keratinocytes and fibroblasts, and bovine collagen type I. On the market for more than 20 years, this product has initially shown in a study of 240 patients to increase healing percentage at 24 weeks when compared with standard of care compression (57% vs 40%, respectively).[36] An acellular product, porcine-derived small intestine submucosa, in a randomized controlled trial compared with compression alone healed 21% more VLUs at 12 weeks (55% vs 34%).

Negative pressure wound therapy

NPWT has been shown to decrease bacterial burden, increase wound perfusion, and by physically stretching cells, aid in granulation tissue formation. Two types of NPWT are currently available, traditional and single use. The advantages of single use NPWT are that it is canisterless, allows for portability, and has shown to both improve wound healing outcomes at 12 weeks and to be more cost effective when compared with traditional NPWT, making it the ideal choice for caring for chronic wounds in the outpatient setting.[37]

Hyperbaric oxygen therapy

Hyperbaric oxygen therapy consists of exposing the body to 100% oxygen at high pressure (2.0–2.4 ATMs or the equivalent of 33–42 feet of sea water). Hyperbaric oxygen therapy has been shown to increase oxygen delivery to wounds, enhance leukocyte activity, promote angiogenesis, and support osteogenesis. The main risks of hyperbaric oxygen therapy are hypoglycemia, oxygen toxicity, barotrauma to the ears or lungs, and a possible increase the rate of cataract growth. Hyperbaric oxygen therapy is now commonly used for the treatment of DFUs and included in most treatment protocols; however, the randomized controlled trials have yet to show conclusive results.[38,39]

Pain Management

Pain, although not always apparent to the clinician, represents an important source of morbidity for the patient, especially those with chronic wounds. Pain management should be discussed and adjusted as needed at each visit using a multimodal approach, where possible. The source of pain should first be identified as inflammatory, neuropathic, or infectious and treated accordingly. In patients with chronic pain, a multimodal approach of topical treatment (topical lidocaine, cool or warm compresses), lifestyle interventions (exercise, nutrition, and sleep), and systemic medications comprises a robust approach to pain. Lifestyle interventions may not only help with pain, but also overall mental health, often affected in chronic wound patients.

A new, nonmedical treatment for pain may be found in virtual reality, during which the patients immerse themselves in an auditory and visual experience using techniques of distraction and positive emotions to treat pain and ease anxiety.[40] Virtual reality may prove especially useful for acute pain and anxiety management during office procedures, such as debridement and biopsies.[41] Other alternative approaches to chronic pain include biofeedback, cognitive behavioral therapy, meditation, among others.

CLINICS CARE POINTS

- Vascular assessment is necessary to determine to exclude arterial disease and to help determine the underlying etiology of various leg ulcers (venous, arterial, or mixed) and to determine severity of disease.

- Adequate arterial perfusion is necessary for wound healing, and revascularization is often necessary, should insufficient arterial perfusion be uncovered.

- Suspect malignancy or an atypical ulcer etiology, especially in nonhealing and chronic wounds warranting the need for biopsy for histology and tissue culture.

- Evidenced-based wound care with management of comorbidities and pain are essential pillars in the management of lower extremity ulcers.

DISCLOSURE

The authors have nothing to disclose.

REFERENCES

1. Sen CK, Gordillo GM, Roy S, et al. Human skin wounds: a major and snowballing threat to public health and the economy. Wound Repair Regen 2009;17(6): 763–71.
2. Vanscheidt W, Laaff H, Wokalek H, et al. Pericapillary fibrin cuff: a histological sign of venous leg ulceration. J Cutan Pathol 1990;17(5):266–8.

3. Mirshahi S, Soria J, Mirshahi M, et al. Expression of elastase and fibrin in venous leg ulcer biopsies: a pilot study of pentoxifylline versus placebo. J Cardiovasc Pharmacol 1995;25(Suppl 2):S101–5.

4. Brown J. The role of the fibrin cuff in the development of venous leg ulcers. J Wound Care 2005;14(7):324–7.

5. Coleridge Smith PD. Pathogenesis of chronic venous insufficiency and possible effects of compression and pentoxifylline. Yale J Biol Med 1993;66(1):47–59.

6. Falanga V, Eaglstein WH. The "trap" hypothesis of venous ulceration. Lancet 1993;341(8851):1006–8.

7. Tang JC, Vivas A, Rey A, et al. Atypical ulcers: wound biopsy results from a university wound pathology service. Ostomy Wound Manage 2012;58(6):20–2, 24, 26-29.

8. Volpe CMO, Villar-Delfino PH, Dos Anjos PMF, et al. Cellular death, reactive oxygen species (ROS) and diabetic complications. Cell Death Dis 2018;9:119.

9. Feldman EL, Nave KA, Jensen TS, et al. New Horizons in diabetic neuropathy: mechanisms, bioenergetics, and pain. Neuron 2017;93:1296.

10. Pecoraro RE, Reiber GE, Burgess EM. Pathways to diabetic limb amputation. Basis for prevention. Diabetes Care 1990;13(5):513–21.

11. Neville RF, Kayssi A, Buescher T, et al. The diabetic foot. Curr Probl Surg 2016; 53(9):408–37.

12. Kelechi TJ, Johnson JJ, Yates S. Chronic venous disease and venous leg ulcers: an evidence-based update. J Vasc Nurs 2015;33(2):36–46.

13. Gerhard-Herman MD, Gornik HL, Barrett C, et al. 2016 AHA/ACC guideline on the management of patients with lower extremity peripheral artery disease: a report of the American College of Cardiology/American Heart Association Task Force on Clinical Practice Guidelines. Circulation 2017;135(12):e726–79.

14. Collins TC, Suarez-Almazor M, Peterson NJ. An absent pulse is not sensitive for the early detection of peripheral arterial disease. Fam Med 2006;38:38–42.

15. Hicks CW, Selvarajah S, Mathioudakis N, et al. Burden of infected diabetic foot ulcers on hospital admissions and costs. Ann Vasc Surg 2016;33:149–58.

16. Lavery LA, Ahn J, Ryan EC, et al. What are the optimal cutoff values for ESR and CRP to diagnose osteomyelitis in patients with diabetes-related foot infections? Clin Orthop Relat Res 2019;477(7):1594–602.

17. Criado E, Farber MA, Marston WA, et al. The role of air plethysmography in the diagnosis of chronic venous insufficiency. J Vasc Surg 1998;27(4):660–70.

18. Khan TH, Farooqui FA, Niazi K. Critical review of the ankle brachial index. Curr Cardiol Rev 2008;4(2):101–6.

19. Panuncialman J, Hammerman S, Carson P, et al. Wound edge biopsy sites in chronic wounds heal rapidly and do not result in delayed overall healing of the wounds. Wound Repair Regen 2010;18(1):21–5.

20. Bergstrom KG. Chronic ulcers: when to consider malignancy? J Drugs Dermatol 2012;11(8):1006–7.

21. Lee YJ, Sadigh S, Mankad K, et al. The imaging of osteomyelitis. Quant Imaging Med Surg 2016;6(2):184–98.

22. Lebrun E, Tomic-Canic M, Kirsner RS. The role of surgical debridement in healing of diabetic foot ulcers. Wound Repair Regen 2010;18(5):433–8.

23. Lipsky BA, Hoey C. Topical antimicrobial therapy for treating chronic wounds. Clin Infect Dis 2009;49(10):1541–9.

24. Naomi R, Fauzi MB. Cellulose/collagen dressings for diabetic foot ulcer: a review. Pharmaceutics 2020;12(9):881.

25. Gohel MS, Barwell JR, Taylor M, et al. Long term results of compression therapy alone versus compression plus surgery in chronic venous ulceration (ESCHAR): randomized controlled trial. BMJ 2007;335(7610):83.
26. O'Meara S, Cullum N, Nelson EA, et al. Compression for venous leg ulcers. Cochrane Database Syst Rev 2012;(11):CD000265.
27. Jull AB, Waters J, Arroll B. Oral pentoxifylline for treatment of venous leg ulcers. Cochrane Database Syst Rev 2000;(2):CD001733.
28. de Oliveira Carvalho PE, Magolbo NG, De Aquino RF, et al. Oral aspirin for treating venous leg ulcers. Cochrane Database Syst Rev 2016;(2):CD009432.
29. Weir GR, Smart H, van Marle J, et al. Arterial disease ulcers, part 2: treatment. Adv Skin Wound Care 2014;27:462–76.
30. Varela C, Acin F, De Haro J, et al. Influence of surgical or endovascular distal revascularization of the lower limbs on ischemic ulcer healing. J Cardiovasc Surg (Torino) 2011;52:381–9.
31. Sieggreen MY, Kline RA. Arterial insufficiency and ulceration: diagnosis and treatment options. Adv Skin Wound Care 2004;17(5 Pt 1):242–51 [quiz 52-3].
32. Stratman S, Schneider C, Kirsner RS. New therapies for the treatment of diabetic foot ulcers: updated review of clinical trials. Surg Technol Int 2020;37:37–47.
33. Armstrong DG, Boulton AJM, Bus SA. Diabetic foot ulcers and their recurrence. N Engl J Med 2017;376(24):2367–75.
34. Herskovitz I, Hughes OB, Macquhae F, et al. Epidermal skin grafting. Int Wound J 2016;13(Suppl 3):52–6.
35. Oualla-Bachiri W, Fernandez-Gonzalez A, Quinones-Vico MI, et al. From grafts to human bioengineered vascularized skin substitutes. Int J Mol Sci 2020;21(21):8197.
36. Zaulyanov L, Kirsner RS. A review of a bi-layered living cell treatment (Apligraf) in the treatment of venous leg ulcers and diabetic foot ulcers. Clin Interv Aging 2007;2(1):93–8.
37. Kirsner RS, Delhougne G, Searle RJ. A cost-effectiveness analysis comparing single-use and traditional negative pressure wound therapy to treat chronic venous and diabetic foot ulcers. Wound Manag Prev 2020;66(3):30–6.
38. Tejada S, Batle JM, Ferrer MD, et al. Therapeutic effects of hyperbaric oxygen in the process of wound healing. Curr Pharm Des 2019;25(15):1682–93.
39. Lalieu RC, Brouwer RJ, Ubbink DT, et al. Hyperbaric oxygen therapy for nonischemic diabetic ulcers: a systematic review. Wound Repair Regen 2020;28(2):266–75.
40. Ahmadpour N, Randall H, Choksi H, et al. Virtual reality interventions for acute and chronic pain management. Int J Biochem Cell Biol 2019;114:105568.
41. Hirt PA, Lev-Tov H. The use of virtual reality for bedside procedures. Br J Dermatol 2019;181(2):393–4.
42. Abbade LPF, Lastória S. Abordagem de pacientes com úlcera da perna de etiologia venosa. An Bras Dermatol 2006;81:509–22.

Cutaneous Manifestations of Diabetes

Alex Hines, MD[a], Afsaneh Alavi, MD[b], Mark D.P. Davis, MD[b],*

KEYWORDS

- Diabetes mellitus • Acanthosis nigricans • Necrobiosis lipoidica
- Diabetic dermopathy • Scleredema diabeticorum • Bullous diabeticorum
- Diabetic foot ulcer • Lipodystrophy

KEY POINTS

- Cutaneous manifestations of DM are common and have been reported in 30% to 79% of individuals with diabetes.
- The characteristic cutaneous manifestations of diabetes include acanthosis nigricans, necrobiosis lipoidica, diabetic dermopathy, skin thickening, and bullous diabeticorum.
- In patients with necrobiosis lipoidica and diabetes, the diabetes diagnosis precedes or occurs concomitantly with NL in 86% of cases.
- Onychomycosis is common in patient with diabetes.
- Clinicians managing patients with diabetes should be familiar with presentations of lipoatrophy and lipodystrophy associated with insulin and insulin pumps, increasing reports of drug induced bullous pemphigoid (BP) caused by new hypoglycemic agents, and contact dermatitis to continuous glucose monitors and insulin pumps.

INTRODUCTION

Diabetes mellitus (DM) is a significant worldwide health concern with an estimated global prevalence of 9.3% in 2019.[1] Global incidence has more than doubled since 1990 and is projected to continue increasing in the future.[2] DM is more prevalent in high-income countries, and the projected prevalence in the United States by 2050 is 21% to 33%.[3] Diabetes negatively impacts quality of life and is associated with a two- to three-fold increase in all-cause mortality.[2] Type 2 DM (T2DM) accounts for approximately 90% of all diabetes.[1]

Cutaneous manifestations of DM are common and have been reported in 30% to 79% of patients with diabetes.[4,5] The spectrum of DM-associated cutaneous disease is vast, and ranges from benign to life-threatening conditions (**Table 1**). Even "benign"

Funding Sources: None.

Conflicts of Interest: None declared.

[a] Department of Internal Medicine, Mayo Clinic, Rochester, MN, USA; [b] Department of Dermatology, Mayo Clinic, Rochester, MN, USA

* Corresponding author. 200 First Street Southwest, Rochester, MN 55905.

E-mail address: davis.mark2@mayo.edu

Med Clin N Am 105 (2021) 681–697

https://doi.org/10.1016/j.mcna.2021.04.008

0025-7125/21/© 2021 Elsevier Inc. All rights reserved.

medical.theclinics.com

Table 1
Characteristics of cutaneous disorders associated with diabetes mellitus

Condition	Prevalence[a]	DM Association	Appearance	Characteristic Distribution	Treatment
Acanthosis nigricans	Intermediate-common	T2DM > T1DM	Velvety, hyperpigmented, hyperkeratotic plaques	Posterior neck, groin, and axilla	Treat underlying cause Retinoids and keratinolytics can improve appearance
Necrobiosis lipoidica	Rare	T1DM > T2DM	Ovoid plaques with yellow-brown atrophic centers and telangiectasis	Pretibial, bilateral	Generally unsatisfactory Topical and intralesional steroids are first line
Diabetic dermopathy	Common	Long-standing (T1 ≈ T2)	Small, brown, round to ovoid atrophic depressions	Pretibial, bilateral, asymmetric	None recommended
Scleredema diabeticorum	Intermediate	Long-standing (T2DM > T1DM)	Skin thickening and induration; ± erythema, peau d'orange appearance	Neck and upper back, symmetric	Generally unsatisfactory PUVA or electron-beam therapy most effective
Scleroderma-like hand changes	Common	Long-standing (T1 and T2)	Symmetric, waxy skin thickening ± limited joint mobility	Bilateral hands	Physical therapy
Bullous diabeticorum	Rare	T1DM > T2DM	Tense bullae on otherwise normal-appearing skin	Acral distal surfaces of lower extremities, unilateral	Conservative (foot offloading) vs drainage Close observation for secondary infection
Bullous pemphigoid	Rare	DPP-4 inhibitors	Tense blisters on normal, erythematous, or urticarial skin	Groin, axilla, flexural areas	Discontinuation of offending medication
Lipohypertrophy	Common	Insulin use	Soft, rubbery, lipoma-like dermal nodules	Insulin injection sites	Rotation of injection sites Avoid injection to areas of lipohypertrophy
Lipoatrophy	Rare	Insulin use	Cutaneous depressions	Insulin injection sites	Same as for lipohypertrophy
Drug-induced BP	Rare	Gliptin	Bulla formation and itching	Generalized	Stop the drug, oral steroid, and doxycycline

Abbreviations: BP, bullous pemphigoid; DPP-4, dipeptidyl peptidase 4; PUVA, psoralen plus ultraviolet A; T1DM, type 1 diabetes mellitus; T2DM, type 2 diabetes mellitus.
[a] Percent of patients with diabetes affected. Rare, <2%; intermediate, 2%–10%; common, >10%.

cutaneous findings are important because they may precede the disease and signal underlying DM in undiagnosed patients, or represent poorly controlled disease in those with known disease. Furthermore, it has been proposed that the visible nature of cutaneous disease may provide motivation for patients to better control their DM.[6] This review describes the dermatologic manifestations of diabetes using the following categories: (1) characteristic skin findings, (2) general skin findings, and (3) findings related to diabetes treatment. The focus of this review is on clinical presentation and diagnosis, pathophysiology, epidemiology, and treatment.

DISCUSSION
Pathophysiology

The pathogenesis of diabetes and its complications are complex, multifactorial, and an area of significant ongoing research. Hyperglycemia is a central feature of diabetes and has a direct effect on keratinocyte and fibroblast function.[7] Hyperglycemia also increases nonenzymatic glycation of proteins, lipids, and nucleic acids, resulting in increased production of advanced glycation end-products. Advanced glycation end-products alter skin structure and skin function, and are involved in the pathogenesis of vascular complications. Vascular disease along with diabetes-associated immune suppression predisposes patients to infection and poor wound healing. Furthermore, hyperinsulinemia alters keratinocyte proliferation, differentiation, and migration, which results in decreased skin barrier function and delays wound healing.[8] The underlying pathophysiology of the conditions discussed in this review is variable, and for many a definitive mechanism remains unknown.

Characteristic Skin Findings

Acanthosis nigricans
Acanthosis nigricans (AN) is characterized by velvety, hyperpigmented, scaly symmetric patches and plaques, most commonly affecting the posterior neck, groin, and axilla (**Fig. 1**). The association of AN with hyperinsulinemic states, such as T2DM, is well established, and pathogenesis involves activation of insulin growth-like receptors leading to keratinocyte and dermal fibroblast hyperproliferation.[6] Patients with AN in

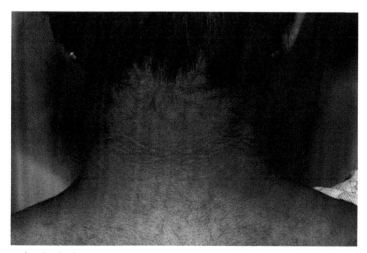

Fig. 1. Acanthosis nigricans.

association with DM are most often overweight and frequently obese. AN can also occur in type 1 DM (T1DM), and is associated with other endocrine disorders (eg, polycystic ovarian syndrome and Cushing syndrome), gastrointestinal malignancy, and certain medications.[7] Diagnosis is typically clinical; however, AN is an important sign of systemic disease and should prompt investigation for the underlying cause. Malignant AN is rare but important paraneoplastic phenomenon commonly associated with gastric adenocarcinoma. The atypical involvement of mucosal surfaces, rapid appearance of extensive AN, and weight loss are the features highly suggestive of internal malignancy.[9]

Management of AN should focus on treating the underlying cause, which has been shown to be effective in diabetes and other causes of AN.[10] It has been proposed that the observable nature of AN may serve as a motivating factor for patients, and in the case of T2DM, AN has been shown to improve with better glycemic control.[6,10] Treatment with retinoids and keratolytics (ie, urea cream) can also improve the appearance of AN.[11]

Necrobiosis lipoidica

Necrobiosis lipoidica (NL) affects between 0.3% and 1.6% of patients with diabetes.[12,13] Previously known as necrobiosis lipoidica diabeticorum, 35% to 89% of patients with NL do not have diabetes, and thus "diabeticorum" has been eliminated from the name.[14,15] Importantly, NL may precede diabetes, and 7% to 42% of patients with NL initially without diabetes subsequently develop impaired glucose tolerance or DM.[14,15]

NL presents initially as well-defined erythematous papules and nodules with red-brown centers.[5] These lesions evolve over time into characteristic, well-defined ovoid plaques with yellow-brown atrophic centers and telangiectasias (**Fig. 2**).[7] Distribution is a particularly useful diagnostic clue, with 88% of patients having a pretibial distribution, and 80% of that group demonstrating bilateral pretibial lesions.[15] NL is a complication of microangiopathy and lesions are typically asymptomatic. However, ulceration occurs in up to 35% of cases and can lead to pain, subsequent secondary infection, or rarely squamous cell carcinoma.[16–18] The overall course is variable, with some patients experiencing spontaneous resolution and others developing chronic disease.[19]

Topical or intralesional steroids are considered first-line treatments; however, results are generally unsatisfactory.[20] Pentoxifylline and antimalarial agents are alternative systemic therapy options.[19] There is insufficient evidence regarding the influence of glycemic control on NL disease course.[21] For ulcerated lesions, treatment should focus on pain control, prevention of secondary infection, and monitoring for development of squamous cell carcinoma, a rare late complication.[5,17]

Diabetic dermopathy

Diabetic dermopathy (DD), also referred to as "shin spots," is often cited as the most common cutaneous manifestation of diabetes, with a reported incidence of 9% to 55%.[22] DD occurs in approximately equal frequencies in T1DM and T2DM and many consider it to be pathognomonic for diabetes.[6,22,23] It occurs most commonly in patients with long-standing diabetes who are greater than 50 years old.[22] Clinically, DD initially presents as red to pink ovoid papules or plaques. Over the course of weeks, these lesions progress to small, brown, round to ovoid atrophic depressions that are characteristic of DD. Lesions characteristically occur on the bilateral pretibial legs and are asymmetric in distribution (**Fig. 3**). DD is asymptomatic and does not require treatment. Spontaneous resolution of individual lesions may occur over several

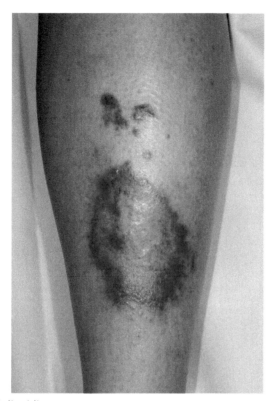

Fig. 2. Necrobiosis lipoidica.

years, although new lesions tend to continuously arise.[22] Importantly, DD is associated with coronary artery disease and microvascular complications (neuropathy, nephropathy, and retinopathy), with the incidence of DD increasing from 21% in patients with diabetes with no microvascular complications to 81% in patients with all three complications.[24]

Diabetic skin thickening
Diabetic skin thickening has been categorized into three distinct types: (1) subclinical and benign generalized skin thickening, (2) scleroderma-like skin changes of the hands, and (3) scleredema diabeticorum (SD).[17,18]

Clinical evidence of skin thickening is present in 22% to 39% of patients with diabetes.[25,26] Furthermore, patients with diabetes without clinical evidence of skin thickening have almost double the skin thickness compared with control subjects.[25] Increased skin thickness is associated with diabetic neuropathy and has been shown to decrease with improved glycemic control.[27,28]

Scleredema is divided into three main variants based on its association with monoclonal gammopathies, infection (typically streptococcal), or DM, although some cases are idiopathic. SD, the most common variant, is the term used in cases associated with DM. It predominately affects men with long-standing diabetes and its overall prevalence in patients with diabetes is between 2.5% and 14%.[29,30] Clinically, SD presents as symmetric skin thickening and induration (**Fig. 4**), sometimes with a peau d'orange appearance. The neck (>90%) and upper back (>80%) are most common

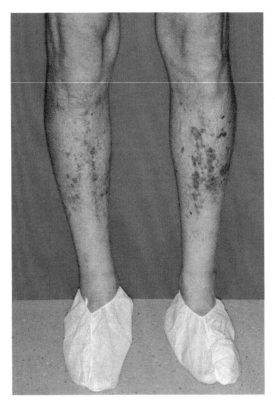

Fig. 3. Diabetic dermopathy.

sites of involvement, but other sites are affected in some cases.[31] The hands and feet are always spared.[31] SD is typically asymptomatic but may be accompanied by pruritus, erythema, and hypoesthesia.[29,31,32] Disease onset is typically insidious with a chronic progression that often goes unnoticed by the patient.[29,31] Importantly, SD can lead to pronounced movement restriction, with 52% to 56% of patients demonstrating limited mobility related to their disease.[31,32] Treatment of SD is generally

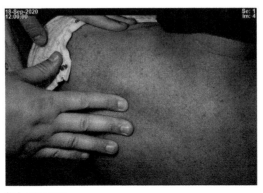

Fig. 4. Scleredema diabeticorum.

unsatisfactory and spontaneous remission is rare.[31,33] In the absence of compelling data, the best available evidence supports the use of phototherapy (particularly psoralen plus ultraviolet A) or electron-beam therapy.[31,33] Although the relationship between glycemic control and SD course is unclear, improved glycemic control is recommended.[31] Physical therapy and tissue massage have also been recommended, particularly for patients with restricted mobility.[31,33]

Scleroderma-like changes of the hands are characterized by symmetric, waxy skin thickening and have been reported in 39% of patients with diabetes.[26] Limited joint mobility (LJM), evidenced by an inability to fully extend the metacarpophalangeal and interphalangeal joints, affects 30% to 40% of patients with diabetes.[18] Useful examination maneuvers for LJM include palm approximation while maintaining wrist flexion ("prayer sign") and flattening the palms against a table ("table top test") (**Fig. 5**).[34] An inability to fully approximate or flatten the palms is evidence of LJM, and physical therapy is the mainstay of treatment. The presence of scleroderma-like changes of the hands and generalized skin thickening are associated with LJM.[26,35] However, these conditions can occur independently, and it remains unclear whether LJM, generalized skin thickening, scleroderma-like changes, and SD share a common pathogenesis.[18]

Bullous diabeticorum
Bullous diabeticorum (BD) affects 0.4% to 2% of patients with diabetes and classically presents as asymptomatic, tense bullae on otherwise normal appearing skin

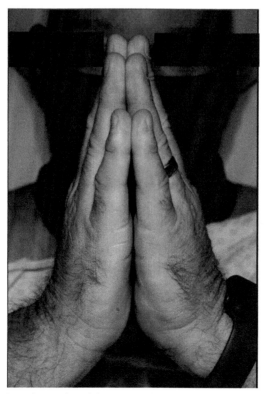

Fig. 5. Diabetic cheiroarthropathy with "prayer sign."

(**Fig. 6**).[4,36–38] Distribution is usually unilateral with involvement of the acral and distal surfaces of the lower extremities.[39,40] Bullae characteristically arise rapidly overnight with no inflammation and resolve without scarring over 2 to 6 weeks; however, development of new lesions in the same or different areas is common.[39,40] There is no clear evidence that glycemic control affects BD; however, many patients in one large case series were noted to have hypoglycemia or highly variable blood glucose at the time of lesion formation.[39] Biopsy findings of BD are nonspecific with a cell-poor subepidermal blister and diagnosis relies on clinical history and examination. Biopsy is useful in ruling out other bullous disorders.

There is agreement that the risk of secondary infection necessitates close observation, and if present requires appropriate treatment with antibiotics and wound care.[5,41] Some advocate leaving blisters intact to allow for spontaneous resolution, whereas others have advocated for more aggressive treatment with drainage, regular wound care, and foot offloading because of the risk for infection and ulceration.[39,40]

General Skin Findings

Diabetic foot ulcer

In patients with diabetes, the lifetime risk of diabetic foot ulcer (DFU) is 15% to 25%, and the 5-year recurrence rate is 50% to 70%.[42] DFU has significant impact on quality of life (equivalent to myocardial infarction and breast cancer), precedes 85% of lower limb amputations, and is the most costly and the most preventable complication of DM.[42] DFU are divided into neuropathic, neuroischemic, and ischemic ulcers. Motor neuropathy alters foot biomechanics and leads to abnormal pressure distribution, sensory neuropathy results in loss of protective sensation, and autonomic neuropathy predisposes to skin dryness and fissuring.[42] Furthermore, impaired immune system function and microvascular and macrovascular disease collectively impair wound healing. Distribution depends on the underlying cause, with neuropathic ulcers occurring over pressure points (**Fig. 7**).

Prevention is the mainstay of therapy, and appropriate screening and subsequent treatment has been estimated to prevent 40% to 85% of amputations.[42] Prevention of DFU is multifactorial and involves regular foot examination (with removal of socks

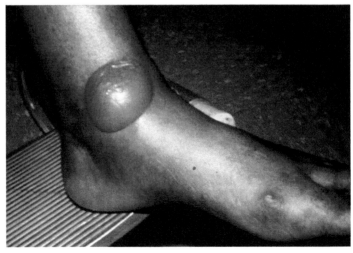

Fig. 6. Diabetic bulla.

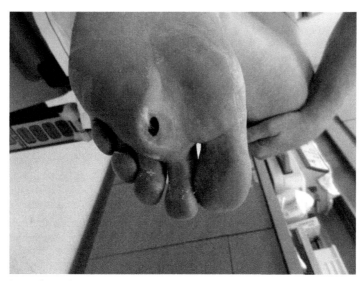

Fig. 7. Diabetic foot ulcer.

and shoes), assessment for peripheral arterial disease, and patient education on regular foot inspection and self-care. Assessment of vascular status should focus on clinical examination and proper vascular studies.

Optimal management of DFUs involves an interdisciplinary approach with physicians, nurses, and foot care specialists. The key areas to address include the vascular system, control of infection, plantar pressure redistribution (orthotics, casts, surgery), wound debridement, and proper moisture balance with selection of an appropriate wound dressing.

More than 50% of DFUs develop infection, most often with gram-positive cocci, although patients with chronic foot ulcers often develop polymicrobial infections.[43] Importantly, diabetes may obscure the typical signs of infection caused by immunopathy, and approximately 50% of patients with a deep diabetic foot infection lack a systemic response (afebrile, normal leukocyte count). All wounds are contaminated and colonized with bacteria. Accordingly, the diagnosis is often clinical and based on an increase in wound size, erythema, edema, warmth, discharge, odor, and pain. Empiric therapy should target the most common culprit organisms, whereas bacterial cultures of the healthy tissue surrounding cleaned and debrided wounds are used to guide antibiotic therapy in patients not responding to empiric treatment. Osteomyelitis is a feared complication of DFU and should be suspected in cases where the ulcer probes to bone. Charcot foot is another complication of diabetes that should be considered in the differential diagnosis along with osteomyelitis. MRI is the gold standard diagnostic test for osteomyelitis.

Dry skin/xerosis
Xerosis is frequently cited as one of the most common dermatologic manifestations of diabetes and exists on a spectrum with mild cases of rough, dry skin, to more severe cases with skin fissuring.[4,36,38] Ichthyosiform changes of the shins can present in both types of diabetes with large bilateral areas of dryness and scaling (fishlike skin), and has been reported in 22% to 48% of patients with T1DM.[44] Xerosis increases the risk of infection and ulceration, and management should focus on skin hygiene and

moisturization.[23,45] Regular emollient application has been shown to significantly improve skin barrier function.[46]

Pruritus

Pruritus affects up to 49% of patients with diabetes and is a predictor of neuropathy.[7] Pruritus is more commonly localized rather than generalized, with localized itching of the scalp, trunk and genitalia commonly reported in patients with diabetes. Pruritus in these patients has been linked to neuropathy rather than transepidermal water loss or diabetic medications.[47] Neuropathic itch should be considered when patients present with unexplained chronic itch or excoriation marks, particularly of the distal limbs.[48] Treatments include topical capsaicin; topical ketamine-amitriptyline-lidocaine; oral anticonvulsants (eg, gabapentin or pregabalin); and, in the case of *Candida* infection, antifungals.

Nail changes and onychomycosis

Onychomycosis is caused by a fungal infection of the nails, most commonly *Trichophyton* or *Candida* species. The most common subtype presents as yellowish discoloration, subungal hyperkeratosis, and onycholysis (**Fig. 8**). Several studies have found higher rates of onychomycosis in patients with diabetes compared with control subjects, with prevalence ranging from 33% to 53%, whereas others have not found increased risk.[49–53] Regardless of the true nature of this association, onychomycosis is a common condition with specific importance for patients with diabetes. Specifically, although treatment of onychomycosis is sometimes optional in elderly patients, in patients with diabetes it is a significant predictor of foot ulceration and treatment is recommended.[54,55] Terbinafine is the first-line oral agent for treatment of onychomycosis because of its generally benign safety profile and favorable long-term cure rate. A meta-analysis of onychomycosis treatment (in the general population) found that compared with azoles, terbinafine had higher rates of mycologic cure (52% vs 68%) and clinical cure (46% vs 58%), with similar rates of recurrence (33% vs 33%) and adverse effects (35% vs 38%).[56] Itraconazole is the second-line oral option for patients who do not achieve cure or tolerate terbinafine. In addition to oral antifungal therapy, treatment should involve physical debridement (ie, clipping or filing of

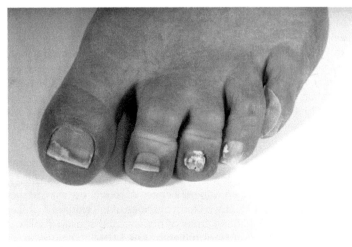

Fig. 8. Onychomycosis.

hypertrophic nails), patient education on proper foot care and self-examination, and treatment with topical antifungal therapy for recurrences of tinea pedis.[57]

Diabetes can predispose to dystrophic toenails in the absence of onychomycosis, and yellow nail (and skin) discoloration is associated with diabetes itself for unclear reasons.[17,18,58] Approximately 40% of patients with diabetes have yellow nails, and 25% to 75% of patients with diabetes with clinically suspected onychomycosis do not have mycologic evidence of infection with KOH or fungal culture.[8,49,59] Accordingly, it is important to confirm onychomycosis before initiating systemic therapy. Diagnosis should be confirmed with a KOH preparation, and if negative, should prompt histopathologic examination of nail clippings with periodic acid–Schiff staining, which is more sensitive than KOH. A positive KOH or periodic acid–Schiff should prompt fungal culture to identify the culprit organism and guide treatment.

Infection

Immune dysfunction, neuropathy, and impaired circulation often accompany diabetes and predispose to typical and atypical infections.[60] Patients with diabetes are two to three times more likely to be hospitalized with infection, and have a two-fold increase in infection-related mortality compared with patients without diabetes.[60–62] A study of administrative claims for a half million patients with diabetes found that 81% (21/26) of the infections analyzed occurred significantly more often in patients with diabetes compared with control subjects with the greatest increases for osteomyelitis (relative risk [RR], 4.39), sepsis (RR, 2.45), postoperative infections (RR, 2.02), and cellulitis (RR, 1.81).[62] Patients with diabetes are more prone to skin and soft tissue infections, are approximately five times more likely to be hospitalized as a result of an infection, and are less likely to achieve treatment success compared with control subjects.[60,63] Cutaneous infections are most often fungal (dermatophyte or *Candida* most commonly).[4,37] Intertrigo or inflammation of skin in folded areas is common in patients with diabetes. The friction, maceration, and heat cause inflammation and irritation of folded skin that is often complicated by infection (fungal, bacterial). In general, prevention and early recognition and treatment when infections occur are crucial for patients with diabetes.

Findings Related to Treatment for Diabetes

The spectrum of dermatologic manifestations with diabetic pharmacotherapies and devices is enormous, and a comprehensive discussion is outside the scope of this article. Instead, this article focuses on some of the commonest adverse effects and recently discovered associations.

Insulin-related adverse events

Lipohypertrophy has been reported in 38% to 44% of patients using insulin and is the most common dermatologic complication of injected insulin.[38,64] Clinically, lipohypertrophy presents as soft, rubbery, lipoma-like dermal nodules at insulin injection sites. Importantly, insulin injection to sites of lipohypertrophy results in erratic absorption, which has been associated with overall worsening of glycemic control and a 10-fold increase in hypoglycemic episodes.[64] Treatment involves rotation of injection sites and avoidance of injection into areas of lipohypertrophy. Conversely, lipoatrophy is characterized by cutaneous depressions at insulin injection sites (**Fig. 9**) and has a prevalence of 0.4% to 2.4% in patients with T1DM.[64] Similar to lipohypertrophy, injection into atrophied sites results in erratic insulin absorption, and treatment involves rotation of injection sites.[64] Lastly, a variety of allergic reactions to insulin or

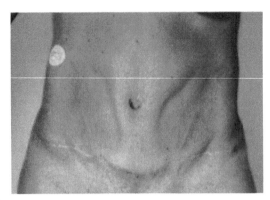

Fig. 9. Lipoatrophy.

components of the insulin preparation can occur; however, the prevalence of such reactions is less than 1% since the advent of recombinant insulin preparations.[18,64]

Glucose monitors and insulin pumps
The use of diabetic devices including continuous glucose monitors (CGM) and insulin pumps (CSII) have increased in recent years. Lipohypertrophy and scarring are common complications of CSII and are managed with rotation of the infusion site.[64] Infusion site infections occur in 17% to 29% of patients with CSII, and management should focus on preventive measures.[64] CSII and CGM can lead to contact dermatitis (irritant or allergic) because of components of the devices themselves or the associated adhesives. Isobornyl acrylate and cyanoacrylate are allergens specifically reported in patients using GCM.[64,65] Diagnosis relies on the presence of a pruritic and dermatitic rash at device sites. Management options involve discontinuation of the offending device or adhesive, patch testing to identify the causative agent, adhesive skin barriers to limit direct skin contact, and topical steroids to address the dermatitis (potentially allowing for continued use).[64]

Drug-induced bullous pemphigoid
Bullous pemphigoid (BP) is autoimmune blistering disorder characterized by tense bullae but may also present with urticarial plaques (**Fig. 10**) or pruritus alone. BP is a rare disorder that may occur spontaneously or be drug-induced. The incidence of BP in patients with diabetes has increased dramatically in recent years and has been attributed to the increasing use of new medications, such as dipetptidyl peptidase 4 (DPP-4) inhibitors.[66,67] Risk estimates vary widely between studies and depend on the specific DPP-4 inhibitor; however, the best available data suggest at least a doubling of the risk of BP in patients with diabetes using DPP-4 inhibitors.[68] Even with DPP-4 inhibitor use the absolute risk of BP remains low, but when suspected management should involve discontinuation of the medication and referral to dermatology for definitive diagnosis with biopsy.

Miscellaneous
There are other conditions with higher prevalence in patients with diabetes listed in **Table 2**. Acquired perforating dermatosis is a skin condition characterized by transepidermal elimination of the connective tissue in the dermis and has been linked to DM, chronic renal failure, and hemodialysis.[45]

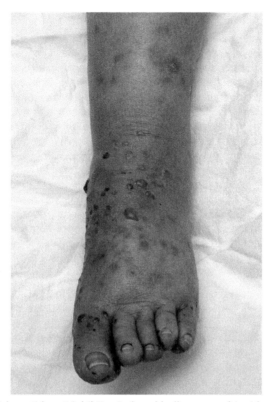

Fig. 10. Dipetptidyl peptidase-4 inhibitor induced bullous pemphigoid.

Table 2 Miscellaneous cutaneous conditions associated with diabetes	
Condition	**Association**[a]
Acrochordons	Definite
Lichen planus	Definite
Psoriasis	Definite
Rubeosis faciei	Definite
Vitiligo	Definite (T1DM)
Acquired perforating dermatosis (Kyrle disease)	Unclear
Granuloma annulare	Unclear

[a] Definite: clear association established. Unclear: conflicting evidence from available studies.

SUMMARY

DM is a common systemic endocrine disease involving millions of people around the world and can affect every organ system including the skin. Cutaneous manifestations are seen in 30% to 79% of patients with diabetes and can signal underlying diabetes in previously undiagnosed patients, indicate suboptimal glycemic control in known patients with diabetes, or occur secondary to diabetic devices and pharmacotherapy. Some of the conditions described in this review are associated with poorly controlled diabetes and several have been linked directly with other complications (ischemia, neuropathy, nephropathy, and retinopathy). Additionally, for some conditions the dermatologic disease improves with better glycemic control, raising the possibility that the visible nature of cutaneous disease could be used as a motivating factor for patients. As the prevalence of diabetes continues to rise, cutaneous manifestations of DM likely will be encountered more frequently by physicians in all disciplines including dermatologists and primary care physicians. Accordingly, knowledge regarding the prevention, diagnosis, and management of cutaneous manifestations is an important aspect in the care of patients with diabetes.

CLINICS CARE POINTS

- Cutaneous manifestations of diabetes are classified in 3 groups: (1) characteristic skin findings, (2) general skin findings, and (3) findings related to diabetes treatment.
- Necrobiosis lipoidica (NL) affects between 0.3% and 1.6% of patients with diabetes. The managment of NL include topical and intralesional steroid followed by pentoxifylline and antimalaria
- Diabetic dermopathy is a marker of coronary artery disease and microvascular complications (neuropathy, nephropathy, and retinopathy).
- Diabetic foot ulcers are the most preventable complication of diabetes.

REFERENCES

1. Saeedi P, Petersohn I, Salpea P, et al. Global and regional diabetes prevalence estimates for 2019 and projections for 2030 and 2045: results from the International Diabetes Federation Diabetes Atlas, 9(th) edition. Diabetes Res Clin Pract 2019;157:107843.
2. Lin X, Xu Y, Pan X, et al. Global, regional, and national burden and trend of diabetes in 195 countries and territories: an analysis from 1990 to 2025. Sci Rep 2020;10(1):14790.
3. Boyle JP, Thompson TJ, Gregg EW, et al. Projection of the year 2050 burden of diabetes in the US adult population: dynamic modeling of incidence, mortality, and prediabetes prevalence. Popul Health Metr 2010;8(1):29.
4. Demirseren DD, Emre S, Akoglu G, et al. Relationship between skin diseases and extracutaneous complications of diabetes mellitus: clinical analysis of 750 patients. Am J Clin Dermatol 2014;15(1):65–70.
5. Sanches MM, Roda A, Pimenta R, et al. Cutaneous manifestations of diabetes mellitus and prediabetes. Acta Med Port 2019;32(6):459–65.
6. Bustan RS, Wasim D, Yderstraede KB, et al. Specific skin signs as a cutaneous marker of diabetes mellitus and the prediabetic state: a systematic review. Danish Med J 2017;64(1):A5316.
7. Lima AL, Illing T, Schliemann S, et al. Cutaneous manifestations of diabetes mellitus: a review. Am J Clin Dermatol 2017;18(4):541–53.

8. Behm B, Schreml S, Landthaler M, et al. Skin signs in diabetes mellitus. J Eur Acad Dermatol Venereol 2012;26(10):1203–11.
9. Schwartz RA. Acanthosis nigricans. J Am Acad Dermatol 1994;31(1):1–19.
10. Higgins SP, Freemark M, Prose NS. Acanthosis nigricans: a practical approach to evaluation and management. Dermatol Online J 2008;14(9):2.
11. Treesirichod A, Chaithirayanon S, Chaikul T, et al. The randomized trials of 10% urea cream and 0.025% tretinoin cream in the treatment of acanthosis nigricans. J Dermatolog Treat 2020;1–6.
12. Muller SA. Dermatologic disorders associated with diabetes mellitus. Mayo Clin Proc 1966;41(10):689–703.
13. Yosipovitch G, Hodak E, Vardi P, et al. The prevalence of cutaneous manifestations in IDDM patients and their association with diabetes risk factors and microvascular complications. Diabetes Care 1998;21(4):506–9.
14. Muller SA. Necrobiosis lipoidica diabeticorum. Arch Dermatol 1966;93(3):265–6.
15. O'Toole EA, Kennedy U, Nolan JJ, et al. Necrobiosis lipoidica: only a minority of patients have diabetes mellitus. Br J Dermatol 1999;140(2):283–6.
16. Lowitt MH, Dover JS. Necrobiosis lipoidica. J Am Acad Dermatol 1991;25(5):735–48.
17. Levy L, Zeichner JA. Dermatologic manifestation of diabetes. J Diabetes 2012;4(1):68–76.
18. Murphy-Chutorian B, Han G, Cohen SR. Dermatologic manifestations of diabetes mellitus: a review. Endocrinol Metab Clin North Am 2013;42(4):869–98.
19. Sibbald C, Reid S, Alavi A. Necrobiosis lipoidica. Dermatol Clin 2015;33(3):343–60.
20. Han G. A new appraisal of dermatologic manifestations of diabetes mellitus. Cutis 2014;94(1):E21–6.
21. Mistry BD, Alavi A, Ali S, et al. A systematic review of the relationship between glycemic control and necrobiosis lipoidica diabeticorum in patients with diabetes mellitus. Int J Dermatol 2017;56(12):1319–27.
22. Morgan AJ, Schwartz RA. Diabetic dermopathy: a subtle sign with grave implications. J Am Acad Dermatol 2008;58(3):447–51.
23. Duff M, Demidova O, Blackburn S, et al. Cutaneous manifestations of diabetes mellitus. Clin Diabetes 2015;33(1):40–8.
24. Shemer A, Bergman R, Linn S, et al. Diabetic dermopathy and internal complications in diabetes mellitus. Int J Dermatol 1998;37(2):113–5.
25. Hanna W, Friesen D, Bombardier C, et al. Pathologic features of diabetic thick skin. J Am Acad Dermatol 1987;16(3):546–53.
26. Fitzcharles MA, Duby S, Waddell RW, et al. Limitation of joint mobility (cheiroarthropathy) in adult noninsulin-dependent diabetic patients. Ann Rheum Dis 1984;43(2):251–4.
27. Forst T, Kann P, Pfutzner A, et al. Association between "diabetic thick skin syndrome" and neurological disorders in diabetes mellitus. Acta Diabetol 1994;31(2):73–7.
28. Lieberman LS, Rosenbloom AL, Riley WJ, et al. Reduced skin thickness with pump administration of insulin. N Engl J Med 1980;303(16):940–1.
29. Cole GW, Headley J, Skowsky R. Scleredema diabeticorum: a common and distinct cutaneous manifestation of diabetes mellitus. Diabetes Care 1983;6(2):189–92.
30. Sattar MA, Diab S, Sugathan TN, et al. Scleroedema diabeticorum: a minor but often unrecognized complication of diabetes mellitus. Diabet Med 1988;5(5):465–8.

31. Rongioletti F, Kaiser F, Cinotti E, et al. Scleredema. A multicentre study of charac-teristics, comorbidities, course and therapy in 44 patients. J Eur Acad Dermatol Venereol 2015;29(12):2399–404.

32. Ray V, Boisseau-Garsaud AM, Ray P, et al. [Obesity persistent scleredema: study of 49 cases]. Ann Dermatol Venereol 2002;129(3):281–5.

33. Miguel D, Schliemann S, Elsner P. Treatment of scleroedema adultorum Buschke: a systematic review. Acta Derm Venereol 2018;98(3):305–9.

34. Papanas N, Maltezos E. The diabetic hand: a forgotten complication? J Diabetes Complications 2010;24(3):154–62.

35. Collier A, Matthews DM, Kellett HA, et al. Change in skin thickness associated with cheiroarthropathy in insulin dependent diabetes mellitus. Br Med J (Clin Res Ed) 1986;292(6525):936.

36. Goyal A, Raina S, Kaushal SS, et al. Pattern of cutaneous manifestations in dia-betes mellitus. Indian J Dermatol 2010;55(1):39–41.

37. Romano G, Moretti G, Di Benedetto A, et al. Skin lesions in diabetes mellitus: prevalence and clinical correlations. Diabetes Res Clin Pract 1998;39(2):101–6.

38. Sawatkar GU, Kanwar AJ, Dogra S, et al. Spectrum of cutaneous manifestations of type 1 diabetes mellitus in 500 South Asian patients. Br J Dermatol 2014; 171(6):1402–6.

39. Larsen K, Jensen T, Karlsmark T, et al. Incidence of bullosis diabeticorum: a controversial cause of chronic foot ulceration. Int Wound J 2008;5(4):591–6.

40. Lipsky BA, Baker PD, Ahroni JH. Diabetic bullae: 12 cases of a purportedly rare cutaneous disorder. Int J Dermatol 2000;39(3):196–200.

41. Sonani H, Abdul Salim S, Garla VV, et al. Bullosis Diabeticorum: A rare presenta-tion with immunoglobulin G (IgG) deposition related vasculopathy. Case report and focused review. Am J Case Rep 2018;19:52–6.

42. Alavi A, Sibbald RG, Mayer D, et al. Diabetic foot ulcers: Part I. Pathophysiology and prevention. J Am Acad Dermatol 2014;70(1):1.e1-18 [quiz: 19–20].

43. Alavi A, Sibbald RG, Mayer D, et al. Diabetic foot ulcers: Part II. Management. J Am Acad Dermatol 2014;70(1):21.e21-4 [quiz: 45–6].

44. Rosen J, Yosipovitch G. Skin manifestations of diabetes mellitus. In: Feingold KR, Anawalt B, Boyce A, et al, editors. Endotext. South Dartmouth (MA): MDText.com, Inc.; 2018. p. 2000. Available at:.

45. Horton WB, Boler PL, Subauste AR. Diabetes mellitus and the skin: recognition and management of cutaneous manifestations. South Med J 2016;109(10): 636–46.

46. Seite S, Khemis A, Rougier A, et al. Importance of treatment of skin xerosis in dia-betes. J Eur Acad Dermatol Venereol 2011;25(5):607–9.

47. Lai CCK, Md Nor N, Kamaruddin NA, et al. Comparison of transepidermal water loss and skin hydration in diabetics and nondiabetics. Clin Exp Dermatol 2020; 46(1):58–64.

48. Steinhoff M, Schmelz M, Szabó IL, et al. Clinical presentation, management, and pathophysiology of neuropathic itch. Lancet Neurol 2018;17(8):709–20.

49. Gupta AK, Konnikov N, MacDonald P, et al. Prevalence and epidemiology of toenail onychomycosis in diabetic subjects: a multicentre survey. Br J Dermatol 1998;139(4):665–71.

50. Chang SJ, Hsu SC, Tien KJ, et al. Metabolic syndrome associated with toenail onychomycosis in Taiwanese with diabetes mellitus. Int J Dermatol 2008;47(5): 467–72.

51. Papini M, Cicoletti M, Fabrizi V, et al. Skin and nail mycoses in patients with dia-betic foot. G Ital Dermatol Venereol 2013;148(6):603–8.

52. Romano C, Massai L, Asta F, et al. Prevalence of dermatophytic skin and nail infections in diabetic patients. Mycoses 2001;44(3–4):83–6.
53. Buxton PK, Milne LJ, Prescott RJ, et al. The prevalence of dermatophyte infection in well-controlled diabetics and the response to Trichophyton antigen. Br J Dermatol 1996;134(5):900–3.
54. Boyko EJ, Ahroni JH, Cohen V, et al. Prediction of diabetic foot ulcer occurrence using commonly available clinical information: the Seattle Diabetic Foot Study. Diabetes Care 2006;29(6):1202–7.
55. Rossaneis MA, Haddad MD, Mantovani MF, et al. Foot ulceration in patients with diabetes: a risk analysis. Br J Nurs 2017;26(6):S6–14.
56. Kreijkamp-Kaspers S, Hawke K, Guo L, et al. Oral antifungal medication for toenail onychomycosis. Cochrane Database Syst Rev 2017;7:CD010031.
57. Rich P. Onychomycosis and tinea pedis in patients with diabetes. J Am Acad Dermatol 2000;43(5 Suppl):S130–4.
58. Nikoleishvili LR, Kurashvili RB, Virsaladze DK, et al. [Characteristic changes of skin and its accessories in type 2 diabetes mellitus]. Georgian Med News 2006;(131):43–6.
59. Gulcan A, Gulcan E, Oksuz S, et al. Prevalence of toenail onychomycosis in patients with type 2 diabetes mellitus and evaluation of risk factors. J Am Podiatr Med Assoc 2011;101(1):49–54.
60. Dryden M, Baguneid M, Eckmann C, et al. Pathophysiology and burden of infection in patients with diabetes mellitus and peripheral vascular disease: focus on skin and soft-tissue infections. Clin Microbiol Infect 2015;21(Suppl 2):S27–32.
61. Bertoni AG, Saydah S, Brancati FL. Diabetes and the risk of infection-related mortality in the U.S. Diabetes Care 2001;24(6):1044–9.
62. Shah BR, Hux JE. Quantifying the risk of infectious diseases for people with diabetes. Diabetes Care 2003;26(2):510–3.
63. Suaya JA, Eisenberg DF, Fang C, et al. Skin and soft tissue infections and associated complications among commercially insured patients aged 0-64 years with and without diabetes in the U.S. PLoS One 2013;8(4):e60057.
64. Jedlowski PM, Te CH, Segal RJ, et al. Cutaneous adverse effects of diabetes mellitus medications and medical devices: a review. Am J Clin Dermatol 2019;20(1):97–114.
65. Corazza M, Scuderi V, Musmeci D, et al. Allergic contact dermatitis caused by isobornyl acrylate in a young diabetic patient using a continuous glucose monitoring system (Freestyle Libre). Contact Dermatitis 2018;79(5):320–1.
66. Gravani A, Gaitanis G, Tsironi T, et al. Changing prevalence of diabetes mellitus in bullous pemphigoid: it is the dipeptidyl peptidase-4 inhibitors. J Eur Acad Dermatol Venereol 2018;32(12):e438–9.
67. Fania L, Di Zenzo G, Didona B, et al. Increased prevalence of diabetes mellitus in bullous pemphigoid patients during the last decade. J Eur Acad Dermatol Venereol 2018;32(4):e153–4.
68. Douros A, Rouette J, Yin H, et al. Dipeptidyl peptidase 4 inhibitors and the risk of bullous pemphigoid among patients with type 2 diabetes. Diabetes Care 2019;42(8):1496–503.

Approach to the Patient with Chronic Pruritus

Zoe M. Lipman, BS, Giuseppe Ingrasci, BS, Gil Yosipovitch, MD*

KEYWORDS

- Chronic pruritus • Itch • Inflammatory itch • Neuropathic itch • Generalized pruritus
- Localized pruritus

KEY POINTS

- Chronic pruritus (pruritus lasting ≥6 weeks) is a common chief complaint that may be the presenting symptom of a broad range of underlying diseases.
- The presence or absence of a primary skin rash associated with itch can help to distinguish between dermatologic versus nondermatologic causes of chronic itch.
- Distinguishing between generalized versus localized itch can often help to differentiate itch that is systemic or neuropathic in origin.
- Localized itch can often be treated with topical treatments, whereas generalized itch often requires systemic treatments.

INTRODUCTION

Itch, or pruritus, is defined as "an unpleasant sensation that elicits the desire or reflex to scratch."[1] It is an extremely common complaint that is responsible for approximately 7 million physician visits per year (about 1% of all physician visits).[2] It has also been estimated that up to 20% of the worldwide population is experiencing itch at any given time.[2,3] Itch is not only extremely bothersome to the patient; chronic pruritus (≥6 weeks) has been shown to have significant impacts on quality of life, mood, sleep, and personal finances.[4,5] In fact, the Global Burden of Disease Study considered chronic pruritus to be within the top 50 most burdensome multidisciplinary symptoms.[6] Despite this high prevalence and burden, correctly diagnosing and successfully treating itch and its associated conditions remains a challenge for both dermatologists and primary care physicians.

In current practice, acute itch (<6 weeks) is a fairly well-managed condition because it often has easily identifiable triggers (recency to exposures), a more abrupt onset (often with a clear temporal relationship to possible exposures), and frequent self-

Dr Phillip Frost Department of Dermatology and Miami Itch Center, University of Miami, University of Miami Hospital, 1600 Northwest 10th Avenue RMSB Building, 10th Street, 2067B Miami, FL, USA
* Corresponding author.
E-mail address: gyosipovitch@med.miami.edu

Med Clin N Am 105 (2021) 699–721
https://doi.org/10.1016/j.mcna.2021.04.007
0025-7125/21/© 2021 Elsevier Inc. All rights reserved.

medical.theclinics.com

resolution or treatment success with traditional antipruritic therapies like emollients, antihistamines, and corticosteroids. Chronic pruritus (>6 weeks), in contrast, is much more complicated and challenging. Part of the reason for this difficulty in diagnosis and treatment of chronic pruritus is the heterogeneity of the conditions for which itch may be a presenting symptom. Although chronic itch can certainly present in a large variety of primary dermatologic conditions, it also may be a symptom of many underlying systemic, neurologic, and psychiatric conditions. Approximately 8% of patients presenting with chronic pruritus do not display any skin changes.[7] Additionally, there are many patients for whom an underlying etiology is never identified, adding to the complicated nature of diagnosing and treating these patients. In the current article, we hope to characterize the many conditions that may present with itch as a chief complaint and minimize some of the present diagnostic challenges by outlining a systematic approach for diagnosis and treatment.

APPROACH

Similar to evaluating a patient with any chief complaint, a thorough history and physical examination is important for determining appropriate diagnostic, management, and treatment steps. This practice is especially important for a nonspecific complaint like itch, where there is a vast list of differential diagnoses that can be explored. The majority of conditions that can produce chronic itch fall into 1 of 5 categories: inflammatory skin conditions, itch secondary to systemic disease, neuropathic pruritus, chronic pruritus of undetermined origin, and psychogenic itch.[8] An extensive, but not exhaustive, list of specific diagnoses and their classifications within these general categories can be found in **Table 1**.

Although all information collected in a history and physical examination can be useful in painting a clearer clinical picture, navigating such an extensive list of differential diagnoses requires a targeted, systematic approach. Therefore, we propose the flowchart presented in **Fig. 1** to help clinicians efficiently navigate clinic visits and guide diagnosis, management, and treatment. As we navigate this flowchart, we plan to highlight some of the most commonly seen itchy diagnoses and their clinical presentations, and keys to management and treatment.

Evaluation

The first step in evaluating a patient with chronic pruritus is determining whether or not the itch can be attributed to a primary dermatologic cause. This process includes a careful skin examination with special focus on the area in which itch is present. Primary skin lesions should be differentiated from lesions secondary to scratching, such as excoriations, nonspecific dermatitis, prurigo nodules, and lichenified skin, which may indicate an underlying nondermatologic etiology or mask more subtle primary dermatologic skin lesions. In addition, xerosis cutis (xeroderma, asteatosis, or dry skin) should be ruled out. A patient with chronic itch who has nonxerosis primary dermatologic skin findings is likely to have an inflammatory skin disease. Using the patient's history, physical examination, and potential skin biopsy, inflammatory skin diseases can be differentiated from one another and treated appropriately. A summary of the basic historical and dermatologic findings of these disorders can be found in **Table 2** and the most common disorders discussed in further detail elsewhere in this article.

Chronic itch with primary dermatologic findings
Xerosis cutis (dry skin). Xerosis, one of the most common skin conditions in the middle-aged and elderly population, has a prevalence estimated to be anywhere

Table 1 Categorization of diagnoses that may present with itch	
Category	**Diagnoses Included**
Inflammatory skin disease	Eczematous dermatitis
	Atopic dermatitis
	Dishydrotic eczema
	Seborrheic dermatitis
	Nummular dermatitis
	Neurodermatitis
	Contact dermatitis (allergic/irritant)
	Venous stasis dermatitis
	Papulosquamous disorders
	Psoriasis
	Lichen planus
	Prurigo nodularis
	Lichen simplex chronicus
	Urticaria
	Infections and infestations
	Scabies
	Tinea infections (corporis, cruris, capitis, pedis)
	Folliculitis
	Skin malignancies
	Cutaneous T-cell lymphoma/mycosis fungoides
	Basal cell carcinoma
	Squamous cell carcinoma
	Autoimmune diseases
	Dermatitis herpetiformis
	Bullous pemphigoid
	Dermatomyositis
	Linear immunoglobulin A disease
	Sjögren syndrome
	Scleroderma
	Systemic lupus erythematosis
	Lichen sclerosis
	Other
	Erythroderma
	Mastocytoma, mastocytosis
	Intertrigo
	Dermal hypersensitivity reaction
	Grovers disease
	Kyrles disease/perforating collagenosis
	Keratoderma with pruritus
	Stasis dermatitis
	Wells syndrome
	Pityriasis rubra pilaris
	PLEVA
	PLC
	Papuloerythroderma of Ofuji
	Pigmented purpuric dermatosis
Pruritus of underdetermined origin	Chronic pruritus of unknown origin
	Chronic pruritus of aging
Neuropathic itch	Itch in the setting of spinal compression, injury, or back pain
	Scalp dysesthesia
	Localized neuropathic itch (scrotal, vulvar, scalp, anal)

(continued on next page)

Table 1 (continued)	
Category	**Diagnoses Included**
	Post-herpetic neuralgia
	Notalgia parasthetica
	Brachioradial pruritus
	Itch associated with diabetic neuropathy
	Multiple sclerosis
	Stroke
	Prion disease
Pruritus secondary to systemic disease	Hematologic
	Polycythemia vera
	Hemochromatosis
	Iron deficiency anemia
	Mastocytosis
	Plasma cell dyscrasias
	Hepatobiliary
	Cholestatic itch
	Cirrhosis
	Biliary cirrhosis
	Chronic pancreatitis
	Drug-induced cholestasis
	Hepatitis (hepatitis C)
	Sclerosing cholangitis
	Infectious disease
	HIV/AIDs
	Infectious hepatitis
	Parasitic infections
	Renal disease
	Chronic kidney disease–associated pruritus
	Endocrine or metabolic disease
	Hyperthyroidism
	Hyperparathyroidism/hypercalcemia
	Diabetes mellitus
	Carcinoid syndrome
	Malignancy
	Leukemia
	Lymphoma
	Multiple myeloma
	Paraneoplastic syndromes secondary to solid tumors
Other	Aquagenic pruritus
	Pruritus owing to stress or hormonal changes
	Autonomic overactivity
	Pruritus gravidarum
	Fibromyalgia
	Pruritus secondary to drug use, biologic and immunotherapies
Psychogenic itch	Anxiety
	Depression
	Somatoform disorders
	Delusional parasitosis
	Obsessive–compulsive disorder

Abbreviation: PCL, pityriasis lichenoides chronica.

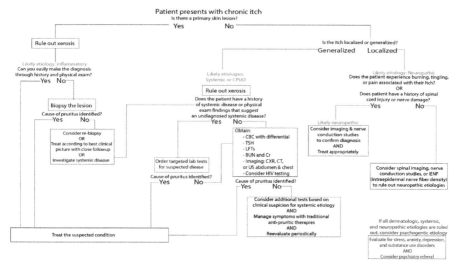

Fig. 1. An algorithm for diagnosing and managing the patient with chronic pruritus.

between 29% and 85% in these age groups.[9–13] Xerosis can present in heterogenous ways that range in visibility from obvious to extremely subtle, as well as localized to generalized. It most often presents with skin scaling, roughness, and/or fissures along with common complaints of itching, burning, skin "tightness," or pain.[14] The most common triggers of dry skin include environmental factors (cold, low humidity/dry indoor heat [commonly described as winter itch] or intense sunlight exposure), and skin cleansing or washing (long, hot showers; alkaline soaps and cleansing agents); if identified, xerosis is easily treated by avoiding triggers and using topical emollients.[13] However, xerosis may also present secondary to other conditions like systemic diseases or it may be drug induced.

Inflammatory skin diseases. This category of itchy diagnoses encompasses a large number of primary dermatologic diseases. With chronic urticaria as an exception, most of these conditions induce pruritus through activation of nonhistaminergic inflammatory pathways within the skin and pruritoceptive C nerve fibers. A summary of the major findings on skin examination of these diseases can be found in **Table 2**.

- Eczematous dermatitis (see also the paper in this issue on Dermatitis)
  - *Atopic dermatitis (traditional "eczema"):* Atopic dermatitis is often simply referred to as the "itch that rashes," because it typically presents as an erythematous or hyperpigmented papular rash on the flexural surfaces (adults), extensor surfaces (children), scalp, and face that appears shortly after itching begins.[15] Patients typically have a personal or family history of other atopic diseases such as asthma, allergic rhinitis, or food allergies. A prominent clinical feature of the disease is alloknesis: a phenomenon in which typically innocuous, benign stimuli (such as water, sweat, or certain fabrics) induces severe itch.[16] If the diagnosis is unclear based on an inspection of the skin lesions, the clinical finding of an infra-auricular fissure can help to identify an atopic patient; this finding has also been shown to be useful marker of disease severity in previously diagnosed atopic patients.[17]
  - *Contact dermatitis:* Contact dermatitis refers to any dermatitis that arises from contact of the skin with a substance and has 2 subtypes: (1) allergic, in which

Table 2
Common inflammatory skin disease clinical presentations

Diagnosis	Dermatologic Features	Key Historical Findings
Atopic dermatitis	Erythematous or hyperpigmented papular rash or plaques on flexor surfaces (adults), scalp or face Presence of an intra-auricular fissure	Personal or family history of atopic diseases (asthma, allergic rhinitis, food allergies)
Contact dermatitis (irritant and allergic)	Sharply demarcated erythematous rash that presents 2–7 d after an exposure	Use of new cosmetics or creams New jewelry item (most commonly nickel) Hobby or occupational exposure to solvents, adhesives, cleaners New animal exposure
Lichen planus	Flat-topped, pink/purple, pearly papules	History of painful lesions on oral mucosa
Psoriasis	Erythematous plaques with silvery scale on extensor surfaces Nail pitting	Arthritis/joint pain (with characteristic "sausage fingers" appearance) Cyclical itch with majority occurring at night
Scabies	Small, excoriated papules or mite burrows in finger webs, genital region, axillae, and/or neck	Close contacts experiencing similar symptoms
Seborrheic dermatitis	Well-demarcated erythematous plaques with greasy-looking, yellowish scale on scalp, center of face, external ears, upper trunk, or intertriginous regions	History of "dandruff" Stress
Tinea infections	Pruritic, red, annular, scaly patch with central clearing and an active boarder	Full or partial resolution with an over-the-counter antifungal medication Worsening of lesion after empiric treatment with topical steroid
Urticaria (chronic)	Intensely pruritic, erythematous welts or wheals often with central pallor Symptomatic dermatographism	Exposure to new medications, supplements, or illicit drugs Self-resolving and/or responsive to antihistamines

contact with a substance triggers an immune response that damages the skin and (2) irritant, in which a substance directly irritates and damages the skin. The erythematous rash can likely be differentiated from other inflammatory rashes owing to its often sharp line of demarcation outlining areas of the skin that came in direct contact with the triggering substance or material. The rash typically presents 2 to 7 days after exposure to the trigger and can persist until the triggering substance is identified and removed. Common triggers include new cosmetics or creams, metals (jewelry; nickel), occupational exposures, and exposure to plants (poison ivy).

  o *Dyshidrotic eczema (palmoplantar dermatitis):* Dyshidrotic eczema is a chronic, recurrent, vesicular eruption on the palms and/or soles that is, extremely pruritic.[18] It is most frequently found on the lateral and dorsal aspects of the fingers. On examination, the vesicles often resemble "tapioca pudding." This condition may worsen or be first noticed after excessive handwashing or hand sanitizer usage.

  o *Seborrheic dermatitis[19]:* Seborrheic dermatitis is an extremely common skin disorder that can occur throughout the lifespan (often referred to as "cradle cap" in infants and "dandruff" in adults when mild and on the scalp). It is characterized physically by well-demarcated, erythematous plaques scales often described to have a yellowish color and a "greasy-looking" texture. It is most commonly seen in areas with a high prevalence of sebaceous glands such as the scalp, center of the face, external ear, upper trunk, and intertriginous areas. Correlations have been found with the increased presence of the fungi genus *Malassezia* (natural members of the skin flora) as well as stress.

  o Other, less common variations of eczematous dermatitis are *nummular eczema* (more common in older patients)[20] and *stasis dermatitis*[21] are summarized in **Table 2**.

- *Chronic urticaria (hives)*[22]: Chronic urticaria presents with an intensely pruritic, transient, erythematous and edematous plaques, often referred to as wheals or welts. These plaques often have a characteristic central pallor and may coalesce with other plaques. A key diagnostic feature is symptomatic dermatographism, in which drawing a blunt but pointed object across the skin results in an immediate, pruritic, linear wheal following the object's path. The plaques can occur on any part of the body and frequently self-resolve over the course of a few hours. Unlike other inflammatory itchy diagnoses, chronic urticaria induces pruritus through the histaminergic pathway and is responsive to antihistaminergic therapies in 40% of the cases. Chronic urticaria can be idiopathic and spontaneous, but also may be associated autoimmune thyroid disease, or the addition of any new medications, supplements, or illicit drugs (eg, angiotensin-converting enzyme inhibitors and opioids).

- *Papulosquamous disorders*

  o *Psoriasis:* Psoriasis is an extremely common, pruritic, inflammatory skin disease that affects more than 7.5 million people in the United States and 125 million people worldwide.[23,24] Its clinical presentation is characterized by erythematous plaques with characteristic silvery scale on extensor surfaces, low back, palms, and soles. Psoriatic itch tends to have a cyclical nature with the worst itch often occurring at night.[25] Patients may present with nail pitting and/or psoriatic arthritis. Psoriasis has also been shown to have a higher prevalence in patients with other medical comorbidities, such as cardiometabolic disease, inflammatory bowel disease, chronic kidney disease, and cutaneous T-cell lymphoma.[26]

    ○ *Lichen planus*[27]: Lichen planus is an intensely pruritic mucocutaneous inflammatory disorder whose etiology is still not fully understood. The characteristic lesions of active disease are flat-topped, pearly, violaceous papules that may leave behind long-term hyperpigmentation after resolution, especially in patients with darker complexions. Lichen planus can also occur on the oral mucosa as symmetric reticular lesions resembling a white "lace-like" network as well as in the anogenital region with findings similar to other skin areas. It is also commonly seen on the scalp, where it may cause severe itching.

- *Infections and infestations* (see also the article on common skin infections)
  - *Dermatophyte/tinea infections*[28]: This category includes tinea corporis (ringworm), tinea capitis (scalp ringworm), tinea cruris ("jock itch"), tinea pedia (athletes foot), and tinea barbae (beard infection in males). These infections are characterized by pruritic, red, annular patches with central clearing and a scaly, centrifugally advancing boarder. These lesions heal completely with proper antifungal treatment, but worsen or persist when steroidal treatment is used either through an over-the-counter purchase of the patient or empiric treatment for a misdiagnosis. In cases where the diagnosis is uncertain, a potassium hydroxide preparation can aid in achieving the diagnosis. A Woods lamp may also be useful in the evaluation of these lesions to rule out other fungal infections.
  - *Scabies*[29]: Scabies is an intensely pruritic mite disorder in which the body produces a delayed hypersensitivity reaction to mite proteins. The itch associated with scabies usually worsens in the evening and can continue for several weeks after the condition is properly treated and the mites are eradicated. Dermatologic findings on examination may show small, excoriated papules and/or mite burrows most frequently seen in intertriginous areas like the fiber webs, genitals, neck, and axillae. Empiric treatment of both the patient and close contacts and housemates are warranted. Patients must also be advised to wash recently worn clothing, used bedsheets, and other items in hot water or seal these items in a bag for 10 days, because mites cannot live for more than 10 days without a human host. If the diagnosis is uncertain, skin scrapings can be used to identify the mite.

Chronic itch without primary dermatologic findings

If the evaluation of the itchy patient's skin does not reveal any primary skin rashes or lesions associated with the itch, the next most important piece of information to learn is whether the itch is generalized throughout or localized to a particular region of the body. Chronic localized itch without any primary skin lesions or rashes suggests a neuropathic etiology, whereas chronic generalized itch without skin changes may suggest either a systemic etiology or a diagnosis that falls into the chronic pruritus of undetermined origin category, such as chronic pruritus of aging. In addition, xerosis should be ruled out in cases of generalized pruritus, because often the characteristic skin findings may be subtle and not grossly visible. Psychogenic itch, which is a diagnosis of exclusion, may present as either generalized or localized itch.

Neuropathic itch. Neuropathic itch makes up 8% to 19% of chronically itchy patients.[30] Defined broadly, neuropathic pruritus refers to any injury or dysfunction of the nerves anywhere along the afferent itch pathway, including both the central and peripheral nervous systems, that results in a sensation to scratch.[31] Damage to the nerves is most commonly due to either physical injury or compression (brachioradial pruritus and notalgia paresthetica) or infection (post-herpetic neuralgia), but can also occur with changes to nerve functioning like in demyelination syndromes (multiple sclerosis) and diabetic neuropathy. Localized itchy complaints are often accompanied with characteristic concurrent burning, tingling, and/or pain that follow the distribution of the affected nerves. As a result of itching, many patients may develop secondary scratch lesions such as lichenification, excoriations, or postinflammatory hyperpigmentation in the affected skin areas. In addition to these common features, specific clinical presentations of the most common forms of neuropathic itch are described here.

- *Spinal nerve compression syndromes*: Compression of spinal nerves may develop as a result of degenerative alterations of the vertebral column (spinal stenosis, spondylolisthesis, etc), anatomic variations, tumors, abscesses, or aneurysms. Compression syndromes can be differentiated by which nerves are affected their associated areas of itching.[32] Brachioradial pruritus involves compression of the cervical spinal cord or spinal ganglia at C5/C7 and results in either unilateral or bilateral pruritus in the proximal or dorsolateral forearms. The "ice pack sign"—symptomatic relief with application of ice to the affected area—is a common clinical finding in these patients.[33] In addition, brachioradial pruritus typically worsens in the summer months, and with prolonged exposure to sunlight, although sunlight's involvement in disease pathology is not yet fully understood.[30] Notalgia paresthetica, in contrast, involves compression of the dorsal branches of thoracic spinal nerves T2 to T6, resulting in pruritus medial to the scapular boarder on the mid or upper back.[32] Brachioradial pruritus is more likely to generalize than notalgia paresthetica.[34] With a known history of spinal disease, the diagnosis of both of these conditions can be made clinically, or confirmed with targeted imaging (preferably with MRI). However, in a patient presenting with a clear notalgia paresthetica or brachioradial pruritus clinical picture without known spinal cord dysfunction, imaging should be ordered to rule out an underlying pathology causing nerve compression.
- *Post-herpetic neuralgia*: Post-herpetic neuralgia is neuropathic symptoms at the site of a prior herpes zoster (shingles) infection, with 30% to 58% of patients experiencing itch.[35,36] This condition is most likely to occur after eruptions on the face, head, and neck. Typically, there is a clear history of prior infection in that region, making diagnosing this condition easier. However, with only a suspected history of infection, a key clinical finding is itch spanning a specific dermatome without crossing the midline.
- *Multiple sclerosis*: An autoimmune demyelination disorder, multiple sclerosis induces itch in about 5% of patients through the activation of artificial synapses in areas of demyelination.[37] Depending on where these areas are, the itch may present as either localized or generalized.
- *Small fiber neuropathies*[38]: Small fiber neuropathies are disorders of small nerve fibers that are associated with autonomic and sensory symptoms, including itch. They may be idiopathic or secondary to more systemic disorders like diabetes or post-herpetic neuropathy. These disorders can be further diagnosed using intraepidermal nerve fiber density testing.

Itch secondary to systemic disease. Systemic disease should be considered in any patient presenting with generalized pruritus without primary dermatologic findings. Typically, the only skin findings present in these patients are skin changes secondary to itching and rubbing. In such patients, a detailed medical history, family medical history, substance use history, and review of systems can provide pertinent information for targeting the workup. In addition, a comprehensive physical examination, including evaluation of the liver, spleen, and lymph nodes should be completed. In the case that both the history and physical examination are unable to suggest an underlying systemic etiology, a comprehensive workup should be begun including a complete blood count with differential, thyroid-stimulating hormone, lever function tests, blood urea nitrogen, and creatinine, and imaging (chest radiograph, computed tomography scan of the chest and abdominal, or ultrasound examination). In addition, HIV testing should be considered in any patient who is at high risk or exhibits signs of immunodeficiency. Subsequent findings should guide any further workup, treatment, and/or referral to specialists. It is important to note that itch may be a presenting symptom of malignancy and may precede any clinical evidence of malignancy by up to several years. A summary of findings, including key features of itch, that may suggest a specific systemic etiology of pruritus can be found in **Table 3**.[39]

- *Hepatobiliary disease*[40]: The broad category of hepatobiliary diseases includes cirrhosis, biliary cirrhosis, sclerosing cholangitis, chronic pancreatitis, drug-induced cholestasis, and hepatitis. All of these diseases are capable of inducing cholestatic pruritus owing to impaired secretion of bile. Although at the time of presentation the patient may complain of generalized pruritus, a history of itch beginning in an acral distribution on the palms and soles is a key finding implying an underlying hepatobiliary etiology.
- *Renal disease*: Uremic pruritus occurs in more than 60% of patients undergoing dialysis and is one of the most disabling symptoms of end stage renal disease.[41] Although unlikely, a patient with undiagnosed end-stage renal disease may present with pruritus; key historical findings would decreased urine output, generalized pruritus that may be more prominent on the back, and itching that frequently worsens at night.[42]
- *Thyroid disease*[43]: Although hypothyroidism is less frequently associated with itch (although, it may cause xerosis), hyperthyroidism, particularly thyrotoxicosis in Graves' disease, is capable of producing generalized pruritus. In a previously undiagnosed patient, clinical signs of Graves' disease include signs of hyperthyroidism (increased heart rate, anxiety, weight loss, heat intolerance, etc) as well as exophthalmos. Graves' dermopathy may also be present with or without associated itch, which includes reddening and thickening of skin on the shins or tops of the feet.
- *Malignancy*: Generalized pruritus may be a presenting sign of both hematologic and solid tumor malignancies and may present up to years before the malignancy is clinically detectable. The resulting pruritus may be part of the disease pathology itself, a consequence of the disease (eg, cholestasis owing to pancreatic carcinoma), or part of a paraneoplastic syndrome (reported in malignant tumors of the breast, stomach, lung, prostate, uterus, colon, nasopharynx, and others). Pruritus is more common in lymphoproliferative disorders such as lymphoma and leukemia. Several of these patients suffer from aquagenic pruritus, which is itch associated with water exposure. Pruritus associated with solid tumors is more likely to be localized, whereas pruritus associated with hematologic malignancies is generalized.
- *Drug-induced pruritus*[44]: Numerous pharmacologic drugs can induce generalized pruritus in patients through a variety of mechanisms, including xerosis, alteration of neural pathways, phototoxicity, cholestatic liver injury, vasodilation, and so on. Although a temporal relationship between the addition of any new drugs and the onset of itch is the clearest way to determine the offending agent,

Table 3
Key distinguishing features of itch secondary to systemic disease

Diagnosis	Distinguishing Itch Features	Key Historical Findings	Key Physical Examination Findings
Hepatobiliary disease	Itch that begins in an acral distribution (palms and soles) and then generalizes	History of alcoholism, IV drug use	Hepatosplenomegaly
Renal disease	Generalized pruritus that may be more prominent on the back, worsens at night	Nausea Malaise Decreased urine output	—
Hyperthyroidism/Graves' disease	Generalized pruritus	Classic hyperthyroid symptoms	Thyromegaly Exophthalmos Graves' dermopathy (reddening and thickening of skin on skins and dorsal feet)
Lymphomas	Itching frequently on lower extremities accompanied by ichthyosiform skin changes Itching may worsen at night	Unexplained weight loss, fever	Lymphadenopathy
Polycythemia vera	Aquagenic pruritus (intractable pruritus within minutes of contact with water) Possible associated stinging, tingling, or burning sensations Most commonly on chest, back, medial upper arms, and anterior legs	Unusual bleeding Orthopnea History of gout	Splenomegaly with or without hepatomegaly
Carcinoid syndrome	Pruritus associated with Intermittent histamine "flush"	Intermittent flushing of skin Diarrhea Rapid heart rate Sudden episodes of lightheadedness/drops in blood pressure	

specific attention should be given to any anticancer treatments such as epidermal growth factor receptor inhibitors, CTLA-4 inhibitors, and programmed cell death-1 inhibitors, because these agents can frequently cause itch with or without a rash.[45]

  ○ *Substance use disorders*[46]: In addition to pruritus secondary to prescribed medications, itch may also be a manifestation of a substance use disorder. Those with opioid use disorders commonly present with generalized pruritus. Additionally, central nervous system stimulant (cocaine, amphetamines) use disorders may present with a delusional parasitosis-like condition, including excoriations and the "matchbox sign," in which patients often bring in boxes of "parasites" that they've pulled from their skin (typically lint, cotton, skin/scabs, or thread). In patients for whom you suspect an underlying substance use disorder, consider ordering a toxicology screen.

- *Chronic pruritus of undetermined origin*:[47] Should the basic laboratory workup proposed for the patient experiencing nondermatologic generalized pruritus, it is possible that they may fall into the category of chronic pruritus of undetermined origin (previously revered to as idiopathic pruritus or generalized pruritus of undetermined origin). In these patients, it is possible that laboratory tests may reveal eosinophilia or mild immunoglobulin E elevation (but <1000 UI/mL); if a biopsy is performed, it may reveal dermal hypersensitivity or spongiotic dermatitis pattern with eosinophils. However, none of these are requirements for diagnosis of this condition.

- *Chronic pruritus of aging* (formerly senile pruritus or mature/old age itch)[48]: Persistent and generalized itching is experienced by more than 50% of individuals in or beyond their 60s. Although the etiology behind this condition is still fairly unknown, it is believed that there may be a component of immunosenescence, age-associated degeneration in peripheral nerve endings, as well as xerosis and skin atrophy.

Psychogenic itch. Psychogenic itch is a diagnosis of exclusion by which all dermatologic, systemic, and neuropathic etiologies must be ruled out. It has an incidence of about 2% in dermatology clinics[49] and may occur comorbidly with prior psychiatric diagnoses (depression, anxiety, or personality disorders), stress, or alone as a distinct clinical entity (such as delusional parasitosis, in which the patient has delusions that they are infested with parasites).[37,50] In the primary care or dermatology clinic setting, a thorough history including sleep, suicidal ideations, and personal and family history of depressive, anxiety, or other psychiatric disorders should be completed in suspected patients. Referral to a mental health professional, psychologist, or psychiatrist for a more thorough evaluation should be considered, but it is not recommended to make the suspected diagnosis of psychogenic itch known to the patient, because they may be less open to receiving outside help. Rather, it is recommended to suggest the help of a mental health expert as an adjunctive treatment for decreasing itch intensity, stress, and anxiety.

TREATMENT

Both pharmacologic and nonpharmacologic treatments are available for use in patients suffering from chronic pruritus. In general, localized pruritus can be treated topically, whereas generalized pruritus often requires more systemic therapies. For all patients presenting with chronic pruritus, targeted treatment of the underlying etiology is the best option. However, in many cases the etiology is not immediately uncovered or takes time to treat and adjunctive itch-specific treatment is necessary for symptom relief. We discuss the many available treatment options for patients with pruritus as well as specific approaches toward managing patients with itch etiologies within the categories described elsewhere in this article.

Nonpharmacologic Interventions

For all patients suffering from chronic pruritus regardless of etiology, proper skin hygiene and the elimination of potential itch triggers is key for mitigating itch. Clinicians should stress the importance of frequent skin moisturization, avoidance of extreme temperatures, and decreasing stress because dryness, extreme heat or cold, and emotional stress are all known exacerbators or triggers of pruritus. Our recommendations for avoiding these triggers are as follows.

- Use of gentle cleansers while bathing is recommended. A gentle cleanser is one that includes a very minimal number of excess ingredients (such as fragrances or color), has a low pH (to help maintain the skin's naturally acidic pH of 5.5), and is typically "soap free" (made from synthetic detergents instead, which are typically gentler than soaps). Liquid soaps are recommended over bar soaps because they often meet more of these criteria.
- Use topical emollients (moisturizing creams, lotions) at least once daily. The skin is able to better absorb moisture while damp, so it should be recommended patients moisturize when they get out of the shower. In addition, there are numerous over-the-counter moisturizing products with anti-itch properties, often containing antipruritic ingredients like promoxine, menthol, or calamine.
- Showers and baths should ideally be lukewarm and limited in time to prevent heat from evaporating skin moisture and irritating skin further.
- Several nutritional supplements such as zinc, vitamin B_{12}, vitamin D, quercetin, and L-theanine claim to be antipruritic; however, at the present time there is not enough research to determine their clinical efficacy and safety. Therefore, we do not currently endorse recommending these supplements to patients.
- Relaxation techniques such as progressive muscle relaxation, meditation, and acupuncture have been shown to decrease itch by decreasing stress.[51] In addition, a referral for adjunctive psychological counseling may be beneficial to any patient appearing or expressing stress and should be considered.[52]

In addition, scratching may perpetuate further itch sensations through the itch–scratch cycle.[53] Patients should be advised to limit scratching their itchy skin, keep fingernails short to mitigate skin damage, and use occlusive dressings on localized areas of itch whenever possible.

Pharmacologic Treatment of Localized Itching

It is responsible for the clinician to minimize patient exposure to systemic treatments whenever possible. As such, many cases of localized itching can be treated effectively with topical or intralesional therapeutic agents. A summary of the available localized therapeutics, when to use them, and when to avoid using them can be found in **Table 4**.

- *Topical and intralesional corticosteroids*: Although they do not treat pruritus directly, corticosteroids are effective for decreasing inflammation in inflammatory skin conditions, which can, in turn, decrease itching. Care should be taken to select the lowest potency steroid that is effective for the patient and limit long-term use to prevent the known main side effects of cutaneous atrophy and

Table 4
Local treatments for pruritus

Medication	Dose	Useful in:	Avoid in:	Notes
Topical corticosteroids	Variable	Inflammatory Skin diseases with visible lesions	Itch secondary to any non-inflammatory etiology	Begin with lower potency doses and only increase as needed. Keep potencies low in children, on face, and in skin folds. Avoid long term use
Topical calcineurin inhibitors	Tacrolimus 0.03% and 0.1% ointment Pimecrolimus 1% cream	Inflammatory skin conditions, particularly facial and anogenital itch	—	May experience transient stinging or burning sensation
Doxepin	5% cream	—	Children, patients on other sedating medications	May cause some sedation
Menthol	1%–3% cream or lotion	Patients who state "cooling" alleviates itch	—	—
Capsaicin	0.025%–0.1% cream	Neuropathic Itch, Pruritus associated with CKD	—	Burning sensation for the first 2 wk
Salicylic acid	2%–6%	Lichen simplex chronicus	Acute inflammatory skin diseases Children	—
Topical PDE4 inhibitors	Crisaborole 2% ointment	Mild to moderate atopic dermatitis	—	Potential burning, stinging, irritation of the skin
Local anesthetics	Lidocaine patch 5% Eutectic mixture of lidocaine 2.5% and prilocaine 2.5% Pramoxine 1%–2.5%	Neuropathic itch Neuropathic itch, post burn itch Face pruritus, Pruritus associated with CKD, genital itch, neuropathic itch	— — —	— Risk of methemglobinemia May experience skin irritation and dryness at the affected area
	Ketamine 5 or 10% + amitriptyline 5% + lidocaine 5%	Many forms of chronic itch	—	—
	5% urea + 3% polidocanol	—	—	Not available in the United States

Abbreviation: CKD, chronic kidney disease.

hypothalamic–pituitary axis suppression, among others.[54] For thick or nodular lesions, intralesional injection may be a more effective choice than topical creams. There is no indication for topical or intralesional steroids in cases of pruritus without evidence of skin inflammation (ie, systemic, neuropathic, chronic pruritus of undetermined origin, and psychogenic etiologies).

- *Topical calcineurin inhibitors*: Tacrolimus and pimecrolimus have been found to be successful in treating multiple inflammatory skin conditions with itch as well as anogenital pruritus, prurigo nodularis, lichen sclerosus, chronic graft-versus-host disease, and chronic hand dermatitis.[55] Patients may experience a burning sensation after application.[56]
- *Topical capsaicin*: Capsaicin (8-methyl-N-vanillyl-6 noneenamide) is a chili pepper–derived substance that activates the transient release potential vanilloid-1 channel to release and deplete substance P and other neuropeptides that can induce pain and itch sensations.[57] In turn, capsaicin has been able to induce lasting desensitization of the neurons to which it is applied, leading to the inhibition of neuronal transmission and mitigation of both pain and pruritus.[31,58,59] This treatment has been found to be particularly successful in forms of neuropathic itch, such as brachioradial pruritus and notalgia paresthetica, as well as other itch disorders like prurigo nodularis, aquagenic pruritus, and chronic kidney disease–associated pruritus.[58] Patients should be warned of a potentially intense burning sensation that may occur immediately after application that may last for up to the next 30 minutes but should decrease after 2 to 3 weeks of use, because this side effect may limit compliance
- *Topical antihistamines*[60]: Because the vast majority of chronically itchy conditions act through pruritic, nonhistaminergic pathways, data are insufficient to support a broad recommendation for the use of topical antihistamines. Topical doxepin, a tricyclic antidepressant with antihistaminergic effects, however, has been studied in several randomized controlled trials and has been found effective in treating pruritus in inflammatory skin disease with side effects of drowsiness and contact dermatitis that limit its use.
- *Topical anesthetics*: Topical anesthetics in various formulations have exhibited antipruritic effects on many different etiologies in both experimental and clinical studies.[61] However, the safety of widespread or long-term use of these agents is currently unknown and toxicity owing to systemic absorption with improper, excessive use. Therefore, it is our recommendation to have patients apply these topicals to as small of an area as needed for itch relief.

Systemic Therapies for Pruritus

Systemic therapies are typically useful in the treatment of generalized pruritus or localized pruritus unresponsive to topical therapies. A summary of the available options can be found in **Table 5**.

- *Antihistamines*: Despite their relative safety, widespread availability, and affordability as both over-the-counter and prescribed oral medications, antihistamines actually have limited efficacy in treating most cases of chronic pruritus. This limitation is because, with the exception of urticaria[62] and mastocytosis, most etiologies of pruritus induce chronic itch through nonhistaminergic pathways.[63] Sedating antihistamines (eg, diphenhydramine, hydroxyzine, doxepin) may be useful in patients who experience pruritus exacerbations at night and could benefit from their sedative effects, but nonsedating antihistamines are not recommended for most etiologies of chronic pruritus.

Table 5
Systemic therapies for chronic pruritus

Drug	Dosage	Useful in:	Avoid in:	Notes:
Antihistamines	Variable	Chronic urticaria, mastocytosis Sedating antihistamines: patients with PM itch exacerbations	Etiologies of chronic itch that act through nonhistaminergic pruritic pathways	–
Neuromodulatory medications	Gabapentin 100–3600 mg/d, usually given in 2–3 divided daily doses Pregabalin 150–300 mg/d	Neuropathic pruritus CKD-associated pruritus Idiopathic pruritus		May cause sedation and weight gain
Antidepressants	*Selective serotonin reuptake inhibitors* Paroxetine 10–40 mg/d	Patients with pruritus with comorbid depressive or anxiety symptoms, paraneoplastic pruritus	Patients with a personal or close family history of bipolar depression, patients on other psychotropic medications	
	Fluvoxamine 25–150 mg/d	Pruritus patients with comorbid depressive or anxiety symptoms, paraneoplastic pruritus		
	Sertraline 75–100 mg/d *Serotonin and norepinephrine reuptake inhibitors*	Cholestatic pruritus		
	Mirtazapine 7.5–15 mg at night	Nocturnal pruritus		

Opioids			
μ-opioid receptor antagonists			
Naltrexone 25–50 mg/d	Intractable pruritus, cholestatic pruritus, CKD-associated pruritus	Patients taking opioids for pain relief (reverses analgesic effect, can precipitate acute withdrawal)	May cause nausea, vomiting, drowsiness
κ-Opioid receptor agonists			
Nalfurafine 2.5–5.0 μg/d	CKD-associated pruritus		Only available in Japan
Difelikefalin	CKD-associated pruritus		Pending US FDA approval
Combination μ-opioid receptor antagonists/κ-opioid receptor agonists			
Butorphanol 1–4 mg intranasally daily	Nocturnal and intractable pruritus	Patients taking opioids for pain relief (reverses analgesic effect, can precipitate acute withdrawal) Patients with a prior substance use disorder/addiction history (has some addictive potential owing to concomitant weak μ-opioid receptor agonist activity)	May cause nausea, vomiting, drowsiness
Substance P antagonist			
Aprepitant 80 mg/d	Pruritus associated with Sézary syndrome Numerous types of chronic itch		Expensive
Thalidomide			
100 mg nightly	Prurigo nodularis	Pregnant women (teratogenic), patients with history of thromboembolic disease	May cause sedation, peripheral neuropathy, thromboembolism, skin eruptions, and dizziness

(continued on next page)

Table 5
(continued)

Drug	Dosage	Useful in:	Avoid in:	Notes:
Biologics and immunosup-pressants	Cyclosporine	Atopic dermatitis, prurigo nodularis, chronic urticaria		
	Methotrexate	Atopic dermatitis, prurigo nodularis, old age itch		
	Dupilumab	Atopic dermatitis Bullous pemphigoid (?) Prurigo nodularis (?)		Anti–IL-4/-13 antibody Great for use in patients with comorbid atopic conditions (eg, asthma, allergic rhinitis)

Abbreviation: FDA, Food and Drug Administration.

- *Neuroactive medications*[64]: The anticonvulsants, gabapentin and pregabalin, have been shown efficacious in many types of pruritus with particular effectiveness in neuropathic itch and uremic pruritus.[65] These agents have also shown some effectiveness in treating patients with idiopathic pruritus. We recommend that patients on the lowest effective dose and titrate up as necessary. These drugs may cause some drowsiness, which may also help patients whose itch is exacerbated at nighttime.
- *Antidepressants*: Selective serotonin reuptake inhibitors, serotonin and norepinephrine reuptake inhibitors, and tricyclic antidepressants have been shown to be effective in the treatment of chronic pruritus in a limited number of randomized controlled trials, case reports/series, and open-label studies.[66] It is suggested that this effectiveness comes from their effects on serotonin and histamine levels, but may also be due to the general reduction of stress and anxiety, which can both exacerbate itch.
- *Opioids*: The use of opioid drugs in the treatment of itch is an emerging field with many new therapeutic agents on their way to the market soon. Opioids effective in treating pruritus antagonize the mu-opioid receptor, agonize the kappa-opioid receptor, or do a combination of both, as activation mu-opioid receptors has been proven to be propruritic and kappa–opioid receptors to be antipruritic.[67–69] These treatments have been shown efficacious in cholestatic pruritus, chronic urticaria, atopic dermatitis, prurigo nodularis, mycosis fungoides, and aquagenic pruritus, among others. In addition, these drugs have been used to manage mu-opioid agonist-induced pruritus.
- *Immunosuppressants and biologics*[65,70]: The effects of many biologic and immunosuppressant drugs on pruritus is likely related to their anti-inflammatory properties and treatment of the underlying inflammatory etiology. Therefore, they are particularly useful in inflammatory skin diseases. A discussion of specific biologics for specific diseases is beyond the scope of this article, but indications for some of the most common ones can be found in **Table 5**.

DISCUSSION

The number of conditions and etiologies that can result in a patient presenting with chronic pruritus is extensive. It is important for clinicians to use a systematic approach to narrow down the long list of potential diagnoses and target further workup, diagnostic steps, and treatment for their patients. For all patients with chronic pruritus, dry skin must be ruled out as a primary cause or exacerbating factor. Proper skin moisturization, avoidance of itchy triggers, and skin hygiene should always be included in a treatment regimen. In addition, caution should be taken in all cases to avoid unnecessary biopsies, laboratory tests, and imaging by making the diagnosis and treating appropriately through the history, visual inspection of the skin, and physical examination. Once a diagnosis is obtained, treating both the itch and the underlying etiology are imperative for achieving the greatest treatment success. Holistic approaches, including stress reduction techniques and psychological support, are greatly encouraged in all patients, but especially those displaying symptoms of stress or anxiety.

In the case of a patient with severe pruritus for which an underlying cause cannot be identified and treated, lifestyle modifications and localized/topical treatments are unlikely to sufficiently mitigate itch. Systemic therapy should be considered beginning with drugs that reduce neural transmission of itch such as low-dose, off-label use of gabapentin (300 mg) and considering upward titration or the addition of low-dose mirtazapine (7.5–15.0 mg) nightly if needed.[8]

SUMMARY

Pruritus is a very broad chief complaint with causative etiologies ranging from inflammatory skin diseases to systemic disease to neuropathic and psychogenic disorders. The 2 most important factors for narrowing a differential diagnosis are (1) the presence of absence of a primary skin rash and (2) whether the itch is localized or generalized, both of which the answers to can then guide the clinician's approach to workup and eventual diagnosis and treatment. Localized topical or intralesional treatments can be useful in patients with localized itch. However, for many patients with severe chronic localized pruritus and generalized pruritus, systemic treatments like anticonvulsants, opioids, antidepressants, immunosuppressants, or biologics are necessary. In addition, lifestyle modifications and proper skin hygiene is imperative to achieving maximum itch mitigation in patients.

CLINICS CARE POINTS

- We suggest taking a systematic approach using the algorithm presented in **Fig. 1** to narrow the broad differential of itch-causing diagnoses and guide targeted workup and management.
- If at any point in patient workup or management the cause of pruritus becomes unclear or a chosen treatment is not effective, we recommend periodic reevaluation of the patient and revisiting the diagnostic algorithm from the beginning to investigate other possible categories.
- Regardless of the diagnostic origin of pruritus, proper skin hygiene and stress management are essential for achieving full treatment success.
- Both topical and systemic treatments are available for the treatment of pruritic conditions and care should be taken in ensuring treatment is targeted for the correct diagnosis.

DISCLOSURE

Dr G. Yosipovitch conducted clinical trials or received honoraria for serving as a member of the Scientific Advisory Board and consultant of, Pfizer, TREVI, Galderma, Regeneron, Sanofi, Novartis, LEO, Kiniksa, and Eli Lilly and received research funds from Pfizer, Sun Pharma, Kiniksa, LEO Foundation, and Novartis.

REFERENCES

1. Ikoma A, Steinhoff M, Ständer S, et al. The neurobiology of itch. Nat Rev Neurosci 2006;7(7):535–47.
2. Shive M, Linos E, Berger T, et al. Itch as a patient-reported symptom in ambulatory care visits in the United States. J Am Acad Dermatol 2013;69(4):550–6.
3. Ständer S, Schäfer I, Phan NQ, et al. Prevalence of chronic pruritus in Germany: results of a cross-sectional study in a sample working population of 11,730. Dermatology 2010;221(3):229–35.
4. Whang KA, Khanna R, Williams KA, et al. Health-related QOL and economic burden of chronic pruritus. J Invest Dermatol 2021;141(4):754–60.
5. Kini SP, DeLong LK, Veledar E, et al. The impact of pruritus on quality of life: the skin equivalent of pain. Arch Dermatol 2011;147(10):1153–6.

6. Hay RJ, Johns NE, Williams HC, et al. The global burden of skin disease in 2010: an analysis of the prevalence and impact of skin conditions. J Invest Dermatol 2014;134(6):1527–34.
7. Weisshaar E, Apfelbacher C, Jäger G, et al. Pruritus as a leading symptom: clinical characteristics and quality of life in German and Ugandan patients. Br J Dermatol 2006;155(5):957–64.
8. Yosipovitch G, Bernhard JD. Chronic Pruritus. N Engl J Med 2013;368(17): 1625–34.
9. Hahnel E, Lichterfeld A, Blume-Peytavi U, et al. The epidemiology of skin conditions in the aged: a systematic review. J Tissue Viability 2017;26(1):20–8.
10. Lichterfeld A, Lahmann N, Blume-Peytavi U, et al. Dry skin in nursing care receivers: a multi-centre cross-sectional prevalence study in hospitals and nursing homes. Int J Nurs Stud 2016;56:37–44.
11. Paul C, Maumus-Robert S, Mazereeuw-Hautier J, et al. Prevalence and risk factors for xerosis in the elderly: a cross-sectional epidemiological study in primary care. Dermatology 2011;223(3):260–5.
12. Smith DR, Atkinson R, Tang S, et al. A survey of skin disease among patients in an Australian nursing home. J Epidemiol 2002;12(4):336–40.
13. Augustin M, Kirsten N, Körber A, et al. Prevalence, predictors and comorbidity of dry skin in the general population. J Eur Acad Dermatol Venereol 2019;33(1): 147–50.
14. Mekić S, Jacobs LC, Gunn DA, et al. Prevalence and determinants for xerosis cutis in the middle-aged and elderly population: a cross-sectional study. J Am Acad Dermatol 2019;81(4):963–9.e2.
15. Pavlis J, Yosipovitch G. Management of itch in atopic dermatitis. Am J Clin Dermatol 2018;19(3):319–32.
16. Mollanazar NK, Smith PK, Yosipovitch G. Mediators of chronic pruritus in atopic dermatitis: getting the itch out? Clin Rev Allergy Immunol 2016;51(3):263–92.
17. Kwatra SG, Tey HL, Ali SM, et al. The infra-auricular fissure: a bedside marker of disease severity in patients with atopic dermatitis. J Am Acad Dermatol 2012; 66(6):1009–10.
18. Calle Sarmiento PM, Chango Azanza JJ. Dyshidrotic eczema: a common cause of palmar dermatitis. Cureus 2020;12(10):e10839.
19. Naldi L, Rebora A. Seborrheic dermatitis. N Engl J Med 2009;360(4):387–96.
20. Leung AK, Lam JM, Leong KF, et al. Nummular eczema: an updated review. Recent Pat Inflamm Allergy Drug Discov 2020;14(2):146–55.
21. Sundaresan S, Migden MR, Silapunt S. Stasis dermatitis: pathophysiology, evaluation, and management. Am J Clin Dermatol 2017;18(3):383–90.
22. Greaves M. Chronic urticaria. J Allergy Clin Immunol 2000;105(4):664–72.
23. Kurd SK, Gelfand JM. The prevalence of previously diagnosed and undiagnosed psoriasis in US adults: results from NHANES 2003-2004. J Am Acad Dermatol 2009;60(2):218–24.
24. Rachakonda TD, Schupp CW, Armstrong AW. Psoriasis prevalence among adults in the United States. J Am Acad Dermatol 2014;70(3):512–6.
25. Dawn A, Yosipovitch G. Treating itch in psoriasis. Dermatol Nurs 2006;18(3):227.
26. Takeshita J, Grewal S, Langan SM, et al. Psoriasis and comorbid diseases: epidemiology. J Am Acad Dermatol 2017;76(3):377–90.
27. Le Cleach L, Chosidow O. Lichen Planus. N Engl J Med 2012;366(8):723–32.
28. Ely JW, Rosenfeld S, Stone MS. Diagnosis and management of tinea infections. Am Fam Physician 2014;90(10):702–10.
29. Chosidow O. Scabies. N Engl J Med 2006;354(16):1718–27.

30. Stumpf A, Ständer S. Neuropathic itch: diagnosis and management. Dermatol Ther 2013;26(2):104–9.
31. Rosen JD, Fostini AC, Yosipovitch G. Diagnosis and management of neuropathic itch. Dermatol Clin 2018;36(3):213–24.
32. Pereira MP, Lüling H, Dieckhöfer A, et al. Brachioradial pruritus and notalgia paraesthetica: a comparative observational study of clinical presentation and morphological pathologies. Acta Derm Venereol 2018;98(1–2):82–8.
33. Bernhard JD, Bordeaux JS. Medical pearl: the ice-pack sign in brachioradial pruritus. J Am Acad Dermatol 2005;52(6):1073.
34. Lipman ZM, Magnolo N, Golpanian RS, et al. Comparison of itch characteristics and sleep in patients with brachioradial pruritus and notalgia paresthetica: a retrospective analysis from 2 itch centers. JAAD Int 2021;2:96–7.
35. Oaklander AL, Bowsher D, Galer B, et al. Herpes zoster itch: preliminary epidemiologic data. J Pain 2003;4(6):338–43.
36. Wood GJ, Akiyama T, Carstens E, et al. An insatiable itch. J Pain 2009;10(8):792–7.
37. Yosipovitch G, Samuel LS. Neuropathic and psychogenic itch. Dermatol Ther 2008;21(1):32–41.
38. Brenaut E, Marcorelles P, Genestet S, et al. Pruritus: an underrecognized symptom of small-fiber neuropathies. J Am Acad Dermatol 2015;72(2):328–32.
39. Krajnik M, Zylicz Z. Understanding pruritus in systemic disease. J Pain Symptom Manage 2001;21(2):151–68.
40. Wang H, Yosipovitch G. New insights into the pathophysiology and treatment of chronic itch in patients with end-stage renal disease, chronic liver disease, and lymphoma. Int J Dermatol 2010;49(1):1–11.
41. Rayner HC, Larkina M, Wang M, et al. International comparisons of prevalence, awareness, and treatment of pruritus in people on hemodialysis. Clin J Am Soc Nephrol 2017;12(12):2000–7.
42. Hashimoto T, Yosipovitch G. Itching as a systemic disease. J Allergy Clin Immunol 2019;144(2):375–80.
43. Kremer AE, Weisshaar E. Endocrine diseases. Pruritus. London, UK: Springer; 2016. p. 267–70.
44. Reich A, Ständer S, Szepietowski JC. Drug-induced pruritus: a review. Acta Derm Venereol 2009;89(3):236–44.
45. Fischer A, Rosen AC, Ensslin CJ, et al. Pruritus to anticancer agents targeting the EGFR, BRAF, and CTLA-4. Dermatol Ther 2013;26(2):135–48.
46. Lipman ZM, Yosipovitch G. Substance use disorders and chronic itch. J Am Acad Dermatol 2021;84(1):148–55.
47. Kim BS, Berger TG, Yosipovitch G. Chronic pruritus of unknown origin (CPUO): uniform nomenclature and diagnosis as a pathway to standardized understanding and treatment. J Am Acad Dermatol 2019;81(5):1223–4.
48. Valdes-Rodriguez R, Stull C, Yosipovitch G. Chronic pruritus in the elderly: pathophysiology, diagnosis and management. Drugs Aging 2015;32(3):201–15.
49. Arnold LM, Auchenbach MB, McElroy SL. Psychogenic excoriation. CNS Drugs 2001;15(5):351–9.
50. Tey H, Yosipovitch G. Targeted treatment of pruritus: a look into the future. Br J Dermatol 2011;165(1):5–17.
51. Bae BG, Ho SO, Park CO, et al. Progressive muscle relaxation therapy for atopic dermatitis: objective assessment of efficacy. Acta Derm Venereol 2012;92(1):57–61.

52. Evers AW, Schut C, Gieler U, et al. Itch management: psychotherapeutic approach. Itch-management in clinical practice. Basel, Switzerland: Karger Publishers; 2016. p. 64–70.
53. Mack MR, Kim BS. The itch–scratch cycle: a neuroimmune perspective. Trends Immunol 2018;39(12):980–91.
54. Ference JD, Last AR. Choosing topical corticosteroids. Am Fam Physician 2009; 79(2):135–40.
55. Ständer S, Schürmeyer-Horst F, Luger TA, et al. Treatment of pruritic diseases with topical calcineurin inhibitors. Ther Clin Risk Manag 2006;2(2):213–8.
56. Pereira U, Boulais N, Lebonvallet N, et al. Mechanisms of the sensory effects of tacrolimus on the skin. Br J Dermatol 2010;163(1):70–7.
57. Cassano N, Tessari G, Vena GA, et al. Chronic pruritus in the absence of specific skin disease: an update on pathophysiology, diagnosis, and therapy. Am J Clin Dermatol 2010;11(6):399–411.
58. Papoiu AD, Yosipovitch G. Topical capsaicin. The fire of a 'hot' medicine is reignited. Expert Opin Pharmacother 2010;11(8):1359–71.
59. Fowler E, Yosipovitch G. Chronic itch management: therapies beyond those targeting the immune system. Ann Allergy Asthma Immunol 2019;123(2):158–65.
60. Eschler DC, Klein PA. An evidence-based review of the efficacy of topical antihistamines in the relief of pruritus. J Drugs Dermatol 2010;9(8):992–7.
61. He A, Kwatra SG, Sharma D, et al. The role of topical anesthetics in the management of chronic pruritus. J Dermatol Treat 2017;28(4):338–41.
62. Greene SL, Reed CE, Schroeter AL. Double-blind crossover study comparing doxepin with diphenhydramine for the treatment of chronic urticaria. J Am Acad Dermatol 1985;12(4):669–75.
63. Yosipovitch G, Bernhard JD. Clinical practice. Chronic pruritus. N Engl J Med 2013;368(17):1625–34.
64. Matsuda KM, Sharma D, Schonfeld AR, et al. Gabapentin and pregabalin for the treatment of chronic pruritus. J Am Acad Dermatol 2016;75(3):619–25.e6.
65. Golpanian RS, Yosipovitch G. Current and emerging systemic treatments targeting the neural system for chronic pruritus. Expert Opin Pharmacother 2020; 21(13):1629–36.
66. Kouwenhoven TA, van de Kerkhof PCM, Kamsteeg M. Use of oral antidepressants in patients with chronic pruritus: a systematic review. J Am Acad Dermatol 2017;77(6):1068–73.e7.
67. Lipman ZM, Yosipovitch G. An evaluation of difelikefalin as a treatment option for moderate-to-severe pruritus in end stage renal disease. Expert Opin Pharmacother 2020;22(5):549–55.
68. Phan NQ, Bernhard JD, Luger TA, et al. Antipruritic treatment with systemic μ-opioid receptor antagonists: a review. J Am Acad Dermatol 2010;63(4):680–8.
69. Phan N, Lotts T, Antal A, et al. Systemic kappa opioid receptor agonists in the treatment of chronic pruritus: a literature review. Acta Derm Venerol 2012;92: 555–60.
70. Pereira MP, Ständer S. Chronic pruritus: current and emerging treatment options. Drugs 2017;77(9):999–1007.

Cellulitis
A Review of Pathogenesis, Diagnosis, and Management

Renajd Rrapi, BA[1], Sidharth Chand, BA[1],
Daniela Kroshinsky, MD, MPH*

KEYWORDS

- Cellulitis • Diagnosis • Treatment • Antibiotic • Skin and soft tissue infection
- Purulence

KEY POINTS

- Cellulitis is a common skin infection, typically presenting with unilateral poorly demarcated erythema, warmth, and tenderness, that has many clinical mimickers.
- Thorough history and clinical examination can narrow the differential diagnosis of cellulitis and minimize unnecessary hospitalization.
- Treatment should be dictated by patient history and risk factors, clinical presentation, and the most likely pathogen culprit, optimizing antibiotic stewardship.

INTRODUCTION

Cellulitis is a common skin infection of the dermis and subcutaneous tissue. There has been a rise in cellulitis incidence and associated cost over the past few decades.[1,2] From 1998 to 2013, cellulitis hospitalizations doubled, and costs increased by nearly 120% to more than $3.7 billion annually.[3] Cellulitis can be challenging to identify given its numerous clinical mimickers and the lack of a gold standard diagnostic test. The inability to confirm the potential microbiological causes of cellulitis can complicate management further when selecting appropriate antibiotics. This review describes the pathophysiology, clinical presentation, and treatment of cellulitis.

PATHOPHYSIOLOGY

Cellulitis is a skin infection typically precipitated by entry of bacteria through a breach in the skin barrier. *Streptococcus pyogenes* is the most common cause of nonpurulent

Funding Sources: None.
Department of Dermatology, Massachusetts General Hospital, 50 Staniford Street, 2nd Floor, Boston, MA 02114, USA
[1] These 2 authors contributed equally to this work.
* Corresponding author.
E-mail address: dkroshinsky@partners.org

Med Clin N Am 105 (2021) 723–735
https://doi.org/10.1016/j.mcna.2021.04.009
0025-7125/21/© 2021 Elsevier Inc. All rights reserved.

medical.theclinics.com

cellulitis, defined as cellulitis lacking pustules or purulent drainage.[4,5] Nonpurulent cellulitis typically does not have a culturable wound source.[4,5] *Staphylococcus aureus* also can cause nonpurulent cellulitis and is the most common cause of purulent cellulitis.[6] Cellulitis can be caused by methicillin-resistant *S aureus* (MRSA) or methicillin-susceptible *S aureus* (MSSA), which can be difficult to clinically distinguish without wound culture and sensitivity testing and has implications for antibiotic selection.[7] MRSA incidence has been increasing in communities, and many patients with MRSA infection present without any risk factors.[7,8] Furthermore, risk factors for MRSA colonization include prior antibiotic use, recent hospitalization or surgery, residence in a long-term facility, human immunodeficiency virus (HIV) infection, injection drug use, incarceration, military service, sharing sporting equipment, and sharing razors.[9–14]

Other potential pathogens besides *Streptococcus pyogenes* and *S aureus* are rarer and should be considered based on clinical context. Cellulitis at the site of a dog bite or cat bite can be due to organisms, such as *Pasteurella*, *Neisseria*, or *Fusobacterium*,[15] whereas organisms to consider in human bites are *Eikenella corrodens* or *Veillonello*.[16] Cellulitis in the setting of an aquatic injury can include *Vibrio*, *Aeromonas,* or *Mycobacterium*.[17] In immunosuppressed patients it is important to investigate the etiology when possible, including nonbacterial causes. *Helicobacter cinaedi* can cause cellulitis in patients with HIV infection or with a recent history of chemotherapy.[18] Patients with systemic lupus erythematosus are susceptible to *Streptococcus pneumoniae* cellulitis.[19] Obtaining patient history relevant to cellulitis infection can elucidate potential casual microorganisms and promote appropriate antibiotic selection and management.

Predisposing factors to cellulitis infection include increasing age, obesity, chronic leg edema, and previous cellulitis infection.[20,21] Lymphedema in particular may harbor bacterial growth,[22] and a retrospective study of more than 165,000 hospital admissions for a primary diagnosis of lymphedema or cellulitis found that 92% of lymphedema cases were associated with cellulitis.[23] Lymphedema, venous insufficiency, and vascular disease have been shown to be predictive of cellulitis recurrence.[24] Furthermore, disruption to skin barrier function from chronic wounds, infection, or trauma is a major modifiable risk factor that can be managed to improve patient outcomes.[21]

CLINICAL PRESENTATION

Cellulitis usually presents with poorly demarcated erythema, edema, tenderness, and warmth of the affected skin (**Fig. 1**). Erysipelas can be considered a type of cellulitis that affects the superficial dermis and present with sharply demarcated erythema.[22,25] Clinical presentation of cellulitis often is distinguished by the presence or absence of purulence. It can be complicated by the formation of cutaneous abscess, a walled collection of pus within the subcutaneous space, which may require surgical intervention. Additional findings can include lymphangitis, lymphadenopathy, vesiculation, or bullae.[6] Fever sometimes is present with incidence estimated widely from approximately 22% to 77%, depending on the clinical setting of the study conducted.[26–29]

Cellulitis can affect any body area, although the lower extremity is the most common site of infection in adults.[26] A retrospective study specifically evaluating lower extremity cellulitis developed the ALT-70 cellulitis score and demonstrated that the clinical factors unilateral cellulitis (+3 if true), age greater than or equal to 70 years old (+2 if true), leukocytosis (white blood cell count ≥10,000/uL) (+1 if true), and tachycardia

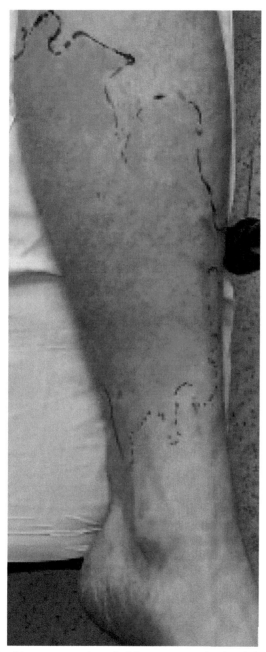

Fig. 1. Photograph of lower extremity cellulitis. Warm, tender, brightly erythematous plaque on left lower extremity suggestive of cellulitis.

(heart rate $\geq$90 beats per minute) (+1 if true) were predictive of true cellulitis.[30] The ALT-70 cellulitis score has a greater than 82% positive predictive value for predicting true cellulitis for scores calculated as greater than or equal to 5.[30] This can be a valuable tool for clinicians when evaluating for lower extremity cellulitis.

Cellulitis often does not present with salient features on laboratory evaluation, and, in general, bloodwork is not required when evaluating uncomplicated cellulitis or patients without comorbidities. Findings tend to be nonspecific and may show leukocytosis in fewer than 50% of patients[31] and elevated inflammatory markers.[32] The Infectious Diseases Society of America (IDSA) 2014 guidelines recommend a Gram stain and culture of purulent cellulitis.[6] Wound culture is not recommended in nonpurulent cellulitis given the lack of a culturable source from swabbing bare skin.[22] Moreover, the IDSA only recommends blood cultures in patients with immunocompromised states, malignancy, signs of systemic infection, or animal bites and recommends acquisition of radiologic imaging in patients with febrile neutropenia.[6] A retrospective study of patients with uncomplicated cellulitis found that a majority of patients underwent radiologic evaluation and blood cultures without meeting IDSA criteria. The evaluation had low clinical utility, seldom changed management, and contributed to more than $226 million in unnecessary costs annually.[33]

DIFFERENTIAL DIAGNOSIS

Cellulitis has many clinical mimickers (**Table 1**). Cellulitis misdiagnosis rate has been estimated to be approximately 30%,[34,35] with some estimations as high as 74%.[31] Thorough history taking and clinical examination can help distinguish cellulitis from its clinical mimickers. If patients with cellulitis fail to improve with appropriate therapy or exhibit features not characteristic of cellulitis, such as bilateral or symmetric findings, it is important to consider alternative diagnoses.

Stasis dermatitis is an inflammatory skin condition of the lower extremities that occurs in patients with chronic venous insufficiency.[36] It is a common clinical mimicker of cellulitis that often can be ruled out given its bilateral presentation in the absence of trauma, although it can uncommonly present unilaterally in the setting of anatomic vein variation or leg injury. Improvement with leg elevation and compression and topical corticosteroid treatment favor a diagnosis of stasis dermatitis over cellulitis.

Contact dermatitis is an inflammatory skin response to an irritant or allergen, and up to 80% of cases tend to be due to an irritant.[37] A distinguishing feature from cellulitis in contact dermatitis is the symptom of pruritus, although pain can be present in severe cases. Although cellulitis and contact dermatitis both can present with erythema, the distribution in contact dermatitis may follow a geometric shape or pattern due to a triggering agent. A thorough history investigating potential triggers, such as detergents, soaps, plants, or fragrances, can clarify the potential etiology. In cases of allergen etiology, patch testing can clarify the offending agent. Removal of the agent, treatment of the skin with topical corticosteroid, and treatment with antihistamine for itching are the mainstays of management.

Necrotizing soft tissue infection, such as necrotizing cellulitis and necrotizing fasciitis, is an important diagnosis to immediately rule out, given its severity and high mortality rate.[38] Patients with signs of systemic toxicity, rapidly progressive erythema or purpura, and pain out of proportion on physical examination require prompt surgical evaluation and antibiotic treatment.[38] Specifically the Laboratory Risk Indicator for Necrotizing Fasciitis (LRINEC) score incorporates C-reactive protein levels; white blood cell count; and hemoglobin, sodium, creatinine, and glucose levels to screen for necrotizing fasciitis when initial clinical suspicion is not high enough to warrant immediate surgical exploration.[39] A meta-analysis demonstrated that an LRINEC greater than or equal to 8 had a specificity of 94.9% for detecting necrotizing fasciitis.[40]

Table 1
Differential diagnosis for cellulitis

Diagnosis	Distinct Clinical Features	Additional Notes
Infectious		
Necrotizing soft tissue infection (ie necrotizing fasciitis)	Rapidly progressive erythema and purpura, signs of systemic toxicity, and pain out of proportion to examination	Immediate surgical evaluation if high clinical suspicion LRINEC score to screen for necrotizing fasciitis[39]
Erythema migrans	History of a tick bite or recent travel to an endemic area. Initially appears as a well-demarcated erythematous macule, patch, or plaque that expands and may develop a targetoid bull's-eye appearance with central clearing	
Herpes zoster	Painful erythematous patch or plaque confined to a dermatome that subsequently develops grouped vesicles without crossing the midline	Polymerase chain reaction–based testing is the preferred diagnostic test for herpes family virus if clinical examination is unclear.[56]
Herpes simplex	Grouped vesicles on an erythematous base that usually appear in the trigeminal or sacral ganglia but may appear at other body locations Can be multifocal	Polymerase chain reaction–based testing is the preferred diagnostic test for herpes family virus if clinical examination is unclear.[56]
Noninfectious, inflammatory		
Contact dermatitis	Pruritus often is a distinguishing symptom. Erythema or vesicles can be seen acutely. Scaling and fissures are seen chronically. Distribution of rash may follow a geometric shape or other nonorganic pattern dependent on allergen exposure.	
Sweet syndrome[a]	Patient with fever higher than 100.4°C and abrupt onset of edematous, painful erythematous to violaceous, sharply demarcated plaques	Meeting both major criteria and 2 of 4 minor criteria is required for diagnosis of Sweet syndrome.[57]
Gout	Acute attack can present as painful, swollen, warm, erythematous skin overlying a joint. It can be accompanied by fever and leukocytosis. Gout nodules can appear as white or yellow.	

(continued on next page)

Table 1 (continued)		
Diagnosis	Distinct Clinical Features	Additional Notes
Erythema nodosum	Initially bright red, tender palpable nodules and plaques seen most commonly along the anterior shins. Over time, lesions may flatten and appear purple.	Lesions typically appear symmetric and can be accompanied by joint pain, but may be singular, large, or isolated.
Vascular		
Stasis dermatitis	Bilateral, chronic history with intermittent exacerbation; improves with leg elevation, compression therapy, and topical corticosteroid use.	Bilateral cellulitis in the absence of bilateral skin trauma is very rare.
Deep vein thrombosis	Unilateral swelling, erythema, or tenderness. Risk factors include prolonged immobilization, prior history of deep vein thrombosis, and active malignancy.	An ultrasound is an inexpensive and highly sensitive and specific tool for diagnosis.
Erythromelalgia	Bilateral, warm, erythematous, extremities with burning paresthesia sensation. Symptoms improve with cooling. Pain is out of proportion to clinical examination.	
Neoplastic		
Carcinoma erysipeloides	Cutaneous metastasis presenting as erythematous, well-demarcated patch or plaque, usually in a region overlying the primary cancer	Carcinoma erysipeloides is associated most often with breast carcinoma.[58] Typically presents unilaterally on the chest

[a] Also referred to as acute febrile neutrophilic dermatosis.

TREATMENT

The systemic inflammatory response syndrome (SIRS) criteria commonly were used to define the severity of sepsis and categorize cellulitis severity for several decades. The score incorporates temperature greater than 38°C or less than 36°C; heart rate greater than 90 beats per minute; respiratory rate greater than 20 breaths per minute or arterial partial pressure of carbon dioxide less than 32 mm Hg; and white blood cell count greater than 12,000/mm^3, less than 4000/mm^3, or greater than 10% immature bands.[41] Mild cellulitis was characterized as without signs of systemic infection, moderate cellulitis as meeting 1 or 2 SIRS criteria, and severe cellulitis as greater than or equal to 2 SIRS criteria plus hypotension, immune compromise, or rapid progression.[22] As discussed later in greater detail, mild cellulitis generally is treated with oral antibiotics and severe cellulitis with intravenous antibiotics.[6] Moderate cellulitis can be treated with oral antibiotics or intravenous antibiotics depending on whether having 1 or 2 SIRS criteria.[22] Nevertheless, the Quick Sequential [sepsis-related] Organ Failure Assessment (qSOFA) score has emerged as the new standard in evaluating sepsis risk.[42] It is scored by respiratory rate greater than or equal to 22 breaths per minute; altered mentation, which can be assessed a Glasgow Coma Scale score less than 15; and systolic blood pressure less than or equal to 100 mm Hg. Given the limited literature evaluating qSOFA scores with cellulitis outcomes, the general principles in characterizing cellulitis based on vital sign abnormalities hold. Mild cellulitis can be characterized as meeting no qSOFA criteria whereas severe cellulitis is characterized by qSOFA score greater than or equal to 2, which is associated with poor sepsis outcomes.[42]

In addition to vital sign abnormalities, the approach to cellulitis treatment is dependent on its clinical presentation as nonpurulent, purulent without cutaneous abscess, or purulent complicated by cutaneous abscess (**Fig. 2**). Cellulitis without cutaneous abscess generally is managed with antibiotic therapy whereas cutaneous abscess is managed surgically (**Table 2**).[6] Antimicrobial stewardship consists of utilizing the narrowest spectrum of antibiotic activity necessary to treat cellulitis. The IDSA recommends initiating treatment of uncomplicated cellulitis with oral antibiotics based on the most likely bacterial culprit.[6] Unnecessary antibiotic coverage can promote drug-resistant organisms, side effects in patients, and increased costs.[43]

Empiric treatment of nonpurulent cellulitis accounts for the most common causal pathogens *Streptococcus pyogenes* and MSSA.[6,22] Patients with mild nonpurulent cellulitis who can tolerate oral therapy and present without MRSA risk factors can be

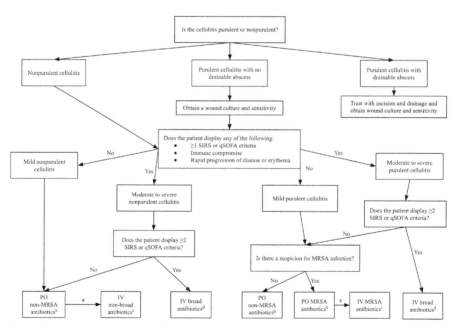

Fig. 2. Characterization of cellulitis and antibiotic treatment algorithm. Details for recommended antibiotic dosing are discussed in **Table 2**. [a]If the patient does not improve, consider transition from oral to intravenous antibiotic treatment. [b]Oral non-MRSA coverage antibiotics include amoxicillin–clavulanic acid, cephalexin, and dicloxacillin. [c]Intravenous MSSA coverage antibiotics include cefazolin, ceftriaxone, and penicillin G. [d]Intravenous broad-spectrum antibiotics include vancomycin plus piperacillin-tazobactam or meropenem. [e]Oral MRSA coverage antibiotics include clindamycin, doxycycline, and trimethoprim-sulfamethoxazole. [f]Intravenous MRSA coverage antibiotics include clindamycin, daptomycin, and vancomycin. IV, intravenous.

Table 2
Cellulitis antibiotic treatment by coverage[6,22]

Route	Antibiotic	Recommended Dose[a]	Comments
Streptococcus and MSSA coverage			
Oral	Amoxicillin–clavulanic acid	875 mg BID	—
	Cephalexin	500 mg QID	Addition of TMP-SMX to cephalexin for empiric MRSA coverage offers no additional beneficial clinical outcomes.[44,45]
	Dicloxacillin	250–500 mg QID	Preferred oral agent for MSSA activity
	Penicillin VK	250–500 mg QID	—
Intravenous	Cefazolin	1 g TID	Alternative for patients with penicillin allergy without history of immediate hypersensitivity reaction
	Ceftaroline	600 mg BID	—
	Ceftriaxone	1–2 g QD	—
	Imipenem	500 mg QID	Administered with cilastatin to prevent rapid inactivation
	Meropenem	1g TID	—
	Nafcillin or oxacillin	1–2g q4h	Preferred parenteral agent for MSSA activity
	Penicillin G	2–4 million U q4–6h	—
	Piperacillin-tazobactam	3.375 g QID	Recommended use with vancomycin for empiric coverage of severe infections
MRSA coverage			
Oral	Clindamycin	300–450 mg QID	Risk of C difficile infection[48] Alternative for patients with penicillin allergy
	Doxycycline or minocycline	100 mg BID	Variable antistreptococcal activity Can administer with amoxicillin for improved streptococcal coverage
	Linezolid	600 mg BID	Alternative for patients with β-lactam allergy Expensive
	TMP-SMX	1–2 DS tablets BID	—
Intravenous	Clindamycin	600 mg TID	—
	Daptomycin	4 mg/kg QD	Alternative for patients who do not tolerate vancomycin
	Linezolid	600 mg BID	—
	Telavancin	10 mg/kg QD	—
	Tigecycline	100 mg, then 50 mg BID	—
	Vancomycin	15 mg/kg BID	Used with piperacillin-tazobactam or imipenem and meropenem for empiric coverage of severe infections

Abbreviations: DS, double-strength; QD, once, a day; TMP-SMX, trimethoprim-sulfamethoxazole; VK, V Potassium.
[a] Recommended dose for standard adult weight and renal function.

treated with an oral antibiotic, such as cephalexin, amoxicillin–clavulanic acid, or dicloxacillin.[6,22] Patients with a true penicillin allergy can be treated with clindamycin.[6] A randomized trial of 153 patients with cellulitis without abscess demonstrated comparable cure rates among patients treated with cephalexin for empiric *Streptococcus pyogenes* and MSSA coverage versus those treated with cephalexin and trimethoprim-sulfamethoxazole for additional empiric MRSA coverage.[44] Similarly, a larger randomized trial of 496 patients with nonpurulent cellulitis demonstrated that the use of cephalexin and trimethoprim-sulfamethoxazole compared with cephalexin alone did not result in higher rates of clinical resolution of cellulitis.[45] Empiric antibiotics against community acquired MRSA in uncomplicated cellulitis does not appear to improve outcomes. Moderate nonpurulent cellulitis without signs of hypotension, immune compromise, or rapid deterioration can be treated with intravenous therapy, such as cefazolin or ceftriaxone, whereas severe nonpurulent cellulitis with any of those features require broad-spectrum antibiotic coverage, such as vancomycin and piperacillin-tazobactam, and consideration for surgical evaluation for necrotizing fasciitis.[6]

Given that purulent cellulitis without abscess commonly is caused by *S Aureus*, antibiotic selection is dependent on MRSA suspicion. Although a wound culture and sensitivity can determine the microbial cause, clinicians often need to treat empirically, because cultures can take up to 5 days to result.[46] Mild purulent cellulitis with no MRSA risk factors can be treated similar to nonpurulent cellulitis with oral antibiotics, such as cephalexin or dicloxacillin. Patients with a suspicion for MRSA infection can be treated with oral antibiotics offering MRSA coverage, such as trimethoprim-sulfamethoxazole or doxycycline. Although oral clindamycin has efficacy comparable to trimethoprim-sulfamethoxazole for treating cellulitis,[47] clindamycin generally is not recommended as a first-line agent in patients without a penicillin allergy given the risk for *Clostridioides difficile* infection.[48] The general principles also apply for moderate and severe purulent cellulitis. Moderate purulent cellulitis with low MRSA suspicion can be treated with intravenous oxacillin or cefazolin. If there is a high suspicion for MRSA infection, intravenous vancomycin or clindamycin is preferred. Severe purulent cellulitis warrants broad intravenous antibiotic coverage and evaluation for necrotizing fasciitis. Antibiotic coverage can be narrowed on clinical improvement and wound culture sensitivities.

Purulent cellulitis with a drainable abscess is treated by incision and drainage. 2014 ISDA guidelines do not recommend antibiotics for mild skin abscesses characterized by the presence of a single drainable abscess in patients without signs of systemic infection or immunocompromise.[6] Nonetheless, 2 recent studies have suggested adjuvant MRSA antibiotic therapy in addition to incision and drainage may result in higher cure rates.[49,50] A multicenter randomized controlled trial of 1247 patients presenting to the emergency department with an abscess greater than or equal to 2 cm in diameter determined that adjuvant trimethoprim-sulfamethoxazole resulted in higher cure rates by approximately 7%, lower subsequent surgical procedures rates by 5.2%, and similar rates of adverse effects.[49] Another multicenter randomized controlled trial of 786 patients in the emergency department or outpatient setting with an abscess less than or equal to 5 cm in diameter similarly demonstrated that adjuvant trimethoprim-sulfamethoxazole or clindamycin resulted in higher cure rates by 12.8% and 14.2%, respectively.[50] In this trial, adjuvant clindamycin also had lower rates of recurrent infection within 1 month compared with placebo by 5.4%. Patients receiving clindamycin, however, had an almost 10% higher rate of experiencing adverse effects such as non–*C difficile*–associated diarrhea.[50] A meta-analysis investigating both these studies and 2 additional smaller randomized controlled trials utilizing adjuvant trimethoprim-sulfamethoxazole replicated the key findings. The adjuvant

MRSA antibiotic group had a 7.4% higher rate of cure and 4.4% higher rate of anti-biotic side effects without long-term sequalae.[51] These results imply a modest benefit in treating uncomplicated abscess with incision and drainage and adjuvant MRSA antibiotics. Additional research is necessary to investigate this topic further.

A patient's clinical response dictates the duration of antibiotic therapy. There is a lack of evidence supporting the use of antibiotic treatment of uncomplicated cellulitis for more than 5 days.[52–54] For uncomplicated cellulitis, the authors recommend pre-scribing an initial antibiotic course for 5 days with close follow-up within 2 days to 3 days to ensure appropriate clinical improvement. A lack of improvement may neces-sitate a change in antibiotic coverage or re-evaluation for pseudocellulitis. For immu-nocompromised patients with cellulitis, treatment duration for 7 days to 10 days and up to 14 days is recommended.[6]

Cellulitis can be a challenging diagnosis, and dermatology assessment can be helpful in management. A randomized controlled trial demonstrated that dermatologists iden-tified pseudocellulitis at a rate of 30.7% in patients with presumed cellulitis compared with a rate of 5.7% by the primary team.[35] Early dermatologic consultation improved outcomes in patients with suspected cellulitis by identifying and managing clinical mim-ickers, treating modifiable risk factors predisposing to cellulitis, and decreasing the length of unwarranted antibiotic treatment.[35] Another study in the United Kingdom demonstrated that early dermatology consultation for presumed cellulitis may be a cost-effective intervention by reducing inappropriate antibiotic use and hospitaliza-tion.[34] Similar findings have been replicated in the United States, where dermatology consultation reduced rates of unnecessary antibiotic use by 74.4% and unnecessary hospitalizations by 85.0% in patients with pseudocellulitis, limiting antibiotic exposure in more than 90,000 patients and saving more than $210 million annually.[55] When avail-able, dermatologist input can help improve patient outcomes for cellulitis.

SUMMARY

Cellulitis is a common skin infection that has resulted in increased hospitalizations and costs. Although cellulitis can be challenging to distinguish from its mimickers, a thor-ough clinical examination can narrow the differential diagnosis and guide appropriate management. Antibiotic selection is determined based on clinical presentation, pa-tient risk factors, and the most likely microbial culprit. Dermatologist evaluation of cellulitis has been associated with improved patient outcomes and can help manage this ubiquitous infection. Additional research is necessary to improve the diagnosis and treatment of cellulitis.

CLINICS CARE POINTS

- Cellulitis usually presents unilaterally and common mimickers such as stasis dermatitis can be ruled out due to their bilateral presentation.

- Mild presentations of cellulitis without vital sign abnormalities, a history of immune compromise, and rapid progression of disease or erythema can be treated with oral antibiotics.

- There are no demonstrated improved outcomes when prescribing oral empiric MRSA coverage in addition to Streptococcus and MSSA coverage for nonpurulent cellulitis.

- Dermatology evaluation has been associated with improved diagnosis and outcomes in patients with cellulitis and may be helpful in patients who fail to improve with initial therapy.

DISCLOSURE

The authors have no conflicts of interest to declare.

REFERENCES

1. Hersh AL. National trends in ambulatory visits and antibiotic prescribing for skin and soft-tissue infections. Arch Intern Med 2008;168(14):1585.
2. Goettsch WG, Bouwes Bavinck JN, Herings RM. Burden of illness of bacterial cellulitis and erysipelas of the leg in the Netherlands. J Eur Acad Dermatol Venereol 2006;20(7):834–9.
3. Peterson RA, Polgreen LA, Cavanaugh JE, et al. Increasing incidence, cost, and seasonality in patients hospitalized for cellulitis. Open Forum Infect Dis 2017;4(1): ofx008.
4. Bernard P. Streptococcal cause of erysipelas and cellulitis in adults. Arch Dermatol 1989;125(6):779.
5. Jeng A, Beheshti M, Li J, et al. The role of β-hemolytic streptococci in causing diffuse, nonculturable cellulitis. Medicine 2010;89(4):217–26.
6. Stevens DL, Bisno AL, Chambers HF, et al. Practice guidelines for the diagnosis and management of skin and soft tissue infections: 2014 update by the Infectious Diseases Society of America. Clin Infect Dis 2014;59(2):e10–52.
7. Miller LG, Remington FP, Bayer AS, et al. Clinical and epidemiologic characteristics cannot distinguish community-associated methicillin-resistant staphylococcus aureus infection from methicillin-susceptible s. aureus infection: a prospective investigation. Clin Infect Dis 2007;44(4):471–82.
8. Fridkin SK, Hageman JC, Morrison M, et al. Methicillin-Resistant Staphylococcus aureus disease in three communities. N Engl J Med 2005;352(14):1436–44.
9. Spindel SJ, Strausbaugh LJ, Jacobson C. Infections caused by Staphylococcus aureus in a Veterans' Affairs nursing home care unit: a 5-year experience. Infect Control Hosp Epidemiol 1995;16(4):217–23.
10. Mathews WC, Caperna JC, Barber RE, et al. Incidence of and risk factors for clinically significant methicillin-resistant Staphylococcus aureus infection in a cohort of HIV-infected adults. J Acquir Immune Defic Syndr 2005;40(2):155–60.
11. Jackson KA, Bohm MK, Brooks JT, et al. Invasive methicillin-resistantstaphylococcus aureusinfections among persons who inject drugs — six sites, 2005–2016. MMWR Morb Mortal Wkly Rep 2018;67(22):625–8.
12. Schneider-Lindner V, Delaney JA, Dial S, et al. Antimicrobial drugs and community-acquired methicillin-resistant Staphylococcus aureus,United Kingdom. Emerging Infect Dis 2007;13(7):994–1000.
13. Begier EM, Frenette K, Barrett NL, et al. A high-morbidity outbreak of methicillin-resistant staphylococcus aureus among players on a college football team, facilitated by cosmetic body shaving and turf burns. Clin Infect Dis 2004;39(10): 1446–53.
14. Aiello AE, Lowy FD, Wright LN, et al. Meticillin-resistant Staphylococcus aureus among US prisoners and military personnel: review and recommendations for future studies. Lancet Infect Dis 2006;6(6):335–41.
15. Abrahamian FM, Goldstein EJC. Microbiology of animal bite wound infections. Clin Microbiol Rev 2011;24(2):231–46.
16. Griego RD, Rosen T, Orengo IF, et al. Dog, cat, and human bites: a review. J Am Acad Dermatol 1995;33(6):1019–29.
17. Finkelstein R, Oren I. Soft tissue infections caused by marine bacterial pathogens. Epidemiol Diagn Management 2011;13(5):470–7.

18. Shimizu S, Shimizu H. Cutaneous manifestations ofHelicobacter cinaedi: a review. Br J Dermatol 2016;175(1):62–8.
19. Jorge P, Parada JNM. Clinical syndromes associated with adult pneumococcal cellulitis. Scand J Infect Dis 2000;32(2):133–6.
20. McNamara DR, Tleyjeh IM, Berbari EF, et al. Incidence of lower-extremity cellulitis: a population-based study in Olmsted county, Minnesota. Mayo Clin Proc 2007;82(7):817–21.
21. Quirke M, Ayoub F, McCabe A, et al. Risk factors for nonpurulent leg cellulitis: a systematic review and meta-analysis. Br J Dermatol 2017;177(2):382–94.
22. Raff AB, Kroshinsky D. Cellulitis. JAMA 2016;316(3):325.
23. Lopez M, Roberson ML, Strassle PD, et al. Epidemiology of Lymphedema-related admissions in the United States: 2012–2017. Surg Oncol 2020;35:249–53.
24. Tay EY, Fook-Chong S, Oh CC, et al. Cellulitis Recurrence Score: a tool for predicting recurrence of lower limb cellulitis. J Am Acad Dermatol 2015;72(1):140–5.
25. Gunderson CG, Martinello RA. A systematic review of bacteremias in cellulitis and erysipelas. J Infect 2012;64(2):148–55.
26. Koutkia P, Mylonakis E, Boyce J. Cellulitis: evaluation of possible predisposing factors in hospitalized patients. Diagn Microbiol Infect Dis 1999;34(4):325–7.
27. Kulthanan K, Rongrungruang Y, Siriporn A, et al. Clinical and microbiologic findings in cellulitis in Thai patients. J Med Assoc Thai 1999;82(6):587–92.
28. Lazzarini L, Conti E, Tositti G, et al. Erysipelas and cellulitis: clinical and microbiological spectrum in an Italian tertiary care hospital. J Infect 2005;51(5):383–9.
29. Hirschmann JV, Raugi GJ. Lower limb cellulitis and its mimics. J Am Acad Dermatol 2012;67(2):163.e1–12.
30. Raff AB, Weng QY, Cohen JM, et al. A predictive model for diagnosis of lower extremity cellulitis: A cross-sectional study. J Am Acad Dermatol 2017;76(4):618–25.e2.
31. Strazzula L, Cotliar J, Fox LP, et al. Inpatient dermatology consultation aids diagnosis of cellulitis among hospitalized patients: a multi-institutional analysis. J Am Acad Dermatol 2015;73(1):70–5.
32. Bruun T, Oppegaard O, Hufthammer KO, et al. Early response in cellulitis: a prospective study of dynamics and predictors. Clin Infect Dis 2016;63(8):1034–41.
33. Ko LN, Garza-Mayers AC, St John J, et al. Clinical usefulness of imaging and blood cultures in cellulitis evaluation. JAMA Intern Med 2018;178(7):994.
34. Levell NJ, Wingfield CG, Garioch JJ. Severe lower limb cellulitis is best diagnosed by dermatologists and managed with shared care between primary and secondary care. Br J Dermatol 2011;164(6):1326–8.
35. Ko LN, Garza-Mayers AC, St John J, et al. Effect of dermatology consultation on outcomes for patients with presumed cellulitis. JAMA Dermatol 2018;154(5):529.
36. Sundaresan S, Migden MR, Silapunt S. Stasis dermatitis: pathophysiology, evaluation, and management. Am J Clin Dermatol 2017;18(3):383–90.
37. Clark SC, Zirwas MJ. Management of occupational dermatitis. Dermatol Clin 2009;27(3):365–83, vii-viii.
38. Stevens DL, Bryant AE. Necrotizing Soft-Tissue Infections. New Engl J Med 2017;377(23):2253–65.
39. Wong CH, Khin LW, Heng KS, et al. The LRINEC (Laboratory Risk Indicator for Necrotizing Fasciitis) score: a tool for distinguishing necrotizing fasciitis from other soft tissue infections. Crit Care Med 2004;32(7):1535–41.
40. Fernando SM, Tran A, Cheng W, et al. Necrotizing soft tissue infection: diagnostic accuracy of physical examination, imaging, and LRINEC score: a systematic review and meta-analysis. Ann Surg 2019;269(1):58–65.

41. Bone RC, Balk RA, Cerra FB, et al. Definitions for sepsis and organ failure and guidelines for the use of innovative therapies in Sepsis. Chest 1992;101(6): 1644–55.
42. Singer M, Deutschman CS, Seymour CW, et al. The third international consensus definitions for sepsis and septic shock (Sepsis-3). JAMA 2016;315(8):801.
43. Timothy, Allison, Ellen, et al. Skin and soft-tissue infections requiring hospitalization at an Academic Medical Center: opportunities for antimicrobial stewardship. Clin Infect Dis 2010;51(8):895–903.
44. Pallin DJ, Binder WD, Allen MB, et al. Clinical trial: comparative effectiveness of cephalexin plus trimethoprim-sulfamethoxazole versus cephalexin alone for treatment of uncomplicated cellulitis: a randomized controlled trial. Clin Infect Dis 2013;56(12):1754–62.
45. Moran GJ, Krishnadasan A, Mower WR, et al. Effect of cephalexin plus trimethoprim-sulfamethoxazole vs cephalexin alone on clinical cure of uncomplicated cellulitis. JAMA 2017;317(20):2088.
46. Rioux J, Edwards J, Bresee L, et al. Nasal-swab results for methicillin-resistant staphylococcus aureus and associated infections. Can J Hosp Pharm 2017; 70(2):107–12.
47. Miller LG, Daum RS, Creech CB, et al. Clindamycin versus trimethoprim–sulfamethoxazole for uncomplicated skin infections. N Engl J Med 2015; 372(12):1093–103.
48. Brown KA, Khanafer N, Daneman N, et al. Meta-analysis of antibiotics and the risk of community-associated clostridium difficile infection. Antimicrob Agents Chemother 2013;57(5):2326–32.
49. Talan DA, Mower WR, Krishnadasan A, et al. Trimethoprim–Sulfamethoxazole versus placebo for uncomplicated skin abscess. N Engl J Med 2016;374(9): 823–32.
50. Daum RS, Miller LG, Immergluck L, et al. A placebo-controlled trial of antibiotics for smaller skin abscesses. N Engl J Med 2017;376(26):2545–55.
51. Gottlieb M, Demott JM, Hallock M, et al. Systemic antibiotics for the treatment of skin and soft tissue abscesses: a systematic review and meta-analysis. Ann Emerg Med 2019;73(1):8–16.
52. Cross ELA, Jordan H, Godfrey R, et al. Route and duration of antibiotic therapy in acute cellulitis: a systematic review and meta-analysis of the effectiveness and harms of antibiotic treatment. J Infect 2020;81(4):521–31.
53. Williams OM, Brindle R. Antibiotic route and duration of therapy for cellulitis: data extracted from a multi-center clinical trial. Int J Antimicrob Agents 2020;56(3): 106076.
54. Brindle R, Williams OM, Barton E, et al. Assessment of antibiotic treatment of cellulitis and erysipelas. JAMA Dermatol 2019;155(9):1033.
55. Li DG, Xia FD, Khosravi H, et al. Outcomes of early dermatology consultation for inpatients diagnosed with cellulitis. JAMA Dermatol 2018;154(5):537.
56. Schmutzhard J. Detection of herpes simplex virus type 1, herpes simplex virus type 2 and varicella-zoster virus in skin lesions. Comparison of real-time PCR, nested PCR and virus isolation. J Clin Virol 2004;29(2):120–6.
57. von den Driesch P. Sweet's syndrome (acute febrile neutrophilic dermatosis). J Am Acad Dermatol 1994;31(4):535–56 [quiz 557-60].
58. Lee DH, Park AY, Seo BK, et al. Primary neuroendocrine carcinoma of the breast with clinical features of inflammatory breast carcinoma: a case report and literature. Review 2015;18(4):404.

Diagnosis and Management of Cutaneous Lymphomas Including Cutaneous T-cell Lymphoma

John A. Zic, MD, MMHC

KEYWORDS

- Cutaneous lymphoma • Cutaneous T-cell lymphoma • Mycosis fungoides
- Sézary syndrome • Lymphomatoid papulosis
- Primary cutaneous CD30+ anaplastic lymphoma

KEY POINTS

- The cutaneous lymphomas often mimic the presentation of common skin diseases.
- Most cutaneous lymphomas have an excellent prognosis due to their indolent course.
- Mycosis fungoides, the most common cutaneous lymphoma, usually presents as fixed, asymptomatic patches or plaques in sun-protected areas.
- In children and patients of color, mycosis fungoides often presents as hypopigmented asymptomatic patches in sun-protected areas.
- Some therapies for cutaneous lymphoma have unique side effects.

INTRODUCTION

The cutaneous lymphomas are great mimickers of other skin diseases and, therefore, all physicians should be acquainted with the more common presentations. The skin is the primary organ of involvement in these malignancies of T-cell and B-cell lymphocytes, which separates them from other lymphomas. Fortunately, most cutaneous lymphomas have a good prognosis due to their indolent nature and slow progression. This review introduces the most common variants of the cutaneous lymphomas and their clinical presentations. In addition, unique side effects of therapies used to treat the cutaneous lymphomas will also be highlighted.

Department of Dermatology, VU Cutaneous Lymphoma Clinic, Vanderbilt University Medical Center, Vanderbilt Dermatology, One Hundred Oaks, 719 Thompson Lane, Suite 26300, Nashville, TN 37204-3609, USA
E-mail address: john.zic@vumc.org

Med Clin N Am 105 (2021) 737–755
https://doi.org/10.1016/j.mcna.2021.04.010
0025-7125/21/Published by Elsevier Inc.

medical.theclinics.com

DEFINITIONS

It is important to have a clear understanding of the descriptive terms used in dermatology to accurately diagnose common skin disease and mimickers such as the cutaneous lymphomas.

- Macule: A change in skin color ≤1.0 cm without elevation that is flat and flush with the surrounding skin.
- Patch: A change in skin color greater than 1.0 cm without elevation that is flat and flush with the surrounding skin.
- Papule: An elevated dome-shaped solid lesion ≤1.0 cm.
- Nodule: An elevated dome-shaped solid lesion greater than 1.0 cm that extends deeper into the dermis. Also labeled as a tumor in mycosis fungoides (MF) and Sézary syndrome (SS).
- Mass/tumor: A solid growth much larger than a nodule (usually >3.0 cm). Also labeled as a tumor in MF and SS.
- Plaque: A raised flat-topped solid lesion larger than 1.0 cm occasionally formed from a confluence of papules or nodules. A thick ulcerated plaque is labeled as a tumor in MF and SS.
- Erythroderma: Widespread ill-defined red patches covering more than 80% body surface area.

CUTANEOUS T-CELL LYMPHOMAS

The cutaneous T-cell lymphomas can be separated into 4 major groups: MF and MF variants, CD30 positive lymphoproliferative diseases, SS, and non-MF variants (**Fig. 1**). Prognosis varies widely within each group and by stage of disease. Cutaneous T-cell lymphomas represent more than 80% of all cutaneous lymphomas worldwide.[1]

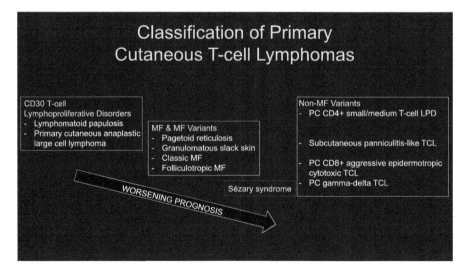

Fig. 1. The cutaneous T-cell lymphomas can be subdivided into 4 groups. SS, PC CD8+ aggressive epidermotropic cytotoxic TCL, and PC gamma-delta TCL have the worst prognoses of the cutaneous T-cell lymphomas. Advanced-stage classic MF and folliculotropic MF both have poor prognoses. LPD, lymphoproliferative disorder; PC, primary cutaneous; TCL, T-cell lymphoma.

Mycosis Fungoides and Mycosis Fungoides Variants

Mycosis fungoides

MF is the most common cutaneous lymphoma with an incidence of approximately 9 to 12 cases per 1,000,000/y. There are estimates of approximately 15,000 patients living with MF in the United States.[2] As with most malignancies, the prognosis varies with stage. Most patients present with fixed asymptomatic patches in sun-protected areas. Many patients ignore the eruption until it progresses or becomes pruritic. On average, patients are diagnosed 1 to 8 years (median 3 years) after the onset of the eruption.[3] Despite this, more than three-quarters of patients have early-stage disease at diagnosis with an excellent prognosis.[4] Patients with the earliest stage, IA, with less than 10% body surface area covered with patches and plaques, have the same life expectancy as patients without the disease.[5] Because patients present with both well-defined and ill-defined patches and plaques, they can mimic the presentation of eczema (ill-defined patches), psoriasis (well-defined plaques, **Fig. 2**), and tinea corporis (well-defined scaly annular patches, **Fig. 3**). Some patients mimic contact dermatitis due to localization in the axillae, on the breasts or buttocks or in the groin. In children and patients of color the most common presentation is scattered hypopigmented patches (**Fig. 4**) that may mimic pityriasis alba and early vitiligo in children and adults, respectively.[6–8] One key to diagnosis is the failure of mid potency topical steroids or antifungal creams to improve the condition. In patients with possible MF, diagnosis is made with multiple skin biopsies from different sites, characteristic skin findings, and occasionally, molecular genetic studies to look for clonal populations of T cells in the biopsy specimens. One caveat of biopsy is that the use of topical corticosteroids can affect the infiltrate observed by the pathologist and if there is suspicion of a T-cell lymphoma, it is preferable to biopsy at a time and site when and where topical corticosteroids have not been used for at least a week. A small percentage of patients progress from patches and plaques to skin tumors (**Fig. 5**) or erythroderma with lymph node and rare visceral organ involvement.[9]

Management of MF varies with stage. Patients are often best managed at regional cutaneous lymphoma clinics using a multidisciplinary approach. Unfortunately, no treatment consistently leads to a clinical cure. Early-stage patients with only patches

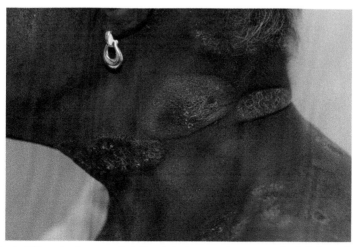

Fig. 2. Classic MF, early stage, well-defined dark gray plaques on the left lateral neck.

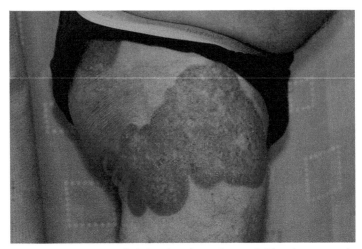

Fig. 3. Classic MF, early stage, well-defined pink patches and thin plaques on the right hip and buttock.

and plaques are treated with skin-directed therapies including ultra-high-potency topical corticosteroids, narrowband ultraviolet B (NBUVB) phototherapy,[10] topical mechlorethamine (also known as nitrogen mustard), topical bexarotene, and/or psoralen and ultraviolet A (PUVA) phototherapy.[11] Skin tumors in patients with advanced-stage MF but no extracutaneous involvement may be treated with localized or total skin electron beam radiotherapy and/or a systemic agent to slow the disease, such as oral bexarotene capsules, vorinostat capsules, and, if necessary, intravenous systemic agents such as brentuximab vedotin, romidepsin, pralatrexate, and others.[12] Advanced-stage patients with lymph node disease or very rare visceral organ involvement require the intravenous systemic agents listed previously for palliation of disease.[13] In young and middle-aged patients with significant extracutaneous disease and few comorbid conditions, allogeneic hematopoietic stem cell transplantation (alloHSCT) may be a viable option.[14]

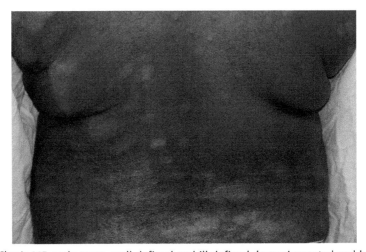

Fig. 4. Classic MF, early stage, well-defined and ill-defined, hypopigmented and hyperpigmented patches on the lower back.

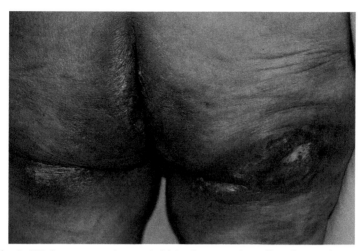

Fig. 5. Classic MF, late stage, ulcerated thick plaque and smaller ulcerated tumor on the right buttock.

Folliculotropic mycosis fungoides

Folliculotropic MF (FMF) is an uncommon variant of MF in which the malignant T cells infiltrate the hair follicle epithelium. Along with the classic patches and plaques of MF, patients with FMF may present with scattered pink patches devoid of hair, clusters of 1-mm to 2-mm follicular-distributed papules, and thick indurated plaques.[15] Unlike classic MF, patients with FMF often present with patches and plaques on the head and neck area (**Fig. 6**). One unusual variant, acneiform FMF, presents with acnelike inflammatory papules on the face that can mimic acne vulgaris and acne rosacea (**Fig. 7**).[16] Once thought to have a uniformly worse prognosis than classic MF, more recent evidence suggests that patients with FMF patches and thin plaques have a much better prognosis than patients with FMF thick plaques and tumors.[17]

Management of FMF varies with stage. Patients are often best managed at regional cutaneous lymphoma clinics using a multidisciplinary approach. Unlike MF, patients with FMF do not respond well to topically applied treatments or NBUVB phototherapy. This is likely due to the deeper infiltrates infiltrating the hair follicle. Unfortunately, no treatment consistently leads to a clinical cure. Early-stage patients with only patches and thin plaques are treated with skin-directed therapies including PUVA phototherapy, localized electron beam radiotherapy, and occasionally oral bexarotene.[18] Skin tumors and thick plaques in patients with more advanced-stage FMF but no extracutaneous involvement may be treated with localized or total skin electron beam radiotherapy and a systemic agent to slow the disease, such as bexarotene capsules, vorinostat capsules, and, if necessary, intravenous systemic agents, such as brentuximab vedotin, romidepsin, pralatrexate, and others. Advanced-stage patients with lymph node disease or very rare visceral organ involvement require intravenous systemic agents and alloHSCT as detailed under management of MF.[18]

Pagetoid reticulosis

Pagetoid reticulosis (PR) is a rare variant of MF that presents on the palms and soles with red plaques or warty nodules mimicking psoriasis,[19] contact dermatitis (**Fig. 8**), dermatophytosis, foot dermatitis,[20] or large verrucae. This variant can be seen in both adults and children and carries a good prognosis.[21]

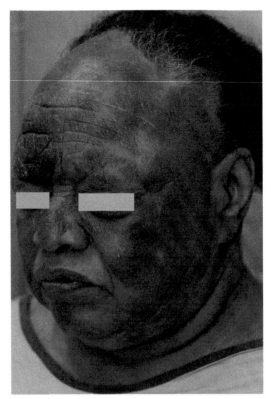

Fig. 6. Folliculotropic MF, ill-defined pink hyperpigmented plaques, milia and loss of eyebrows on the face.

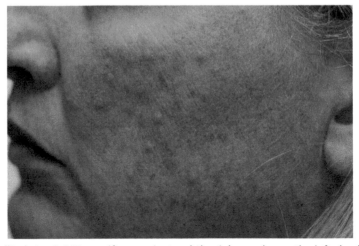

Fig. 7. Folliculotropic MF, acneiform variant, subtle pink papules on the left cheek.

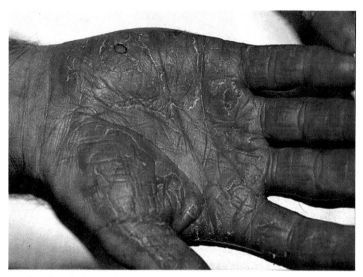

Fig. 8. PR, well-defined pink red plaque on the right palm.

Management of PR will often respond to skin-directed therapy because of its localized nature on the palms and soles. Treatment options include ultra-potent topical steroids, topical mechlorethamine, topical bexarotene, topical tazarotene, hand and foot phototherapy, and localized electron beam radiotherapy.[19]

Granulomatous slack skin
Granulomatous slack skin (GSS) is a rare variant of MF that presents with deep red patches and plaques on the proximal arms and medial thighs, which over time evolve into pendulous skin folds (**Fig. 9**).[22] Some patients are misdiagnosed with cellulitis and treated unsuccessfully with antibiotics. Other cases have been reported to mimic borderline leprosy.[23] Skin biopsies show deep granulomatous inflammation and destruction of elastic fibers that lead to pendulous skin folds. Early studies of patients with GSS suggested an increased risk for Hodgkin lymphoma in up to 25% of patients.[24,25]

Management of GSS is similar to the management of FMF due to the deep nature of the malignant T-cell infiltrate and granulomatous inflammation. Treatment options include PUVA phototherapy and both localized and total skin electron beam radiotherapy.[26]

CD30-Positive Lymphoproliferative Disorders

Lymphomatoid papulosis
Lymphomatoid papulosis (LyP) is one of 2 cutaneous T-cell lymphoma variants characterized by the presence of numerous atypical CD30-positive T cells. LyP presents with crops of 4-mm to 10-mm red papules that may mimic arthropod bites or folliculitis (**Fig. 10**).[27] Unique to LyP, the crops of papules ulcerate before resolving spontaneously within 1 to 2 months.[28] Recurrence is common and variable. Although lymphomatoid papulosis is considered among the most indolent of the cutaneous T-cell lymphomas, it is associated with an increased risk of other lymphomas, such as MF, anaplastic large cell lymphoma, and other non-Hodgkin and Hodgkin lymphomas.[29,30]

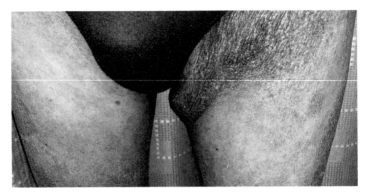

Fig. 9. GSS, pendulous, pink atrophic plaque on the left upper medial thigh.

Because of its indolent course, mild cases of LyP may be observed without treatment. High-potency topical corticosteroids may hasten resolution of inflammatory papules. Most patients with more active disease will respond well to low-dose methotrexate[31] or phototherapy; however, these treatments merely suppress the disease.[32]

Primary cutaneous CD30-positive anaplastic large cell lymphoma

Primary cutaneous CD30-positive anaplastic large cell lymphoma (PCALCL) is the more aggressive CD30-positive lymphoproliferative disorder that presents with 1-cm to 4-cm pink nodules rather than the smaller papules of LyP (**Fig. 11**). In addition, fewer than 25% of patients with PCALCL show spontaneous regression of their nodules. Uncommonly, patients may develop peripheral lymph node involvement.[33] If this occurs early in the disease, it may be difficult to distinguish PCALCL from systemic node-based ALCL.

Fortunately, most patients with PCALCL have an excellent prognosis and are often treated with localized radiotherapy to individual nodules. Patients with more extensive

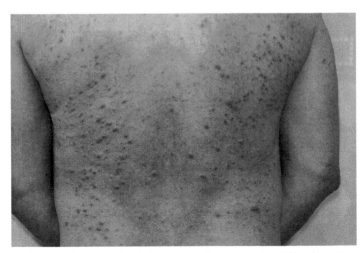

Fig. 10. Lymphomatoid papulosis, pink 3-mm to 6-mm papules diffusely scattered on the back.

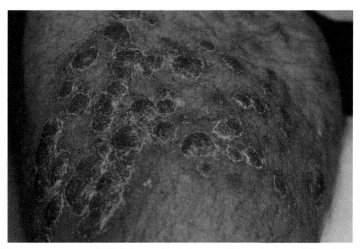

Fig. 11. Primary cutaneous CD30 (+) anaplastic large cell lymphoma, pink red 1-cm to 3-cm nodules on the right anterior thigh.

disease require systemic therapy, such as intermediate-dose methotrexate or brentuximab vedotin, a monoclonal antibody fusion protein targeting the CD30 antigen.[34]

Sézary Syndrome

SS is the second most common variant of the cutaneous T-cell lymphomas. Often referred to as the leukemic variant of cutaneous T-cell lymphoma (CTCL), SS is characterized by erythroderma (**Fig. 12**) and significant blood involvement with malignant T cells.[35] Patients suffer with intense itching and occasional skin pain. It is not unusual for patients to develop bulky peripheral adenopathy. This advanced CTCL has a poor prognosis with a median survival of less than 5 years.[36] In patients with a history of heart disease, erythroderma may lead to high-output cardiac failure. SS is one of many causes of erythroderma. Other causes of erythroderma include drugs, psoriasis, atopic eczema, pityriasis rubra pilaris, graft-versus-host disease, internal malignancy, and crusted scabies. Skin biopsies in patients with SS are often nondiagnostic because of the presence of significant inflammation. The diagnosis is made via flow cytometry of peripheral blood to identify large atypical T-cell populations expressing CD4+CD7- and/or CD4+CD26- immunophenotypes. Lymph node biopsies also may be helpful in establishing the diagnosis.

Because of its more aggressive course, patients with SS are treated with systemic therapies including photopheresis plus low-dose subcutaneous interferon, mogamulizumab infusions, and/or romidepsin infusions.[37,38]

Non–Mycosis Fungoides Variants

Primary cutaneous small-medium pleomorphic T-cell lymphoproliferative disorder
Primary cutaneous small-medium pleomorphic T-cell lymphoproliferative disorder is an uncommon variant of CTCL that usually presents with a solitary pink nodule of less than 6 months' duration. When it occurs in sun-exposed areas, it may mimic nonmelanoma skin cancers such as basal cell carcinoma, Merkel cell carcinoma, or extra digital glomus tumors. Recurrence is uncommon, and treatment options include intralesional steroids, localized radiotherapy, and simple excision.[39]

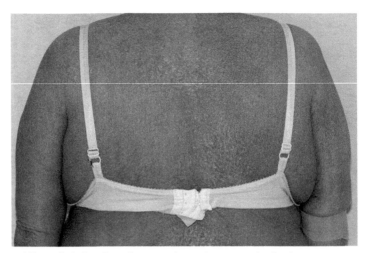

Fig. 12. SS, diffuse ill-defined confluent scaly erythema on the back.

Subcutaneous panniculitis-like T-cell lymphoma

Subcutaneous panniculitis-like T-cell lymphoma (SPTL) is an uncommon variant of CTCL that presents with slightly tender subcutaneous and slightly exophytic nodules often on the extremities (**Fig. 13**). This presentation can mimic other types of panniculitis including erythema nodosum and lupus erythematosus panniculitis. In contrast to other types of panniculitis, deep skin biopsies of SPTL usually show CD8+ atypical lymphocytes rimming adipocytes. Distinguishing SPTL from lupus panniculitis can be a clinical and pathologic challenge.[40] The prognosis is favorable with rare extracutaneous progression and uncommon hemophagocytic syndrome.[41] Unlike other forms of CTCL, patients with SPTL respond to oral anti-inflammatory agents such as prednisone, methotrexate, bexarotene, and cyclosporine.[42]

Primary cutaneous gamma-delta T-cell lymphoma

Primary cutaneous gamma-delta T-cell lymphoma (PCGDTCL) is a rare aggressive variant of CTCL.[43] Patients may present with several different primary skin lesions, such as purplish patches, plaques, nodules, and subcutaneous tumors.[44] Skin biopsies show atypical T-cell infiltrates composed of gamma-delta T cells rather than the more common alpha-beta T cells.[44] Prognosis is poor with median survival of 1 to 2 years and a higher risk of hemophagocytic syndrome than patients with SPTL from which it must be distinguished. Because of its more worrisome course, patients with PCGDTCL are treated with aggressive systemic therapies, such as brentuximab vedotin and other anticancer agents in preparation for alloHSCT.[45,46]

Primary cutaneous aggressive CD8+ epidermotropic T-cell lymphoma

Primary cutaneous aggressive CD8+ epidermotropic T-cell lymphoma (PCAETCL) is a rare aggressive variant of CTCL. Patients often present with rapidly progressive disease characterized by psoriasislike plaques (**Fig. 14**) to punched-out ulcerations on the trunk and extremities causing significant pain.[47] Patients show brief periods of stable disease between cycles of traditional systemic chemotherapy. Occasionally, classic MF will show a CD8+ predominant phenotype rather than the usual CD4+ predominant phenotype. Such patients should be watched closely for evidence of rapidly progressive disease.[48]

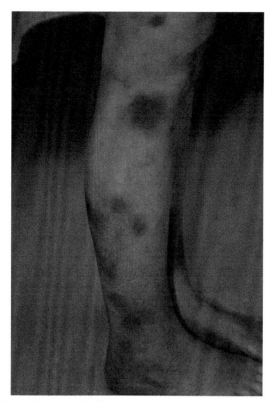

Fig. 13. SPTL, tender, pink to purple, firm subcutaneous plaques and nodules on the lower legs.

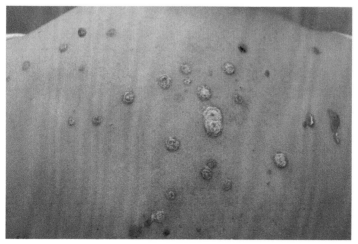

Fig. 14. Primary cutaneous aggressive CD8(+) epidermotropic T-cell lymphoma, well-defined pink plaques with psoriasislike thick scale on the upper back.

CUTANEOUS B-CELL LYMPHOMAS
Primary Cutaneous Follicle Center Cell Lymphoma

Primary cutaneous follicle center cell lymphoma (PCFCCL) is an indolent B-cell lymphoma in which the skin is the primary organ of involvement. PCFCCL often presents as 1 or 2 pink to purple small nodules on the head (**Fig. 15**). A solitary nodule may mimic a nonmelanoma skin cancer such as basal cell carcinoma or Merkel cell tumor. Because it may be difficult to distinguish PCFCCL from a metastasis to the skin from node-based follicle center cell lymphoma, imaging studies are indicated to rule out node-based disease.[49] The prognosis is excellent with uncommon relapse after skin-directed radiotherapy.[50]

Primary Cutaneous Marginal Zone Lymphoma

Primary cutaneous marginal zone lymphoma (PCMZL) is an indolent B-cell lymphoma where the skin is the primary organ of involvement. PCMZL often presents as multiple pink papules to small pink nodules on the extremities and trunk where they can mimic basal cell carcinomas and arthropod bites (**Fig. 16**).[51] Imaging studies are indicated to rule out node base disease. Unlike PCFCCL, relapse is common in PCMZL. Despite this, the prognosis is excellent. Management often involves observation, occasionally topical or intralesional steroids, localized radiotherapy, and less commonly intralesional or systemic rituximab.[52]

Primary Cutaneous Large B-cell Lymphoma, Leg Type

Primary cutaneous large B-cell lymphoma, leg type (PCLBLL) is the most aggressive subtype of the cutaneous B-cell lymphomas. The classic presentation is seen in elderly individuals (>70 years old) in whom tender pink to purple nodules and masses develop on one or both lower extremities over a period of less than 12 to 24 months (**Fig. 17**). The initial nodules may mimic erythema nodosum, Kaposi sarcoma, or an infectious nodule.[53,54] Most patients will respond to rituximab + CHOP chemotherapy followed by localized electron beam radiotherapy.[38] However, relapses are common and some patients go on to develop regional lymphadenopathy.[55]

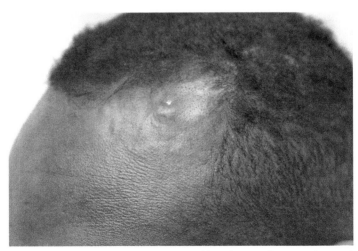

Fig. 15. Primary cutaneous follicle center cell B-cell lymphoma, alopecia, clustered pink nodules and plaques on the left frontal hairline.

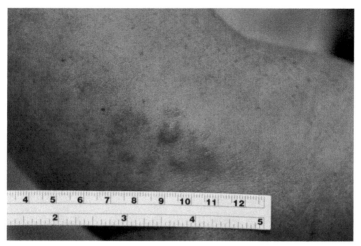

Fig. 16. Primary cutaneous marginal zone B-cell lymphoma, clustered pink papules and thin plaques on the right lateral elbow.

UNIQUE SIDE EFFECTS TO THERAPIES FOR CUTANEOUS LYMPHOMA
Contact Dermatitis Due to Topical Mechlorethamine

Mechlorethamine (nitrogen mustard) is an alkylating agent used topically to treat early stages of MF. Depending on the vehicle, allergic contact dermatitis may develop in 10% to 25% of patients.[56] Occasionally, the increased pruritic erythema is mistaken for progressive disease prior to the diagnosis of allergic contact dermatitis to mechlorethamine.[57] The allergic contact dermatitis may require a slow prednisone taper or high-potency topical steroids for resolution.

Central Hypothyroidism Due to Bexarotene Capsules

Bexarotene is a unique retinoid that binds to the RXR receptor. The oral capsules are used to treat refractory early-stage and advanced-stage MF and other variants of CTCL. Bexarotene induces central hypothyroidism in most patients. Laboratory studies showing low thyroid-stimulating hormone and low free T4 levels establish the diagnosis. Patients may complain of cold intolerance and fatigue, which may be attributed to other causes. Occasionally, physicians may misinterpret the low thyroid-stimulating hormone level as an indication to lower thyroid supplementation doses. Once central hypothyroidism is established there is no need to monitor thyroid-stimulating hormone levels but rather, only free T4 levels.[58,59]

Hyperlipidemia Due to Bexarotene Capsules

Bexarotene, like most oral retinoids, may lead to hyperlipidemia. The hyperlipidemia induced by bexarotene is usually much more severe than induced by other oral retinoids such as isotretinoin or acitretin. Specifically, patients may develop marked hypertriglyceridemia, elevated low-density lipoprotein (LDL) levels and low high-density lipoprotein levels. The hypertriglyceridemia may be managed with omega-3 fatty acid fish oil capsules and other agents such as fenofibrate.[60] The elevated LDL levels may be managed with statins, though bexarotene may reduce levels of statins through induction of CYP3A4.[61] Occasionally, dose reduction of bexarotene is necessary to improve the hyperlipidemia to less worrisome levels.

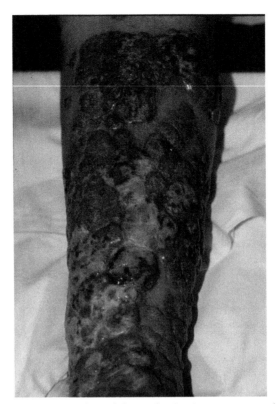

Fig. 17. PCLBLL, diffuse pink purple nodules coalescing into masses on the left shin.

Peripheral Neuropathy Due to Intravenous Brentuximab Vedotin

Brentuximab vedotin is a monoclonal antibody to the CD30 antigen coupled with a spindle cell inhibitor, vedotin. The drug is administered intravenously every 3 weeks to manage advanced cutaneous T-cell lymphoma including those cases with peripheral adenopathy, bulky skin tumors, and refractory PCALCL. More than 60% of patients will develop peripheral sensory neuropathy of the fingers and toes that will

Table 1 CTCLs: The great imitators	
Cutaneous Lymphoma	**May Resemble....**
Classic MF	Eczema, psoriasis, tinea corporis
Folliculotropic MF	Eczema, acne
Pagetoid reticulosis	Warts, hand dermatitis
Granulomatous slack skin	Cellulitis
Subcutaneous Panniculitislike TCL	Erythema nodosum
PC gamma-delta TCL	Eczema, psoriasis
PC CD4+ small/medium T-cell LPD	Basal cell carcinoma

Abbreviations: CTCLs, cutaneous T-cell lymphomas; LPD, lymphoproliferative disorder; MF, mycosis fungoides; PC, primary cutaneous; TCL, T-cell lymphoma.

start with paresthesias and may progress to numbness.[62,63] Fortunately, most patients will have improvement after stopping the drug, but a minority will have permanent neurologic impairment.

SUMMARY

Patients with cutaneous lymphoma often present with skin manifestations mimicking other more common skin diseases. See **Table 1**. It is important for physicians who treat common skin diseases to be aware of the cutaneous lymphomas, especially when patients fail standard therapy for common skin diseases, such as eczema, psoriasis, or tinea corporis. Although most patients with cutaneous lymphoma have a good prognosis, a small minority of patients may progress and die of the disease.

CLINICS CARE POINTS

- Consider MF in any patient with a chronic asymptomatic eruption of patches and plaques in sun-protected areas.
- Consider MF in children or patients of color who present with scattered hypopigmented patches in sun-protected areas.
- Consider SS in any patient with an evolving erythroderma, especially with palpable lymphadenopathy.
- Evaluate patients with erythroderma via flow cytometry of peripheral blood to look for abnormal populations of T cells.
- Expand your differential diagnosis of subcutaneous nodules to include SPTL and PCGDTCL.
- Consider the diagnosis of the indolent cutaneous B-cell lymphomas (PCFCCL and PCMZL) in patients that present with pink to purple nodules on the skin.
- Before embarking on an expensive work-up for newly diagnosed central hypothyroidism consider bexarotene-induced central hypothyroidism.
- Patients on bexarotene capsules will often require aggressive lipid-lowering management.
- Patients on brentuximab require careful monitoring for progressive peripheral sensory neuropathy.

DISCLOSURE

The author has no disclosures to report.

REFERENCES

1. Dobos G, Pohrt A, Ram-Wolff C, et al. Epidemiology of cutaneous T-Cell lymphomas: a systematic review and meta-analysis of 16,953 patients. Cancers (Basel) 2020;12(10):2921.
2. Pujol RM, Gallardo F. Cutaneous Lymphomas - Part I: mycosis fungoides, sezary syndrome, and CD30(+) cutaneous lymphoproliferative disorders. Actas Dermosifiliogr 2021;112(1):14–23.
3. Scarisbrick JJ, Quaglino P, Prince HM, et al. The PROCLIPI international registry of early-stage mycosis fungoides identifies substantial diagnostic delay in most patients. Br J Dermatol 2019;181(2):350–7.
4. Maguire A, Puelles J, Raboisson P, et al. Early-stage mycosis fungoides: epidemiology and prognosis. Acta Derm Venereol 2020;100(1):adv00013.

5. Kim YH, Jensen RA, Watanabe GL, et al. Clinical stage IA (limited patch and plaque) mycosis fungoides. A long-term outcome analysis. Arch Dermatol 1996; 132(11):1309–13.

6. Hodak E, Amitay-Laish I, Feinmesser M, et al. Juvenile mycosis fungoides: cutaneous T-cell lymphoma with frequent follicular involvement. J Am Acad Dermatol 2014;70(6):993–1001.

7. Valencia Ocampo OJ, Julio L, Zapata V, et al. Mycosis fungoides in children and adolescents: a series of 23 cases. Actas Dermosifiliogr 2020;111(2):149–56.

8. Geller S, Lebowitz E, Pulitzer MP, et al. Outcomes and prognostic factors in African American and black patients with mycosis fungoides/Sezary syndrome: retrospective analysis of 157 patients from a referral cancer center. J Am Acad Dermatol 2020;83(2):430–9.

9. Quaglino P, Pimpinelli N, Berti E, et al. Time course, clinical pathways, and long-term hazards risk trends of disease progression in patients with classic mycosis fungoides: a multicenter, retrospective follow-up study from the Italian Group of Cutaneous Lymphomas. Cancer 2012;118(23):5830–9.

10. Marka A, Carter JB. Phototherapy for cutaneous T-Cell lymphoma. Dermatol Clin 2020;38(1):127–35.

11. Quaglino P, Prince HM, Cowan R, et al. Treatment of early-stage mycosis fungoides: results from the PROspective Cutaneous Lymphoma International Study (PROCLIPI study). Br J Dermatol 2021;184(4):722–30.

12. Patrawala SA, Broussard KC, Wang L, et al. Tumor stage mycosis fungoides: a single-center study on clinicopathologic features, treatments, and patient outcome. Dermatol Online J 2016;22(5). 13030/qt1q15b903.

13. Quaglino P, Maule M, Prince HM, et al. Global patterns of care in advanced stage mycosis fungoides/Sezary syndrome: a multicenter retrospective follow-up study from the Cutaneous Lymphoma International Consortium. Ann Oncol 2017; 28(10):2517–25.

14. Dumont M, Peffault de Latour R, Ram-Wolff C, et al. Allogeneic Hematopoietic Stem Cell Transplantation in Cutaneous T-Cell Lymphomas. Cancers (Basel) 2020;12(10):2856.

15. Malveira MIB, Pascoal G, Gamonal SBL, et al. Folliculotropic mycosis fungoides: challenging clinical, histopathological and immunohistochemical diagnosis. An Bras Dermatol 2017;92(5 Suppl 1):73–5.

16. Shamim H, Riemer C, Weenig R, et al. Acneiform presentations of folliculotropic mycosis fungoides. Am J Dermatopathol 2021;43(2):85–92.

17. van Santen S, Jansen PM, Quint KD, et al. Plaque stage folliculotropic mycosis fungoides: histopathologic features and prognostic factors in a series of 40 patients. J Cutan Pathol 2020;47(3):241–50.

18. Kalay Yildizhan I, Sanli H, Akay BN, et al. Folliculotropic mycosis fungoides: Clinical characteristics, treatments, and long-term outcomes of 53 patients in a tertiary hospital. Dermatol Ther 2020;33(4):e13585.

19. Wang SC, Mistry N. Woringer-Kolopp disease mimicking psoriasis. CMAJ 2015; 187(17):1310.

20. Yao Y, Mark LA. Woringer-Kolopp disease mimicking foot dermatitis. Cutis 2012; 90(6):307–9, 316.

21. Corbeddu M, Ferreli C, Pilloni L, et al. Pagetoid reticulosis (Woringer-Kolopp disease) in a 2-year-old girl-Case report and review of the literature. JAAD Case Rep 2019;5(1):104–7.

22. Swoboda R, Kaminska-Winciorek G, Wesolowski M, et al. Granulomatous slack skin variant of mycosis fungoides: clinical and dermoscopic follow-up of a very rare entity. Dermatol Ther 2021;34(2):e14822.
23. Pratchyapruit W, Vashrangsi N, Tagami H. Granulomatous slack skin clinically and histologically masquerading as borderline leprosy in its early stages. Eur J Dermatol 2009;19(1):88–9.
24. Noto G, Pravata G, Miceli S, et al. Granulomatous slack skin: report of a case associated with Hodgkin's disease and a review of the literature. Br J Dermatol 1994;131(2):275–9.
25. Carton de Tournai D, Deschamps L, Laly P, et al. [Granulomatous slack skin associated with metastatic testicular seminoma]. Ann Dermatol Venereol 2017; 144(6–7):446–9.
26. Vakeva L, Kovanen PE, Pulliainen L, et al. Granulomatous slack skin: an unusual variant of cutaneous T-cell lymphoma. Int J Dermatol 2017;56(1):29–31.
27. Verheyden MJ, Venning VL, Khurana S, et al. Follicular lymphomatoid papulosis - not a simple folliculitis. Australas J Dermatol 2020. https://doi.org/10.1111/ajd. 13493.
28. Sica A, Vitiello P, Sorriento A, et al. Lymphomatoid papulosis. Minerva Med 2020; 111(2):166–72.
29. Melchers RC, Willemze R, Bekkenk MW, et al. Frequency and prognosis of associated malignancies in 504 patients with lymphomatoid papulosis. J Eur Acad Dermatol Venereol 2020;34(2):260–6.
30. Molgo M, Espinoza-Benavides L, Rojas P, et al. Mycosis Fungoides, Lymphomatoid Papulosis and Hodgkin's lymphoma in the same patient: apropos of a possible monoclonal origin. Indian J Dermatol 2020;65(1):57–60.
31. Bruijn MS, Horvath B, van Voorst Vader PC, et al. Recommendations for treatment of lymphomatoid papulosis with methotrexate: a report from the Dutch Cutaneous Lymphoma Group. Br J Dermatol 2015;173(5):1319–22.
32. Fernandez-de-Misa R, Hernandez-Machin B, Servitje O, et al. First-line treatment in lymphomatoid papulosis: a retrospective multicentre study. Clin Exp Dermatol 2018;43(2):137–43.
33. Di Raimondo C, Parekh V, Song JY, et al. Primary cutaneous CD30+ lymphoproliferative disorders: a comprehensive review. Curr hematologic malignancy Rep 2020;15(4):333–42.
34. Enos TH, Feigenbaum LS, Wickless HW. Brentuximab vedotin in CD30(+) primary cutaneous T-cell lymphomas: a review and analysis of existing data. Int J Dermatol 2017;56(12):1400–5.
35. Illingworth A, Johansson U, Huang S, et al. International guidelines for the flow cytometric evaluation of peripheral blood for suspected Sezary syndrome or mycosis fungoides: assay development/optimization, validation, and ongoing quality monitors. Cytometry 2021;100:156–82.
36. Scarisbrick JJ. Survival in mycosis fungoides and sezary syndrome: how can we predict outcome? J Invest Dermatol 2020;140(2):281–3.
37. Olsen EA, Rook AH, Zic J, et al. Sezary syndrome: immunopathogenesis, literature review of therapeutic options, and recommendations for therapy by the United States Cutaneous Lymphoma Consortium (USCLC). J Am Acad Dermatol 2011;64(2):352–404.
38. Mehta-Shah N, Horwitz SM, Ansell S, et al. NCCN guidelines insights: primary cutaneous lymphomas, version 2.2020. J Natl Compr Canc Netw 2020;18(5): 522–36.

39. Surmanowicz P, Doherty S, Sivanand A, et al. The clinical spectrum of primary cutaneous CD4+ small/medium-sized pleomorphic T-cell lymphoproliferative disorder: an updated systematic literature review and case series. Dermatology 2020;1–11. https://doi.org/10.1159/000511473.
40. Arps DP, Patel RM. Lupus profundus (panniculitis): a potential mimic of subcutaneous panniculitis-like T-cell lymphoma. Arch Pathol Lab Med 2013;137(9): 1211–5.
41. Khemani UN, Pardeshi SS. Treatment considerations in case of subcutaneous panniculitis like T cell lymphoma with hemophagocytic syndrome. Dermatol Ther 2021;34(2):e14742.
42. Lopez-Lerma I, Penate Y, Gallardo F, et al. Subcutaneous panniculitis-like T-cell lymphoma: clinical features, therapeutic approach, and outcome in a case series of 16 patients. J Am Acad Dermatol 2018;79(5):892–8.
43. Goyal A, Goyal K, Bohjanen K, et al. Epidemiology of primary cutaneous gamma-delta T-cell lymphoma and subcutaneous panniculitis-like T-cell lymphoma in the U.S.A. from 2006 to 2015: a Surveillance, Epidemiology, and End Results-18 analysis. Br J Dermatol 2019;181(4):848–50.
44. Guitart J, Weisenburger DD, Subtil A, et al. Cutaneous gammadelta T-cell lymphomas: a spectrum of presentations with overlap with other cytotoxic lymphomas. Am J Surg Pathol 2012;36(11):1656–65.
45. Lastrucci I, Grandi V, Gozzini A, et al. Complete remission with brentuximab vedotin in a case of primary cutaneous gamma-delta T-cell lymphoma relapsed after allogeneic stem cell transplantation. Int J Dermatol 2021;60:778–80.
46. Isufi I, Seropian S, Gowda L, et al. Outcomes for allogeneic stem cell transplantation in refractory mycosis fungoides and primary cutaneous gamma Delta T cell lymphomas. Leuk Lymphoma 2020;61(12):2955–61.
47. Onsun N, Dizman D, Emiroglu N, et al. Challenges in early diagnosis of primary cutaneous CD8+ aggressive epidermotropic cytotoxic T-cell lymphoma: a case series of four patients. Eur J Dermatol 2020;30(4):358–61.
48. Jaque A, Mereniuk A, Walsh S, et al. Influence of the phenotype on mycosis fungoides prognosis, a retrospective cohort study of 160 patients. Int J Dermatol 2019;58(8):933–9.
49. Guinard E, Alenezi F, Lamant L, et al. Staging of primary cutaneous follicle centre B-cell lymphoma: bone marrow biopsy, CD10, BCL2 and t(14;18) are not relevant prognostic factors. Eur J Dermatol 2019. https://doi.org/10.1684/ejd.2018.3489.
50. Oertel M, Elsayad K, Weishaupt C, et al. De-escalated radiotherapy for indolent primary cutaneous B-cell lymphoma. Strahlenther Onkol 2020;196(2):126–31.
51. Gibson SE, Swerdlow SH. How i diagnose primary cutaneous marginal zone lymphoma. Am J Clin Pathol 2020;154(4):428–49.
52. Porkert S, Mai P, Jonak C, et al. Long-term therapeutic success of intravenous rituximab in 26 patients with indolent primary cutaneous B-cell Lymphoma. Acta Derm Venereol 2021;101(2):adv00383.
53. Ibrahim S, Jain A, Pai K. A case of false identity: primary cutaneous diffuse large B-cell lymphoma masquerading as Madura Foot. Trop Doct 2021. https://doi.org/10.1177/0049475521991339.
54. Long V, Liang MW, Lee JSS, et al. Two instructive cases of primary cutaneous diffuse large B-cell lymphoma (leg type) mimicking cellulitis and sporotrichosis. JAAD Case Rep 2020;6(9):815–8.
55. Sumida H, Sugaya M, Miyagaki T, et al. Frequent relapse and irradiation strategy in primary cutaneous diffuse large B-cell lymphoma, leg-type. Acta Derm Venereol 2013;93(1):97–8.

56. Liner K, Brown C, McGirt LY. Clinical potential of mechlorethamine gel for the topical treatment of mycosis fungoides-type cutaneous T-cell lymphoma: a review on current efficacy and safety data. Drug Des Devel Ther 2018;12:241–54.

57. Gilmore ES, Alexander-Savino CV, Chung CG, et al. Evaluation and management of patients with early-stage mycosis fungoides who interrupt or discontinue topical mechlorethamine gel because of dermatitis. JAAD Case Rep 2020;6(9): 878–81.

58. Pattan V, Schaab K, Sundaresh V. Bexarotene: a rare cause of misleading thyroid function tests. Cureus 2020;12(11):e11591.

59. Makita N, Manaka K, Sato J, et al. Bexarotene-induced hypothyroidism: characteristics and therapeutic strategies. Clin Endocrinol 2019;91(1):195–200.

60. Cabello I, Servitje O, Corbella X, et al. Omega-3 fatty acids as adjunctive treatment for bexarotene-induced hypertriglyceridaemia in patients with cutaneous T-cell lymphoma. Clin Exp Dermatol 2017;42(3):276–81.

61. Wakelee HA, Takimoto CH, Lopez-Anaya A, et al. The effect of bexarotene on atorvastatin pharmacokinetics: results from a phase I trial of bexarotene plus chemotherapy in patients with advanced non-small cell lung cancer. Cancer Chemother Pharmacol 2012;69(2):563–71.

62. Gao S, Zhang M, Wu K, et al. Risk of adverse events in lymphoma patients treated with brentuximab vedotin: a systematic review and meta-analysis. Expert Opin Drug Saf 2020;19(5):617–23.

63. Fargeot G, Dupel-Pottier C, Stephant M, et al. Brentuximab vedotin treatment associated with acute and chronic inflammatory demyelinating polyradiculo-neuropathies. J Neurol Neurosurg Psychiatry 2020;91(7):786–8.

Recognition and Management of Cutaneous Connective Tissue Diseases

Kylee J.B. Kus, BS[a,b], Avery H. LaChance, MD, MPH[c,*],
Ruth Ann Vleugels, MD, MPH, MBA[d,*]

KEYWORDS

- Lupus erythematosus • Discoid lupus erythematosus
- Subacute cutaneous lupus erythematosus • Dermatomyositis
- Clinically amyopathic dermatomyositis • Systemic sclerosis • Scleroderma
- Vasculitis

KEY POINTS

- Cutaneous manifestations may be an early indication of underlying connective tissue disease, prompting crucial work-up.
- It is critical to screen patients with connective tissue disease for possible systemic involvement and, in some cases, malignancy because early detection and management can improve outcomes.
- Management of connective tissue diseases frequently entails systemic pharmacotherapy with associated risks and need for monitoring, and comorbidities should be taken into consideration when determining the particular treatment modality.

INTRODUCTION

Connective tissue diseases (CTDs) present with an expansive range of diverse clinical signs and symptoms, often posing a challenge to achieve an accurate and timely diagnosis. The multisystem involvement and variable disease course of CTDs are often best suited for interdisciplinary care. Frequently, patients with CTD initially present to internists or primary care physicians, providing a crucial opportunity for early

Funding Sources: None.

Conflicts of Interest: None declared.

[a] Department of Dermatology, Brigham and Women's Hospital, Harvard Medical School, 221 Longwood Avenue, Boston, MA 02115, USA; [b] Oakland University William Beaumont School of Medicine, 586 Pioneer Drive, Rochester, MI 48309-4482, USA; [c] Connective Tissue Disease Clinic, Department of Dermatology, Brigham and Women's Hospital, Harvard Medical School, 221 Longwood Avenue, Boston, MA 02115, USA; [d] Autoimmune Skin Disease Program, Department of Dermatology, Brigham and Women's Hospital, Harvard Medical School, 221 Longwood Avenue, Boston, MA 02115, USA

* Corresponding authors and Co-senior authors.

E-mail addresses: alachance@bwh.harvard.edu (A.H.L.); rvleugels@bwh.harvard.edu (R.A.V.)

https://doi.org/10.1016/j.mcna.2021.04.011
medical.theclinics.com

detection, thus facilitating appropriate diagnosis, management, and improved prognosis.[1] In this article, we provide an overview of the cutaneous findings of and most salient details pertinent to the diagnosis and work-up of lupus erythematosus (LE), dermatomyositis (DM), systemic sclerosis (SSc), and vasculitis.

LUPUS ERYTHEMATOSUS

LE is an autoimmune disease with a broad spectrum of clinical symptoms, ranging from skin-limited disease to severe systemic involvement. The pathogenesis of LE is not fully elucidated; however, current theories suggest LE has a multifactorial cause that encompasses polygenic genetic susceptibility, autoimmune induction, and immune system damage.[2] Cutaneous LE (CLE) and systemic LE (SLE) can occur together or separately, with CLE occurring two to three times more frequently than SLE. The incidence of CLE is estimated to be approximately 4.3 cases per 100,000 persons in the United States with a female to male ratio of 3:1 and an average age of diagnosis around 54 years.[3,4] SLE is more common in Asian and Black patients than in white patients and more frequently affects women than men across all ages and ethnic groups.[5,6]

Diagnosis

Subsets of CLE are defined by clinical symptoms, duration of symptoms, and histologic findings. The LE-specific cutaneous manifestations are divided into three major subtypes including: acute CLE (ACLE), subacute CLE (SCLE), and chronic CLE (CCLE), with discoid LE (DLE) being the most common form of CCLE.[2,7] Importantly, different types of CLE are associated with varying levels of risk of development of SLE over the course of a patient's lifetime. Recognizing the different cutaneous manifestations of lupus and their likelihood of being associated with SLE is key to helping guide diagnosis, work-up, counseling, and management.

ACLE typically presents during the third decade of life and is almost invariably associated with SLE.[8,9] Approximately 95% of patients with ACLE are antinuclear antibody (ANA) positive, and anti-dsDNA and anti-Smith antibodies are common.[10]

There are localized and generalized forms of ACLE, with localized disease being more common. The localized form is characterized by the pathognomonic malar rash or "butterfly" erythema that extends over the bilateral malar cheeks and nasal bridge with striking sparing of the nasolabial folds. The eruption is classically sun-induced.[11,12] The differential diagnosis includes erysipelas; DM; acne/rosacea; drug-induced phototoxic reactions; and contact, atopic, and seborrheic dermatitis.[11] Of note, malar rashes are reported in up to 52% of patients with SLE at the time of diagnosis, and clinical activity of the malar rash often parallels that of the systemic disease.[13] The generalized form of ACLE is typically characterized by widespread erythematous macules and papules. Lesions may appear more prominently in a photodistributed pattern. The differential diagnosis of generalized ACLE is broad, however, and includes viral exanthems.

SCLE is reported most frequently in young to middle aged white women.[12] Approximately 15% to 20% of patients with SCLE have lesions consistent with another type of CLE, and nearly 50% of patients with SCLE fulfill the American College of Rheumatology (ACR) criteria for SLE, but rarely develop severe systemic disease. Approximately 60% to 80% of patients with SCLE are ANA positive, 70% display the anti-Ro/SSA antibody, and 30% to 50% exhibit the anti-La/SSB antibody, frequently overlapping with the anti-Ro/SSA antibody.[14]

Patients with SCLE are exquisitely photosensitive, and lesions mainly appear on sun-exposed areas (**Fig. 1**).[12,14] The two morphologic variants of SCLE are annular

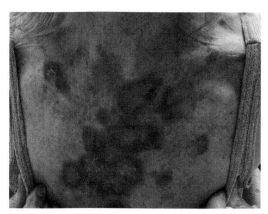

Fig. 1. Subacute cutaneous lupus erythematosus.

and papulosquamous. The annular type is characterized by annular erythematous to violaceous plaques or papules, which may coalesce into a widespread polycyclic pattern, often with a fine superimposed trailing scale.[12] The papulosquamous form may resemble psoriasis, most classically, or even lichen planus, eczema, or pityriasis rosea.[15] Lesions heal without scarring, but often cause long-lasting postinflammatory pigmentary changes.[14,16]

Several drugs have been implicated as triggers for SCLE, referred to as drug-induced SCLE. A case-control study concluded that more than one-third of SCLE cases could be attributed to exposure to drugs, such as terbinafine, tumor necrosis factor-α inhibitors, antiepileptics, and proton pump inhibitors, among many others.[17] Drug-induced SCLE is reversible and often resolves clinically within 1 to 3 months following withdrawal of the inciting drug. For suspected SCLE diagnoses, it is important to thoroughly review medical history for drugs initiated in the weeks to months leading up to symptom onset, particularly given that drug-induced cases cannot be distinguished from idiopathic cases based on antibodies or skin biopsy.[18]

CCLE encompasses DLE, LE panniculitis (LEP), chilblain LE, and LE tumidus. DLE is the most common subtype of CCLE, occurring more frequently in women during the fourth and fifth decade of life.[12] Approximately 5% to 10% of patients with localized disease and 25% of patients with disseminated disease develop SLE.[19,20] Akin to SCLE, DLE is notably photosensitive. DLE has a predilection for the head and neck and can also prominently affect mucosal surfaces.[21,22] Serologically, patients with DLE have a positive ANA in approximately one-third of cases.

Localized disease is characterized by lesions above the neck, predominantly located on the scalp and ears, and is observed in 60% to 80% of patients with DLE (**Fig. 2**). Generalized disease involves lesions above and below the neck and affects 20% to 40% of patients with DLE.[21,23] Lesions begin as erythematosus to violaceous macules or papules with scale that gradually expand peripherally into larger plaques that heal with atrophic scars and pigmentary changes. Given that the inflammation in DLE extends from the epidermis to the middermis and extends around the cutaneous adnexa, including the hair follicles, there is a high risk for scarring alopecia without prompt recognition and treatment.[2,7]

The histologic features of CLE include vacuolar interface dermatitis and mucin deposition. In DLE specifically, there may be thickening of the basement membrane and follicular plugging.

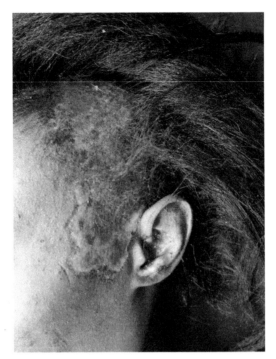

Fig. 2. Discoid lupus erythematosus.

LEP is an uncommon panniculitis featuring firm, painful subcutaneous nodules, some of which have overlying DLE. Over time, previous areas of inflammation develop substantial contour change or depressions in the skin, resulting in cosmetic disfigurement in many patients. LEP is primarily located on areas with increased fat deposition including the cheeks, breasts, upper arms, thighs, and buttocks. Ultraviolet exposure seems to have minimal influence in this subset. The disease course of LEP is chronic, with alternating remission and flares. Histologically, LEP displays lobular panniculitis with a dense lymphocytic infiltrate. Lesions can resemble subcutaneous lymphoma, emphasizing the importance of biopsy and, occasionally, T-cell markers and gene rearrangements to determine the diagnosis.[24]

Chilblain LE lesions are painful, erythematous to violaceous papules and plaques presenting in cold-exposed areas, most classically the feet and hands. Typically, a history of cold-exposure is elicited; however, in some patients with more severe disease, lesions are present year-round.

LE tumidus is characterized by severe photosensitivity and a tendency to occur in men. Lesions are erythematous, edematous, annular plaques that lack associated scale, predominantly located on the face and other photodistributed locations. Histologically these lesions demonstrate dense perivascular and periadnexal infiltrate, but lack the typical interface dermatitis seen in ACLE, SCLE, and DLE.

Classification of SLE is complex because of the lack of universal, uniform criteria. Two major classification systems are the Systemic Lupus International Collaborating Clinics 2012 criteria and the joint European League Against Rheumatism and ACR 2019 criteria (**Table 1**). A study comparing the two systems observed that they detect nonoverlapping patients, suggesting a combination should be used to maximize the capture and representation of patients.[25]

Table 1
Comparison of SLICC 2012 criteria and the joint EULAR/ACR 2019 criteria for SLE

	SLICC 2012[a]	EULAR/ACR 2019[b]
Authors	52	64
Patients	1392	2218
Entry criterion	None	Positive ANA
Clinical criteria (weight)	Acute cutaneous lupus Chronic cutaneous lupus Oral/nasal ulcers Nonscarring alopecia Synovitis 2+ joints Serositis Renal Neurologic Hemolytic anemia Leukopenia (<4000/mm^3) Thrombocytopenia (<100,000/mm^3)	Constitutional Fever (2) Hematologic Leukopenia (3) Thrombocytopenia (4) Autoimmune hemolysis (4) Neuropsychiatric Delirium (2) Psychosis (3) Seizure (5) Mucocutaneous Nonscarring alopecia (2) Oral ulcers (2) Subacute cutaneous or discoid lupus (6) Acute cutaneous lupus (6) Serosal Pleural/pericardial effusion (5) Acute pericarditis (6) Musculoskeletal Joint involvement (6) Renal Proteinuria >0.5 g/24 h (4) Renal biopsy class II or V lupus nephritis (8) Renal biopsy class III or IV lupus nephritis (10)
Immunologic criteria (weight)	ANA Anti-DNA Anti-Sm Antiphospholipid Ab Low complement (C3, C4, CH50) Direct Coombs test in the absence of hemolytic anemia	Antiphospholipid antibodies Anticardiolipin (2) Anti-β2GP1 (2) Lupus anticoagulant (2) Complement proteins Low C3 or low C4 (3) Low C4 and low C4 (4) SLE-specific antibodies Anti-dsDNA (6) Anti-Smith (6)

Abbreviations: EULAR/ACR, European League Against Rheumatism and American College of Rheumatology; SLICC, Systemic Lupus International Collaborating Clinics.
[a] SLICC classification for SLE requires fulfillment of 4+ criteria, including at least one clinical and one immunologic criterion. Biopsy-proven lupus nephritis in the presence of ANA or anti-dsDNA can also be classified as SLE.
[b] EULAR/ACR classification for SLE requires fulfillment of 1+ clinical criterion and ≥10 points. Only the highest weighted criteria from each domain is counted toward the total score.

Cutaneous involvement is common in patients with SLE, with more than 80% exhibiting skin findings during their disease course. For 20% to 25% of patients diagnosed with SLE, cutaneous symptoms were the first manifestation of SLE.[13,26,27] During the first 3 years following a diagnosis of CLE, 18% of patients are diagnosed with SLE, and

24% of patients diagnosed with CLE have a prior SLE diagnosis.[4] A study of 260 patients with SLE found LE-specific cutaneous manifestations in 23% of patients and LE-nonspecific cutaneous manifestations in 43% of patients. The most common LE-specific findings were DLE (11%), SCLE (8%), and ACLE (4%), whereas the most common LE-nonspecific features were Raynaud phenomenon (RP; 25%), non-scarring alopecia (9%), and vasculitis (8%).[28]

Work-Up

To properly diagnose and treat CLE, it is critical to correctly recognize and diagnose the presenting disease subtype and subsequently perform a work-up for underlying systemic involvement (**Table 2**). Diagnosis and disease classification should be determined by findings in the patient history, physical examination, laboratory studies, serology, and histology. In most cases clinical and histologic findings are adequate to make a diagnosis. Efforts should be made to avoid solely relying on ACR criteria for diagnosis, because these were designed for clinical trial purposes and may miss a subset of patients with disease.[2]

Detailed skin examination and careful assessment of disease morphology is essential to identifying the CLE subtype. Blood tests, such as complete blood count with differential (CBC), are used to evaluate for cytopenias, which may raise suspicion for SLE. Serum creatinine, blood urea nitrogen, and urinalysis are also important in screening for renal disease. Antibody studies are another integral part of classifying disease. Testing should begin with an ANA screen, with a negative ANA being rare for patients with SLE, and a positive ANA being observed in one-to two-thirds of patients with CLE with or without systemic disease.[2] Of note, a positive ANA is seen in up to 35% of normal individuals at a 1:40 dilution, particularly in elderly persons. Hence, routine ordering of ANA without a reasonable suspicion for CTD should be avoided.[29] Additional autoantibody profiling may yield positives for dsDNA, Sm, or ribosomal P, which are highly specific for SLE. Patients with SLE may also be positive for autoantibodies to Ro, La, U1RNP, and ssDNA, but these are not disease-specific.[2]

When morphology is unclear, lesional skin biopsy is extremely helpful for CLE diagnosis because it distinguishes CLE from nearly all skin mimickers other than DM.

Table 2 Recommended work-up for patients with cutaneous lupus erythematosus	
Medical history	Associated symptoms Family history
Physical examination	Total body skin examination Disease morphology Anatomic location
Assessment of skin disease	Biopsy of lesion with histopathologic evaluation Direct immunofluorescence for some cases
Routine studies	Complete blood count, comprehensive metabolic panel, urinalysis Renal function: serum creatinine, blood urea nitrogen
Additional studies	Antinuclear antibody Autoantibody profile: anti-dsDNA, anti-Sm, anti-ribosomal P, anti-Ro, anti-La, anti-U1RNP, antihistone, anti-ssDNA Complement levels (C3 and C4)

Improved serum lupus serologies have essentially made the lupus band test all but obsolete for aiding SLE diagnosis.[13] The lupus band test is occasionally used in patients with CLE, but false-positives are known to occur in sun-damaged skin and routine use is not common.

Goals of Management

Currently, CLE is managed, but not cured. Patient education, smoking cessation, topical and systemic therapies, and avoidance of triggers, such as sun exposure and culprit medications, should all be considered pillars of disease management.[2,7] Treatment of CLE is similar across subsets, consisting of strict sun protection, smoking cessation, local therapy with topical corticosteroids or calcineurin inhibitors, and, often, antimalarials.[30] Antimalarials are considered to be the first-line systemic agent, with hydroxychloroquine being the drug of choice. Antimalarials often require 2 to 3 months to reach maximum efficacy.[2] Many cases, particularly those that are extensive or refractory, require additional systemic treatment. For cases recalcitrant to antimalarials, methotrexate, mycophenolate mofetil (MMF), thalidomide, lenalidomide, oral retinoids, azathioprine, dapsone, or rituximab, among other options is considered, weighing the benefits and potential adverse effects in a particular patient.[7,30]

The management of SLE should aim to enhance long-term survival, prevent organ damage, and optimize health-related quality of life by controlling disease activity and minimizing adverse effects of drug toxicity. Lifestyle habits, such as smoking cessation, physical activity, and vitamin D supplementation, have been shown to reduce cardiovascular risk and improve fatigue and mental health.[31–33] Similar to CLE treatment, antimalarials are the cornerstone of SLE therapy with alternatives consisting of MMF, azathioprine, cyclophosphamide, cyclosporine A, tacrolimus, rituximab, and belimumab, among others. Systemic glucocorticoids are used to achieve acute control of SLE and are often used in lower doses longer term, but use should be minimized as much as possible with the use of steroid-sparing agents. Multiple ongoing studies are evaluating novel therapeutic options for SLE.

DERMATOMYOSITIS

DM is a rare inflammatory disease characterized by distinct cutaneous features and varying degrees of systemic involvement. It is more commonly observed in adults older than the age of 40 but can occur at any age. Juvenile DM (JDM) impacts children, with a peak incidence between ages 5 and 12.[34] DM affects both genders and all ethnic groups, but it is more common in women and African Americans.[35] The pathogenetic factors of DM are complex, and encompass genetic predisposition, environmental stressors, and immune- and nonimmune-mediated mechanisms.[36] Adult patients with DM have an increased risk of concomitant malignancy, stressing the importance of early and accurate diagnosis of DM so that patients can undergo timely screening for cancer.[37]

Diagnosis

Because of the diverse array of presentations and phenotypes, DM is challenging to diagnose. Most patients with DM are diagnosed with classic DM (CDM), which presents with a combination of distinct cutaneous findings and progressive, symmetric, proximal muscle weakness. The myopathy is often painless with an acute or subacute onset. A smaller portion of patients are diagnosed with clinically amyopathic DM, which presents with similar cutaneous findings but lacks the muscle involvement observed in CDM. The clinically amyopathic DM diagnosis encompasses patients who are amyopathic, lacking clinical or laboratory evidence of muscle disease, or hypomyopathic, demonstrating subclinical evidence of myositis on electrophysiologic, laboratory, or radiologic evaluation despite the absence of clinical symptoms.[37] In more than half of patients with DM, skin manifestations precede muscle involvement by months or years, underscoring their utility in achieving a timely diagnosis.[36] Patients may present with one or multiple DM-associated skin findings. Cutaneous features may be categorized as pathognomonic, characteristic, less common, rare, and nonspecific.[34,35]

Pathognomonic findings include Gottron papules, Gottron sign, and the heliotrope eruption. Gottron papules are characterized by pink-violaceous papules or plaques on the dorsal hands, often found overlying the metacarpophalangeal and interphalangeal joints (**Fig. 3**). They may have associated scale and tend to leave dyspigmentation, atrophy, or scarring on resolution. Gottron sign is defined by erythematous or violaceous macules or papules overlying the extensor surfaces of the elbows, knees, or other joints. The heliotrope eruption consists of a pink to violaceous eruption, with or without concomitant edema, that most often affects the upper eyelids, but can also affect the lower eyelids.[34-36]

Characteristic features include midfacial erythema, nailfold changes, shawl or V-sign, scalp involvement, and holster sign. Patients with DM frequently have midfacial erythema involving the nasolabial folds. This is helpful in distinguishing the facial erythema of DM from the malar rash of SLE, which classically spares the nasolabial folds. Typical nailfold abnormalities include periungual telangiectasias, characterized by dilated and tortuous nailfold capillaries, with associated dystrophic cuticles and small hemorrhagic infarcts (**Fig. 4**). The shawl sign refers to photodistributed poikiloderma, consisting of hyperpigmentation and hypopigmentation, telangiectasia, and superficial atrophy, overlying the upper back, whereas the V-sign represents similar findings on the upper chest. The holster sign is characterized by poikiloderma of the lateral thighs and is highly characteristic of DM. Scalp involvement is characterized by pink to violaceous erythema, poikiloderma, and associated scaling, often with nonscarring hair loss. It is often misdiagnosed as seborrheic dermatitis or psoriasis.[35-37]

Less common findings include calcinosis cutis; cutaneous vasculitis; and vesiculobullous, necrotic, or ulcerative lesions. Calcinosis cutis refers to calcified deposits in the skin and subcutaneous tissues, and is more common in JDM, affecting adult

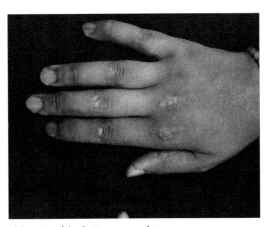

Fig. 3. Dermatomyositis, atrophic Gottron papules.

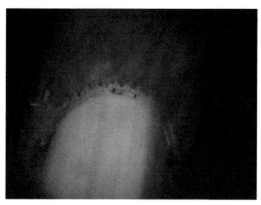

Fig. 4. Dermatomyositis, nailfold capillary change, and microhemorrhage.

patients less frequently. Cutaneous vasculitis may include petechial macules, palpable purpura, or cutaneous ulceration, and is more common in patients with JDM. Ulcerative lesions generally develop on extensor surfaces of joints, over the Gottron papules, or on the lateral nailfolds, and on sun-exposed areas, such as the anterior chest. Skin ulceration may be associated with malignancy or interstitial lung disease (ILD).[34,36,38]

There are a variety of rare manifestations of cutaneous DM, including flagellate erythema, follicular hyperkeratosis, panniculitis, mucinosis, erythroderma, oral mucosal changes, and mechanic's hands. Mechanic's hands refer to hyperkeratotic, scaly, or fissured plaques on the lateral or ventral fingers or palms and are most commonly seen as part of the antisynthetase syndrome, which is characterized by ILD, myositis, polyarthritis, fever, and RP.[34,35,39,40] RP, photosensitivity, and pruritus are considered nonspecific findings, but are common in patients with DM.[34–36]

Aside from the skin manifestations and muscle involvement, DM can also present with a constellation of systemic findings. Clinicians should be aware of the risk of potential ILD, arthralgia with or without arthritis, esophageal involvement (often presenting as dysphagia or gastroesophageal reflux), and myocarditis, among other systemic features.[34] Patients with DM also have an increased risk of malignancy. Studies support that approximately 10% to 25% of patients with DM have an associated cancer, depending on the cohort. One study found that 6.8% of patients in their DM cohort had an undiagnosed malignancy at the time of DM diagnosis and that 59% of these cancers were asymptomatic, suggesting that timely diagnosis of DM can substantially impact patient outcomes.[41]

Work-Up

Initial evaluation should include a total body skin examination, assessment of muscle strength, laboratory testing, and clinical history taking (**Table 3**). Serum muscle enzymes including creatine kinase, lactate dehydrogenase, aspartate aminotransferase, alanine aminotransferase, and aldolase should be measured. Of note, creatine kinase is normal in some patients with DM and elevated in patients who do not have DM.[42] Cases that remain ambiguous may benefit from skin or muscle biopsy, T2-weighted MRI of the bilateral thighs with a myositis protocol, or electromyography.[43] Additionally, creatine kinase elevations are seen in patients following exercise. Myositis-specific antibodies (MSAs) are antibodies distinctly associated with an idiopathic inflammatory myopathy diagnosis and various clinical features. MSAs

Table 3
Recommended work-up for patients with dermatomyositis

Medical history	Prior malignancy Associated symptoms Occupational and recreational exposures, toxins, infections, travel, vaccinations, substance use
Physical examination	Total body skin examination Women: pelvic and breast examination Men: rectal and prostate examination

Assessment of muscle
    involvement
	Serum muscle enzymes: creatinine kinase, aldolase,
	    lactate dehydrogenase, aspartate aminotransferase,
	    alanine aminotransferase
	Electromyography
	Muscle tissue biopsy
	MRI

Assessment of skin disease	Biopsy of lesion with histopathologic evaluation Immunofluorescence
Routine studies	Complete blood count, comprehensive metabolic panel, urinalysis Thyroid function tests Electrocardiogram Fasting glucose and lipids (pediatric patients)
Screening for malignancy	Stool occult blood testing, colonoscopy Gastrointestinal endoscopy Cancer antigen 19-9 Women: Papanicolaou smear, cancer antigen 125

Imaging	Chest radiograph, possible
	    high-resolution computed
	    tomography of the chest
	Computed tomography scan of chest,
	    abdomen, and pelvis
	Women: pelvic ultrasound, mammography

Pulmonary
    evaluation
	Pulmonary function tests with diffusion
	    capacity studies

Esophageal evaluation	Barium swallow, manometry, cineradiography

Additional studies	Echocardiogram
	Autoantibody profile: anti-Mi2, anti-MDA5,
	    aanti-NXP2/anti-MJ, anti-TIF1γ, anti-SAE,
	    among others
	Holter monitor
	Esophagogastroduodenoscopy in Asian patients

unique to DM include anti-Mi2, antimelanoma differentiation-associated protein 5 (MDA5), anti-NXP2 (also known as anti-MJ), antitranscription intermediary factor-1-gamma (TIF1γ), and anti-small ubiquitin-like modifier activating enzyme (SAE), among others. Although these antibodies can guide management and help prognosticate patients with DM, they are not routinely used for diagnosis at this time, particularly given that many laboratories do not have reliable testing for MSAs.[44–46]

Once the diagnosis of DM is confirmed, patients should be evaluated to identify potential systemic manifestations. All patients with DM should be screened for ILD using pulmonary function tests with diffusion capacity of carbon monoxide.

A high-resolution chest computed tomography (CT) with ILD protocol is indicated for patients with symptoms suggestive of ILD or asymptomatic patients with decreased diffusion capacity or restrictive physiology demonstrated on pulmonary function testing. If ILD is absent on initial assessment, patients are monitored clinically with repeat testing if new or worsening pulmonary symptoms arise or if their clinical presentation or MSA subtype (eg, MDA5, which carries a high risk of associated ILD) suggests more frequent screening. Patients with ILD should undergo urgent pulmonary evaluation and require specific therapies.[47] Further assessment for systemic involvement should be guided by the patient's targeted review of symptoms and, potentially, their MSA profile.[48]

Adult patients with DM should also undergo work-up for malignancy because of the increased risk of cancer, particularly within 3 years of diagnosis. Patients with JDM need a full physical examination, but do not require further evaluation for malignancy because cancer risk is not considered to be elevated in this population. No standard guidelines for malignancy screening in adult patients with DM currently exist. Experts often agree that reasonable testing should include CT of the chest, abdomen, and pelvis and a full physical examination and age-appropriate cancer screenings. Many also suggest a transvaginal pelvic ultrasound, mammography, and Papanicolaou smear in women. Tumor markers including cancer antigen 125 and cancer antigen 19-9 are used in some centers. Consideration is given to colonoscopy if age-appropriate. In patients from Southeast Asia, an esophagogastroduodenoscopy is recommended given an increased risk of nasopharyngeal carcinoma. Similar to assessment for systemic involvement, MSA profiles may aid in consideration of the likelihood of malignancy risk; however, at this time, all adult patients should undergo cancer screening. Age is the strongest predictor of malignancy in patients with DM, with older patients more at risk than younger. The ideal reimaging interval for high-risk patients who initially have a negative work-up for malignancy has yet to be established, although many centers consider screening annually for 3 years from the initiation of clinical symptoms to be adequate.[48,49]

Goals of Management

DM manifestations can vary greatly among patients necessitating individualized therapeutic plans based on the presence and severity of muscle disease, extent of systemic involvement, presence of malignancy, existing comorbidities, and disease impact on the patient's quality of life. Cutaneous aspects of DM are often chronic, debilitating, refractory to therapy, and negatively impact quality of life. Management of skin disease in DM aims to control symptoms and address associated pruritus, photosensitivity, and appearance of skin lesions. Initial therapy should incorporate aggressive photoprotection to prevent cutaneous flares; bland emollients to minimize xerosis; antipruritic agents; and topical anti-inflammatory medications, such as corticosteroids or calcineurin inhibitors. In nearly all patients, treatment of cutaneous DM often involves systemic medications including antimalarials, methotrexate, MMF, and/or intravenous immunoglobulin (IVIG), among others.[37] Antimalarials are useful for their photoprotective and anti-inflammatory properties, but cause a drug eruption in one-third of patients with DM.[37,50] Selection of systemic agents should be shaped by other DM manifestations, such as myositis and pulmonary involvement and patient comorbidities.

Regarding the active muscle disease of DM, systemic corticosteroids are first-line therapy; however, their adverse side effect profile limits their long-term utility, and they should always be paired with a corticosteroid-sparing agent. Such medications as methotrexate, MMF, azathioprine, IVIG, and rituximab are frequently used corticosteroid-sparing agents for DM muscle disease.[34] Corticosteroids should be administered at higher doses until muscle disease is dormant, and then slowly tapered over several months according to improvement in clinical examination and reduction in muscle enzyme levels. Intravenous pulse methylprednisolone may be used in cases of severe muscle disease or involvement of internal organs.[36] Patients with CDM should also be recommended to have physical therapy because multiple trials have demonstrated enhanced muscle strength and improved functional outcomes with the use of exercise and rehabilitation, including during periods of active muscle disease.[51,52]

SYSTEMIC SCLEROSIS

SSc is a complex multisystem autoimmune CTD characterized by diffuse vasculopathy and immune dysregulation, which ultimately results in chronic and progressive fibrosis of the skin and internal organs. It occurs more frequently in women, with age of onset peaking in the fifth decade of life.[53] The exact cause of SSc is yet to be elucidated but is thought to result from environmental triggers in genetically predisposed hosts. Disease pathogenesis involves endothelial cell dysfunction leading to immune activation, inflammation, and subsequent tissue fibrosis.[54] Although the pathogenesis is thought to be similar across the disease spectrum, disease phenotype and degree of different organ involvement can vary substantially between patients.[55]

Diagnosis

Initial presenting signs of SSc can be subtle and may include puffy and swollen fingers or hands, distal skin tightening, fatigue, RP, or gastroesophageal reflux. Thus, keeping a high index of suspicion for SSc in patients who present with new-onset RP and puffy fingers or hands later in life is key to allow for early diagnosis. Nailfold changes are often present and can help confirm the clinical diagnosis. Some patients present early with systemic organ involvement, such as pulmonary fibrosis, pulmonary arterial hypertension (PAH), renal complications, or severe gastrointestinal symptoms; however, these may also develop later in the disease course.[56]

The ACR and 2013 European League Against Rheumatism classification criteria is a useful tool in helping to guide SSc diagnosis (**Table 4**). Candidate items are clustered and arranged in a multicriteria additive point system with a threshold to classify cases as SSc. Item clusters include skin thickening, fingertip lesions, telangiectasia, abnormal nailfold capillaries, pulmonary involvement, RP, and various SSc-related autoantibodies.[57] Given the predominance of cutaneous features in these criteria, conducting a thorough skin examination for patients with suspected SSc is essential. However, these criteria were designed for research purposes, and not all patients with SSc meet these criteria.

Subsets of SSc are distinguished by differing clinical features and antibodies.[56] Diffuse cutaneous SSc (dcSSc) tends to have an aggressive course, characterized by induration and cutaneous sclerosis that extends proximal to elbows or knees (frequently extending onto the trunk), and is often associated with prominent internal organ fibrosis. Cutaneous fibrosis in patients with dcSSc can result in joint contractures and lead to significant impairment in mobility. Additionally, renal crisis, cardiac complications, and pulmonary fibrosis are more common in patients with dcSSc.[58]

Limited cutaneous SSc (lcSSc) is classically associated with a slower disease course and cutaneous sclerosis limited to the extremities distal to the elbow and knees. Many patients with lcSSc present with symptoms consistent with CREST syndrome, characterized by calcinosis, RP, esophageal dysmotility, sclerodactyly, and

Table 4 Overview of weighted items from the 2013 American College of Rheumatology and European League against Rheumatism classification criteria for systemic sclerosis	
Items and Subitems	**Score[a]**
Skin thickening of fingers of both hands (extending proximal to MCP joints)	9

Skin thickening of the fingers
  Puffy fingers
  Sclerodactyly of the fingers
    (distal to MCP joints but
    proximal to PIP joints)
	-
	2
	4

Fingertip lesions
  Digital tip ulcers
  Fingertip pitting scars
	-
	2
	3

Telangiectasia	2
Abnormal nailfold capillaries	2

Pulmonary arterial hypertension or
  interstitial lung disease
  Pulmonary arterial hypertension
  Interstitial lung disease
	-
	2
	2

Raynaud phenomenon	3

SSc-related autoantibodies
  Anticentromere
  Antitopoisomerase I
  Anti-RNA polymerase III
	-
	3
	3
	3

Abbreviations: MCP, metacarpophalangeal; PIP, proximal interphalangeal.

[a]The total score is the sum of the maximum scores from each category. A patient with a score ≥ 9 is classified as having systemic sclerosis.

Data from: Van Den Hoogen F, Khanna D, Fransen J, et al. 2013 classification criteria for systemic sclerosis: An American College of Rheumatology/European League Against Rheumatism collaborative initiative. *Ann Rheum Dis.* 2013;72(11):1747-1755.[57]

matt telangiectasia. Although patients with lcSSc traditionally are considered to have higher risk for PAH than pulmonary fibrosis, they can develop both. Systemic sclerosis sine scleroderma is often considered to be a part of the lcSSc spectrum.[58] These cases often present with gastrointestinal dysmotility and/or PAH.

Characteristic cutaneous findings commonly seen in patients with both disease subtypes include dilated nailfold capillaries, sclerosis of the distal digits, matt telangiectasias, dyspigmentation, and facial involvement leading to microstomia (**Fig. 5**). Diffuse pruritus is commonly reported in patients with SSc and can have a major impact on quality of life. Hand function in patients with either subtype is impacted by progressive sclerodactyly from skin induration and digital ulcers in the setting of refractory RP, with the potential for tissue loss and distal gangrene (**Fig. 6**).[56]

SSc overlap syndromes consist of combinations of SSc with clinical signs of various CTDs, particularly polymyositis, DM, rheumatoid arthritis, Sjögren syndrome, or SLE.[58]

Work-Up

Appropriate screening strategies aid timely recognition of internal complications and initiation of therapies to cease progression.[53] Initial work-up should include an in-depth clinical history and physical examination with attention to cutaneous findings

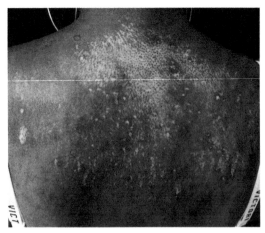

Fig. 5. Systemic sclerosis, salt and pepper dyspigmentation.

and musculoskeletal involvement. Evaluation of skin involvement paired with assessment of serologic status has shown to reliably predict clinical outcome and prognosis.[59]

Detection of ANA is an instrumental part of SSc work-up and is achieved through a variety of laboratory methods; however, indirect immunofluorescence is considered the gold standard method for the screening of ANA, and most autoantibodies clinically relevant to SSc. There are three main ANA staining patterns seen in patients with SSc: (1) centromere, (2) speckled, and (3) nucleolar. The centromere pattern is indicative of anticentromere antibodies, which are associated with lcSSc. The speckled pattern is more commonly seen in patients with antitopoisomerase I (anti-Scl-70) and anti-RNA polymerase III antibodies, the two most common autoantibodies in patients with dcSSc. Importantly, patients with anti-RNA polymerase III have been found to be at greater risk for severe renal involvement and underlying malignancy.[60] Therefore, detection of anti-RNA polymerase III in any patient with SSc should prompt close monitoring of renal involvement and a careful review of systems to evaluate for

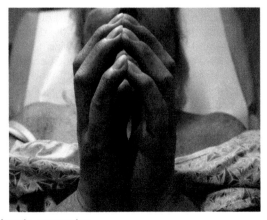

Fig. 6. Systemic sclerosis, prayer sign.

symptoms to suggest underlying malignancy. A speckled ANA can also be seen along with several less common antibodies, such as anti-U11/U12 RNP, anti-Ku, anti-U1 RNP, and anti-RuvBL1/2. The nucleolar pattern often accompanies the presence of anti-U3 RNP, anti-Th/To, anti-NOR 90, and anti-PM/Scl. Antibodies are usually detected at disease onset and are unlikely to change over the course of disease.[58]

Baseline evaluation is critical to identifying any underlying organ involvement.[56] Routine pulmonary function testing with measurement of diffusing capacity for carbon monoxide is commonly advised at baseline and every 6 months during the first several years of follow-up to screen for ILD.[61] High-resolution CT of the lungs with an ILD protocol is used if abnormalities are found on pulmonary function testing or routinely in some centers. Echocardiography is recommended yearly to screen for early evidence of PAH. Right heart catheterization may be used to confirm PAH in select cases. For gastrointestinal evaluation, investigations should be symptom-based, and most commonly include barium swallows and gastric-emptying studies.[56] Because of the risk of scleroderma renal crisis (SRC), patients are encouraged to monitor their blood pressure regularly and have creatinine clearance and urinalysis assessed at regular intervals. Investigation for possible associated malignancy may also be appropriate in cases that raise clinical suspicion, including in cases with recent weight loss, concerning review of symptoms, older age of onset, or the presence of RNA polymerase III antibodies.[56]

Goals of Management

Management of SSc should take into consideration the classification of SSc, disease duration and severity, and presence of any clinical features that overlap with another CTD. There are currently no established standard of care guidelines for the treatment of SSc, and therapy is usually tailored on the presence of organ involvement and, more recently, autoantibody and molecular gene expression profiles.[56]

SSc-ILD can range from mild and self-limiting to rapidly progressive. Large clinical trials have supported the use of cyclophosphamide or MMF as treatment options, with MMF being the safer of the two.[62] In these trials, MMF also demonstrated efficacy for cutaneous sclerosis in SSc, and many centers of excellence use MMF first-line in most patients with SSc given its demonstrated benefit in skin and lung disease. Although the efficacy of rituximab for SSc-ILD has mixed supportive evidence with some studies observing stabilized lung function, whereas others have found no significant improvement, it is also used for SSc-ILD in many centers.[63] Rituximab can also help cutaneous sclerosis in some patients. IVIG and tocilizumab have also demonstrated benefit for cutaneous sclerosis in SSc.[64–66] Additionally, it is crucial for patients with cutaneous sclerosis to participate in occupational and physical therapy to improve and maintain mobility, particularly hand mobility.[67,68] Antifibrotic treatment can improve microstomia and there are limited data to support the use of hyaluronidase injections for local treatment.[69] Pruritis is another common symptom in patients with SSc. In general, improved cutaneous sclerosis can decrease symptoms of itch as shown in a small cohort of patients, which demonstrated improvement of SSc-related pruritus in patients treated with rituximab.[70]

SSc-PAH is often characterized by rapid progression and poor prognosis, necessitating aggressive treatment. The combination of an endothelin receptor antagonist plus a phosphodiesterase 5 inhibitor has shown to reduce the risk of a clinical failure event by 50% compared with monotherapies.[71] This combination has also demonstrated improved right and left ventricle function in SSc-PAH.[72] In patients with less severe disease, a phosphodiesterase 5 inhibitor is often used as monotherapy.

The prognosis of SRC has remained poor because of lack of tangible improvement with available treatment options. Angiotensin-converting enzyme inhibitors are the mainstay of treatment once a definite diagnosis is made, but there is a lack of consistent evidence to support the use of angiotensin-converting enzyme inhibitors as a prophylactic measure before SRC involvement. In contrast, there is some evidence suggesting the prevalent use vasodilators in SSc may have contributed to the decline of SRC incidence in the last few decades.[63]

For articular and muscular involvement in patients with overlap disease, methotrexate remains a frequently used agent. IVIg can also be considered in patients with associated myositis, exhibiting significant reduction of creatine phosphokinase levels in patients with SSc.[73] Biologics used for other inflammatory articular diseases have yielded observational data in patients with SSc but lack randomized controlled trials.[63]

Treatment of gastrointestinal involvement heavily relies on proton-pump inhibitors, antacids, and prokinetics despite the lack of evidence-based data.[63] Weight loss and malnutrition are additional manifestations to consider, and in severe cases, enteral or parenteral feeding supplementations may be indicated.[74]

Recent randomized controlled trials in SSc have shifted focus to small molecules and biologics including abatacept, nintedanib, riociguat, and tocilizumab among others. Hematopoietic stem cell transplantation has also been examined as a possible disease-modifying approach for patients with early and rapidly progressive dcSSc and evident organ involvement.[63]

Patients with SSc nearly all suffer from RP, which is often severe in patients with SSc and can result in digital ulcers, gangrene, and tissue loss. First-line treatments include calcium channel blockers and/or sildenafil.[75] Other therapeutic agents include aspirin, selective serotonin reuptake inhibitors, α-blockers, and angiotensin II receptor blockades.[76] RP and digital ulcers have also been demonstrated to improve with botulinum toxin.[77]

CUTANEOUS VASCULITIS

Vasculitis is the inflammation and resultant compromise or destruction of the blood vessel wall leading to a broad spectrum of clinical manifestations. Vasculitis affects all ages, but is seen more frequently in adults rather than children and females slightly more often than males. The vast mosaic of clinical and histologic findings paired with diverse attributable triggers suggests that various vasculitides are likely a product of differing pathogenic mechanisms.[78] For cutaneous vasculitis in particular, disease is thought to be largely influenced by enhanced expression of vascular adhesion molecules attracting and activating neutrophils, which propagate ongoing inflammation.[79] The approach to patients with cutaneous vasculitis should incorporate classifying the vasculitis, working the patient up for systemic involvement, identifying triggers and associated comorbidities, and starting appropriate therapy.

Diagnosis

Currently, the most widely accepted vasculitis classification systems are the Chapel Hill Consensus Conference, based on pathologic criteria, and the ACR criteria, predominantly based on clinical findings. Neither system is without flaws, because both criteria were developed to compare categories of affected patients rather than to serve as diagnostic criteria. Both systems help to distinguish between primary and secondary vasculitis, recognize the dominant blood vessel size involved, and integrate pathophysiologic markers.[78,80] Importantly, small-vessel vasculitides typically present with palpable purpura and occasionally nonpalpable purpura, whereas medium-vessel vasculitides classically present with subcutaneous nodules, ulcers,

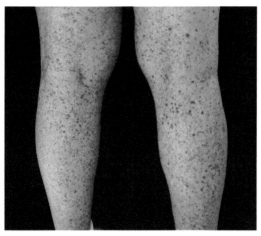

Fig. 7. Leukocytoclastic vasculitis.

livedo racemosa, and/or gangrene. Hence, the clinical skin examination can give the clinician excellent clues as to whether the patient has a small- versus medium-vessel vasculitis.

Small-vessel vasculitis includes cutaneous leukocytoclastic angiitis (CLA), Henoch-Schönlein purpura (HSP) or IgA vasculitis, urticarial vasculitis (UV), cryoglobulinemic vasculitis (CV), and drug- or infection-induced vasculitides, among others.

CLA typically affects middle-aged adults with a clinical presentation classically featuring palpable purpura over the lower extremities associated with pruritus, tenderness, or burning (**Fig. 7**).[81,82] Lesions generally resolve within 3 to 6 weeks; however, they often leave residual hyperpigmentation. In rare cases, CLA exhibits hemorrhagic bullae, erosions, or ulcerations on the lower legs (**Fig. 8**).[80] Occasionally, patients may

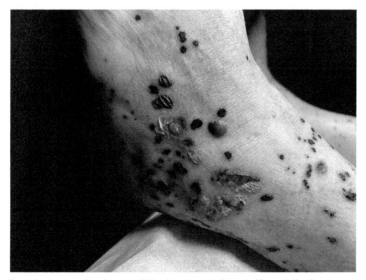

Fig. 8. Bullous leukocytoclastic vasculitis. (*Courtesy* of Dr. Jeffrey Callen).

present with recurrent or chronic disease, particularly when an underlying disease trigger exists. Patients with CLA can experience constitutional symptoms of fever, weight loss, malaise, arthralgia, or arthritis, whereas less than 10% of patients with CLA are found to have renal and/or gastrointestinal involvement.[83]

HSP is an IgA-associated vasculitis that comprises nearly 10% of all cutaneous vasculitis cases and accounts for almost 90% of vasculitis cases in children.[78,84] In 50% of patients, an upper respiratory tract infections precedes presentation. The clinical tetrad of HSP consists of cutaneous vasculitis, arthritis, gastrointestinal involvement, and/or nephritis; however, patients do not necessarily exhibit all four manifestations. Skin involvement with palpable purpura is a universal finding, whereas nephritis is the least frequently observed. Classically, the cutaneous lesions of HSP extend past the lower legs, often involving the thighs and buttocks, but this is not pathognomonic and can occur in multiple other vasculitides. HSP is generally self-limited, with full recovery occurring within weeks to months. Relapses are typically mild, often not requiring treatment, and can affect up to 40% of patients.[80,85] Akin to CLA, a minority of cases can become chronic and recurrent requiring long-term therapy.

UV affects women more frequently than men, particularly during the fourth or fifth decade of life.[84] Patients typically exhibit burning or pruritic papules or plaques that classically persist for greater than 24 hours (unlike urticaria) and up to 72 hours, often leaving residual bruise-like purpura or hyperpigmentation. UV is often misdiagnosed as urticaria, which by contrast lasts less than 24 hours, classically is more pruritic than invoking a burning sensation, and resolves without residual hyperpigmentation. Other UV symptoms can include low-grade fever, angioedema, arthralgia, arthritis, and abdominal pain.[80] All patients with UV should have complement studies performed because hypocomplementemic UV is associated with a more challenging disease course and with a risk of SLE.

CV vasculitis is defined as cutaneous vasculitis occurring in the presence of cryoglobulins, which are cold-precipitating immunoglobulins. CV presents with purpura triggered by cold exposure, and patients may have associated arthralgia. Cutaneous manifestations include palpable purpura, retiform purpura, ulcers, splinter hemorrhages, and palmar erythema. Systemic disease can involve glomerulonephritis, neuropathy, hemoptysis, or dyspnea. Patients with CV often have elevated rheumatoid factor titers and low C4 levels. Serum cryoglobulins are crucial in confirming diagnosis; however, appropriate testing can prove challenging in some laboratories. Careful instructions should be provided to the laboratory to ensure serum is incubated at 37°C immediately after the sample is collected to avoid cryoprecipitation of cryoglobulins before testing.

Approximately 20% of cutaneous vasculitis cases represent an adverse drug eruption, exhibiting small-vessel neutrophilic vasculitis or lymphocytic vasculitis of the superficial blood vessels in the dermis.[78,84] The time interval between exposure and symptom onset is highly varied, ranging from hours to years, with vasculitis occurring after drug dosage increases or after rechallenge. Offending drugs are divided into an antineutrophil cytoplasmic antibody (ANCA)-associated group consisting of propylthiouracil, hydralazine, allopurinol, minocycline, penicillamine, and phenytoin, and an ANCA-negative group encompassing colony-stimulating factors, isotretinoin, and methotrexate. The former group can induce systemic life-threatening visceral involvement within months to years following exposure, whereas the latter group is primarily limited to cutaneous involvement alone that presents within days to weeks following exposure. Of note, virtually every pharmacologic class has been implicated in drug-induced vasculitis.[86] Identification of the offending drug is essential to treatment, because discontinuation is followed by rapid improvement in most cases.

Roughly 22% of cutaneous vasculitis cases are associated with infection. Sources and agents of infection can include viruses, bacteria, fungi, protozoa, or helminths.[78,84] Septic vasculitis is a variant of infection-induced vasculitis that is frequently caused by infective endocarditis or septicemia from gonococci, meningococci, pseudomonads, staphylococci, streptococci, or certain rickettsial infections.[84] Skin lesions of septic vasculitis include purpura, petechiae, ecchymoses, vesiculopustules signifying potential necrosis, hemorrhagic bullae, and rarely ulceration. Patients with chronic gonococcemia or chronic meningococcemia often have a triad of intermittent fever, arthralgia, and fewer cutaneous lesions, mainly consisting of petechiae surrounded by erythema and vesiculopustules with a gray necrotic roof distributed over the extremities.[80]

In addition to small-vessel vasculitis, there are several vasculitides that can affect medium vessels of the skin. A form of polyarteritis nodosa (PAN), known as cutaneous PAN (CPAN), predominantly affects medium vessels of the skin without systemic organ involvement. ANCA-associated vasculitides, such as granulomatosis with polyangiitis (GPA), eosinophilic granulomatosis with polyangiitis (EGP), and microscopic polyangiitis, can affect small and medium vessels. Vasculitis secondary to CTD can also involve small or medium vessels.

CPAN should be suspected in patients who present with painful nodules, livedo racemosa, ulcers, acral gangrene, and/or neuropathy. Nodules most commonly occur on the lower extremities.[80] CPAN generally follows a benign disease course primarily confined to cutaneous manifestations; however, severe cases can involve constitutional symptoms, mononeuropathy multiplex, and arthralgia/arthritis.[87] Additionally, nearly half of patients with systemic PAN exhibit skin involvement, underscoring the necessity of a thorough work-up to distinguish CPAN from potential systemic PAN.[88] Work-up for systemic PAN includes serum creatinine and BUN, urinalysis, muscle enzymes, liver function tests, hepatitis B and C serologies, and blood cultures to exclude endovascular infection. Assays, such as ANCA, ANA, C3, C4, and cryoglobulins, can also help narrow the differential diagnosis.[89]

GPA is known for affecting the upper and lower respiratory tracts in the form of necrotizing granulomatous inflammation and the kidneys as glomerulonephritis.[84] Nearly 15% of patients with GPA present with cutaneous lesions, and approximately 50% develop cutaneous lesions at some point in their disease course. Palpable or nonpalpable purpura caused by small-vessel neutrophilic vasculitis is observed in 60% of patients with GPA with cutaneous disease. Subcutaneous nodules, ulcers, or gangrene secondary to medium-vessel vasculitis is found in 31%. Polymorphic lesions consisting of rheumatoid papules, malignant pyoderma, urticaria, vesiculobullous lesions, or gingival hyperplasia are present in 17% of patients.[84]

EGP is characterized by asthma, other allergic symptoms, peripheral and tissue eosinophilia, and systemic vasculitis. Renal disease is less prevalent in EGP when compared with GPA; however, peripheral nerve, cutaneous, and cardiac manifestations are more common. Skin findings include palpable purpura, petechiae, ecchymoses, hemorrhagic bullae, dermal and subcutaneous papules and nodules, urticarial lesions, erythematous macules, and livedo reticularis. The dermal and subcutaneous papules/nodules are observed in 30% of patients, and are often located on the scalp or symmetrically distributed over the extremities.[84,90]

Microscopic polyangiitis is characterized by a systemic, neutrophilic, vasculitis without extravascular granulomas or asthma. It is frequently associated with focal segmental necrotizing glomerulonephritis, skin involvement, and p-ANCA antibodies. Cutaneous lesions include palpable purpura and petechiae in more than three-quarters of patients, and splinter hemorrhages, nodules, palmar erythema, and livedo reticularis. Patients may experience systemic symptoms including fever, weight loss, myalgias, or arthralgias in the months to years leading up to disease presentation.[80,84]

Approximately 12% of cutaneous vasculitides are associated with CTD, and vasculitis secondary to CTD should be considered in patients who present with such symptoms as dry eyes, dry mouth, arthritis, sclerosis, photosensitivity or serologic evidence of ANA, rheumatoid factor, antiphospholipid, or anti-DNA, anti-Ro, or anti-La antibodies. CTD vasculitis is most frequently observed in SLE, rheumatoid arthritis, and Sjögren syndrome, and less commonly in DM, SSc, and relapsing polychondritis.[78,84] Compared with CLA, CTD vasculitis exhibits more widespread organ involvement and variation in caliber of affected vessels. Skin manifestations include purpura, vesiculobullous lesions, urticaria, and splinter hemorrhages. Arterial involvement should be suspected if cutaneous ulcers, nodules, digital gangrene, livedo racemosa, punctate acral scars, or malignant pyoderma are present, increasing the patient's probability of visceral vasculitis. The coexistence of small- and medium-vessel vasculitis within the same biopsy specimen is characteristic of CTD vasculitis. Additionally, patients with CTD may display p-ANCA or c-ANCA by indirect immunofluorescence.[80]

Work-Up

The initial step in management is to establish that cutaneous vasculitis is present via skin biopsy and to eliminate potential mimics, particularly vasculopathy, which is any noninflammatory obliterative disorder affecting the blood vessels. Once the presence of vasculitis is confirmed, clinicians may use findings from patient history, physical examination, laboratory evaluation, and biopsy features to characterize the type of vasculitis, assess extent of systemic involvement, and guide treatment. In all cases, patients should be initially screened for systemic disease and then periodically monitored for systemic involvement or newly identifiable treatable etiologies.[85]

Regarding patient history, it is important to determine chronicity of the condition and screen for various exposures. Symptoms indicative of systemic disease, malignancy, or consistent with CTDs should also be investigated. Physical examination is useful for identifying the size of vessel involvement and suggesting diagnosis. Palpable purpura, pinpoint papules, vesicles, petechiae, splinter hemorrhages, vesicopustules, or urticarial lesions may suggest small-vessel vasculitis. Subcutaneous nodules, ulcers, livedo racemose, papulonecrotic lesions, or digital infarcts may imply medium-vessel vasculitis.[85]

Recommended laboratory testing is influenced by clinical findings. Patients with suspected chronic vasculitis or possible systemic disease should have several studies performed including CBC with differential, blood urea nitrogen/creatinine, liver function panel, urinalysis, stool guaiac, hepatitis B and C serologies, cryoglobulins, complement levels, and rheumatoid factor.[85] Febrile patients with a heart murmur warrant blood cultures and echocardiography, and children or adults with a history of cardiac septal defect should have anti–streptolysin O titers performed. In patients with suspected medium-sized vessel involvement or CTD, ANA and ANCAs should be assessed.[85] For most patients, chest radiography paired with CBC with differential is sufficient screening for malignancy; however, patients with high fever, weight loss, severe anemia, cryoglobulinemia, or RP in the absence of CTD should prompt more thorough evaluation for malignancy.[91]

Tissue biopsy can reveal the size of vessels involved and the presence of granulomatous inflammation or lymphocytic infiltrate.[92] Timing of the biopsy should be less than 48 hours following the appearance of a lesion, because specimens taken too late may resemble the pathology of repair more than that of the initial injury.[93] Biopsies should generally be taken from the most tender, erythematous, or purpuric lesions and should include subcutaneous fat to assess deeper vessels. Serial section may be necessary to identify the key involved vessels.

Goals of Management

Treatment of cutaneous vasculitis involves avoidance of triggers and initiation of therapies as necessary to achieve disease control. Nonulcerative, purpuric lesions (eg, leukocytoclastic vasculitis [LCV]) may be treated with topical corticosteroids and compression stockings, whereas systemic vasculitis or severe cutaneous disease with ulcers or infarcts may require pulses of cyclophosphamide, rituximab, or other agents.[78,94]

In some cases, cutaneous vasculitis is self-limited, and is relieved by leg elevation, compression stockings, and topical corticosteroids. Identification of the underlying cause of vasculitis and its respective treatment is often the most effective management. Resolution of pruritus or burning can often be achieved with topical corticosteroids, nonsteroidal anti-inflammatory drugs, or antihistamines. These therapies have not been shown to alter the disease course, but can provide symptomatic relief.[80]

For patients with mild, limited cutaneous vasculitis that is persistent, recurrent, or symptomatic, using colchicine or dapsone, separately or combined, can often prompt rapid resolution.[94] It is important to remember to check a glucose-6-phosphate dehydrogenase level for any patient before initiation of therapy with dapsone. For moderate-to-severe skin disease, systemic corticosteroids may be required in addition to a corticosteroid-sparing agent, such as methotrexate, MMF, or azathioprine.[80] Standard therapy for systemic vasculitis with severe internal organ involvement entails a combination of systemic corticosteroids and cyclophosphamide or rituximab.

SUMMARY

CTDs have a wide array of clinical presentations and manifestations. The potential for systemic involvement often necessitates interdisciplinary care to best manage these patients. In many cases, cutaneous features may serve as an early indication of disease and a careful skin examination can guide diagnosis, work-up, and management. Evaluation often entails careful history taking, combined with physician examination, laboratory testing, and possible biopsy. CTDs can have several disease subtypes or classifications, and proper identification is critical to optimize management strategies. Treatment often takes an escalating stepwise approach determined by disease severity and acuity and patient comorbidities. As research progresses and the pathogenic mechanisms of CTDs are better elucidated, treatment modalities will continue to be further refined and more targeted.

CLINICS CARE POINTS

- A careful skin examination is crucial in differentiating between various cutaneous connective tissue diseases.
- Patients with CTD should be screened for possible systemic involvement and malignancy, because early detection and management can improve outcomes.
- Several pharmacotherapies used in the management of CTDs have potential for toxicity, requiring high-risk medication monitoring, which should be considered when selecting appropriate treatment options at each phase of management.

REFERENCES

1. Khanna D, McLaughlin V. Screening and early detection of pulmonary arterial hypertension in connective tissue diseases: it is time to institute it! Am J Respir Crit Care Med 2015;192(9):1032–3.
2. Okon LG, Werth VP. Cutaneous lupus erythematosus: diagnosis and treatment. Best Pract Res Clin Rheumatol 2013;27(3):391–404.
3. Durosaro O, Davis MDP, Reed KB, et al. Incidence of cutaneous lupus erythematosus, 1965-2005 a population-based study. Arch Dermatol 2009;145(3):249–53.
4. Grönhagen CM, Fored CM, Granath F, et al. Cutaneous lupus erythematosus and the association with systemic lupus erythematosus: a population-based cohort of 1088 patients in Sweden. Br J Dermatol 2011;164(6):1335–41.
5. Rees F, Doherty M, Grainge MJ, et al. The worldwide incidence and prevalence of systemic lupus erythematosus: a systematic review of epidemiological studies. Rheumatology (United Kingdom) 2017;56(11):1945–61.
6. Chiu YM, Lai CH. Nationwide population-based epidemiologic study of systemic lupus erythematosus in Taiwan. Lupus 2010;19(10):1250–5.
7. Grönhagen C, Nyberg F. Cutaneous lupus erythematosus: an update. Indian Dermatol Online J 2014;5(1):7.
8. Ng PPL, Tan SH, Koh ET, et al. Epidemiology of cutaneous lupus erythematosus in a tertiary referral centre in Singapore. Australas J Dermatol 2000;41(4):229–33.
9. Fabbri P, Cardinali C, Giomi B, et al. Cutaneous lupus erythematosus: diagnosis and management. Am J Clin Dermatol 2003;4(7):449–65.
10. Tebbe B, Mansmann U, Wollina U, et al. Markers in cutaneous lupus erythematosus indicating systemic involvement. A multicenter study on 296 patients. Acta Derm Venereol 1997;77(4):305–8.
11. Obermoser G, Sontheimer RD, Zelger B. Overview of common, rare and atypical manifestations of cutaneous lupus erythematosus and histopathological correlates. Lupus 2010;19(9):1050–70.
12. Walling H, Sontheimer R. Cutaneous lupus erythematosus: issues in diagnosis and treatment. Am J Clin Dermatol 2009;10(6):365–81.
13. Rothfield N, Sontheimer RD, Bernstein M. Lupus erythematosus: systemic and cutaneous manifestations. Clin Dermatol 2006;24(5):348–62.
14. Lin JH, Dutz JP, Sontheimer RD, et al. Pathophysiology of cutaneous lupus erythematosus. Clin Rev Allergy Immunol 2007;33(1–2):85–106.
15. Caproni M, Cardinali C, Salvatore E, et al. Subacute cutaneous lupus erythematosus with pityriasis-like cutaneous manifestations. Int J Dermatol 2001;40(1):59–62.
16. Kuhn A, Sticherling M, Bonsmann G. Clinical manifestations of cutaneous lupus erythematosus. J Ger Soc Dermatol 2007;5(12):1124–37.
17. Grönhagen CM, Fored CM, Linder M, et al. Subacute cutaneous lupus erythematosus and its association with drugs: a population-based matched case-control study of 234 patients in Sweden. Br J Dermatol 2012;167(2):296–305.
18. Callen JP. Drug-induced subacute cutaneous lupus erythematosus. Lupus 2010;19(9):1107–11.
19. Chong BF, Song J, Olsen NJ. Determining risk factors for developing systemic lupus erythematosus in patients with discoid lupus erythematosus. Br J Dermatol 2012;166(1):29–35.
20. Crowson AN, Magro C. The cutaneous pathology of lupus erythematosus: a review. J Cutan Pathol 2001;28(1):1–23.

21. Cardinali C, Caproni M, Bernacchi E, et al. The spectrum of cutaneous manifestations in lupus erythematosus: the Italian experience. Lupus 2000;9(6):417–23.
22. Lee HJ, Sinha AA. Cutaneous lupus erythematosus: understanding of clinical features, genetic basis, and pathobiology of disease guides therapeutic strategies. Autoimmunity 2006;39(6):433–44.
23. Vera-Recabarren MA, García-Carrasco M, Ramos-Casals M, et al. Comparative analysis of subacute cutaneous lupus erythematosus and chronic cutaneous lupus erythematosus: clinical and immunological study of 270 patients. Br J Dermatol 2010;162(1):91–101.
24. Magro CM, Neil Crowson A, Harnst TJ. Atypical lymphoid infiltrates arising in cutaneous lesions of connective tissue disease. Am J Dermatopathol 1997;19(5):446–55.
25. Adamichou C, Nikolopoulos D, Genitsaridi I, et al. In an early SLE cohort the ACR-1997, SLICC-2012 and EULAR/ACR-2019 criteria classify non-overlapping groups of patients: use of all three criteria ensures optimal capture for clinical studies while their modification earlier classification and treatment. Ann Rheum Dis 2020;79(2):232–41.
26. Zečević RD, Vojvodić D, Ristić B, et al. Skin lesions: an indicator of disease activity in systemic lupus erythematosus? Lupus 2001;10(5):364–7.
27. Werth VP. Clinical manifestations of cutaneous lupus erythematosus. Autoimmun Rev 2005;4(5):296–302.
28. Grönhagen CM, Gunnarsson I, Svenungsson E, et al. Cutaneous manifestations and serological findings in 260 patients with systemic lupus erythematosus. Lupus 2010;19(10):1187–94.
29. Marin GG, Cardiel MH, Cornejo H, et al. Prevalence of antinuclear antibodies in 3 groups of healthy individuals: blood donors, hospital personnel, and relatives of patients with autoimmune diseases. J Clin Rheumatol 2009;15(7):325–9.
30. Jessop S, Whitelaw DA, Delamere FM. Drugs for discoid lupus erythematosus. Cochrane Database Syst Rev 2009;(4):CD002954.
31. Guan SY, Cai HY, Wang P, et al. Association between circulating 25-hydroxyvitamin D and systemic lupus erythematosus: a systematic review and meta-analysis. Int J Rheum Dis 2019;22(10):1803–13.
32. Parisis D, Bernier C, Chasset F, et al. Impact of tobacco smoking upon disease risk, activity and therapeutic response in systemic lupus erythematosus: a systematic review and meta-analysis. Autoimmun Rev 2019;18(11):102393.
33. Margiotta DPE, Basta F, Dolcini G, et al. Physical activity and sedentary behavior in patients with systemic lupus erythematosus. PLoS One 2018;13(3):e0193728.
34. Bogdanov I, Kazandjieva J, Darlenski R, et al. Dermatomyositis: current concepts. Clin Dermatol 2018;36(4):450–8.
35. DeWane ME, Waldman R, Lu J. Dermatomyositis: clinical features and pathogenesis. J Am Acad Dermatol 2020;82(2):267–81.
36. Mainetti C, Terziroli Beretta-Piccoli B, Selmi C. Cutaneous manifestations of dermatomyositis: a comprehensive review. Clin Rev Allergy Immunol 2017;53(3):337–56.
37. Cobos GA, Femia A, Vleugels RA. Dermatomyositis: an update on diagnosis and treatment. Am J Clin Dermatol 2020;21(3):339–53.
38. Gallais V, Crickx B, Belaich S. Prognostic factors and predictive signs of malignancy in adult dermatomyositis. Ann Dermatol Venereol 1996;123(11):722–6.
39. Katzap E, Barilla-Labarca ML, Marder G. Antisynthetase syndrome. Curr Rheumatol Rep 2011;13(3):175–81.

40. Bowerman K, Pearson DR, Okawa J, et al. Malignancy in dermatomyositis: a retrospective study of 201 patients seen at the University of Pennsylvania. J Am Acad Dermatol 2020;83(1):117–22.

41. Leatham H, Schadt C, Chisolm S, et al. Evidence supports blind screening for internal malignancy in dermatomyositis: data from 2 large US dermatology cohorts. Medicine (Baltimore) 2018;97(2):e9639.

42. Thompson C, Piguet V, Choy E. The pathogenesis of dermatomyositis. Br J Dermatol 2018;179(6):1256–62.

43. Ran J, Ji S, Morelli JN, et al. T2 mapping in dermatomyositis/polymyositis and correlation with clinical parameters. Clin Radiol 2018;73(12):1057.e13–8.

44. Mariampillai K, Granger B, Amelin D, et al. Development of a new classification system for idiopathic inflammatory myopathies based on clinical manifestations and myositis-specific autoantibodies. JAMA Neurol 2018;75(12):1528–37.

45. Best M, Jachiet M, Molinari N, et al. Distinctive cutaneous and systemic features associated with specific antimyositis antibodies in adults with dermatomyositis: a prospective multicentric study of 117 patients. J Eur Acad Dermatol Venereol 2018;32(7):1164–72.

46. Wolstencroft PW, Fiorentino DF. Dermatomyositis clinical and pathological phenotypes associated with myositis-specific autoantibodies. Curr Rheumatol Rep 2018;20(5):1–11.

47. Vij R, Strek ME. Diagnosis and treatment of connective tissue disease-associated interstitial lung disease. Chest 2013;143(3):814–24.

48. Waldman R, DeWane ME, Lu J. Dermatomyositis: diagnosis and treatment. J Am Acad Dermatol 2020;82(2):283–96.

49. Yang H, Peng Q, Yin L, et al. Identification of multiple cancer-associated myositis-specific autoantibodies in idiopathic inflammatory myopathies: a large longitudinal cohort study. Arthritis Res Ther 2017;19(1):1–9.

50. Femia AN, Vleugels RA, Callen JP. Cutaneous dermatomyositis: an updated review of treatment options and internal associations. Am J Clin Dermatol 2013;14(4):291–313.

51. Alexanderson H, Munters LA, Dastmalchi M, et al. Resistive home exercise in patients with recent-onset polymyositis and dermatomyositis: a randomized controlled single-blinded study with a 2-year followup. J Rheumatol 2014;41(6):1124–32.

52. Habers GEA, Takken T. Safety and efficacy of exercise training in patients with an idiopathic inflammatory myopathy: a systematic review. Rheumatology (Oxford) 2011;50(11):2113–24.

53. Allanore Y, Simms R, Distler O, et al. Systemic sclerosis. Nat Rev Dis Prim 2015;1(1):1–21.

54. Cutolo M, Soldano S, Smith V. Pathophysiology of systemic sclerosis: current understanding and new insights. Expert Rev Clin Immunol 2019;15(7):753–64.

55. Asano Y. Systemic sclerosis. J Dermatol 2018;45(2):128–38.

56. Denton CP, Khanna D. Systemic sclerosis. Lancet 2017;390(10103):1685–99.

57. Van Den Hoogen F, Khanna D, Fransen J, et al. 2013 classification criteria for systemic sclerosis: an American College of Rheumatology/European League Against Rheumatism collaborative initiative. Ann Rheum Dis 2013;72(11):1747–55.

58. Stochmal A, Czuwara J, Trojanowska M, et al. Antinuclear antibodies in systemic sclerosis: an update. Clin Rev Allergy Immunol 2020;58(1):40–51.

59. Srivastava N, Hudson M, Tatibouet S, et al. Thinking outside the box: the associations with cutaneous involvement and autoantibody status in systemic sclerosis are not always what we expect. Semin Arthritis Rheum 2015;45(2):184–9.

60. Lynch B, Stern E, Ong V, et al. UK Scleroderma Study Group (UKSSG) guidelines on the diagnosis and management of scleroderma renal crisis. Clin Exp Rheumatol 2016;34:106–9.

61. Domsic RT, Nihtyanova SI, Wisniewski SR, et al. Derivation and external validation of a prediction rule for five-year mortality in patients with early diffuse cutaneous systemic sclerosis. Arthritis Rheumatol 2016;68(4):993–1003.

62. Tashkin DP, Roth MD, Clements PJ, et al. Mycophenolate mofetil versus oral cyclophosphamide in scleroderma-related interstitial lung disease (SLS II): a randomised controlled, double-blind, parallel group trial. Lancet Respir Med 2016;4(9):708–19.

63. Zanatta E, Codullo V, Avouac J, et al. Systemic sclerosis: recent insight in clinical management. Jt Bone Spine 2020;87(4):293–9.

64. Gomes JP, Santos L, Shoenfeld Y. Intravenous immunoglobulin (IVIG) in the vanguard therapy of systemic sclerosis. Clin Immunol 2019;199:25–8.

65. Shima Y, Kuwahara Y, Murota H, et al. The skin of patients with systemic sclerosis softened during the treatment with anti-IL-6 receptor antibody tocilizumab. Rheumatology 2010;49(12):2408–12.

66. Sakkas LI. Spotlight on tocilizumab and its potential in the treatment of systemic sclerosis. Drug Des Devel Ther 2016;10:2723–8.

67. Zanatta E, Rodeghiero F, Pigatto E, et al. Long-term improvement in activities of daily living in women with systemic sclerosis attending occupational therapy. Br J Occup Ther 2017;80(7):417–22.

68. Horváth J, Bálint Z, Szép E, et al. Efficacy of intensive hand physical therapy in patients with systemic sclerosis. Clin Exp Rheumatol 2017;106(4):159–66.

69. Melvin OG, Hunt KM, Jacobson ES. Hyaluronidase treatment of scleroderma-induced microstomia. JAMA Dermatol 2019;155(7):857–9.

70. Giuggioli D, Lumetti F, Colaci M, et al. Rituximab in the treatment of patients with systemic sclerosis. Our experience and review of the literature. Autoimmun Rev 2015;14(11):1072–8.

71. Coghlan JG, Galiè N, Barberà JA, et al. Initial combination therapy with ambrisentan and tadalafil in connective tissue disease-associated pulmonary arterial hypertension (CTD-PAH): subgroup analysis from the AMBITION trial. Ann Rheum Dis 2017;76(7):1219–27.

72. Sato T, Ambale-Venkatesh B, Lima JAC, et al. The impact of ambrisentan and tadalafil upfront combination therapy on cardiac function in scleroderma associated pulmonary arterial hypertension patients: cardiac magnetic resonance feature tracking study. Pulm Circ 2018;8(1). 2045893217748307.

73. Sanges S, Rivière S, Mekinian A, et al. Intravenous immunoglobulins in systemic sclerosis: data from a French nationwide cohort of 46 patients and review of the literature. Autoimmun Rev 2017;16(4):377–84.

74. Bharadwaj S, Tandon P, Gohel T, et al. Gastrointestinal manifestations, malnutrition, and role of enteral and parenteral nutrition in patients with scleroderma. J Clin Gastroenterol 2015;49(7):559–64.

75. Blagojevic J, Abignano G, Avouac J, et al. Use of vasoactive/vasodilating drugs for systemic sclerosis (SSc)-related digital ulcers (DUs) in expert tertiary centres: results from the analysis of the observational real-life DeSScipher study. Clin Rheumatol 2020;39(1):27–36.

76. Chung L. Therapeutic options for digital ulcers in patients with systemic sclerosis. J Dtsch Dermatol Ges 2007;5(6):460–5.
77. Motegi S, Yamada K, Toki S, et al. Beneficial effect of botulinum toxin A on Raynaud's phenomenon in Japanese patients with systemic sclerosis: a prospective, case series study. J Dermatol 2016;43(1):56–62.
78. Carlson JA, Ng BT, Chen KR. Cutaneous vasculitis update: diagnostic criteria, classification, epidemiology, etiology, pathogenesis, evaluation and prognosis. Am J Dermatopathol 2005;27(6):504–28.
79. Belmont HM, Abramson SB, Lie JT. Pathology and pathogenesis of vascular injury in systemic lupus erythematosus Interactions of inflammatory cells and activated endothelium. Arthritis Rheum 1996;39(1):9–22.
80. Chen KR, Carlson JA. Clinical approach to cutaneous vasculitis. Am J Clin Dermatol 2008;9(2):71–92.
81. Kelly RI, Opie J, Nixon R. Golfer's vasculitis. Australas J Dermatol 2005; 46(1):11–4.
82. Ramelet AA. Exercise-induced vasculitis. J Eur Acad Dermatol Venereol 2006; 20(4):423–7.
83. Blanco R, Martínez-Taboada VM, Rodríguez-Valverde V, et al. Cutaneous vasculitis in children and adults: associated diseases and etiologic factors in 303 patients. Medicine (Baltimore) 1998;77(6):403–18.
84. Carlson JA, Chen KR. Cutaneous vasculitis update: small vessel neutrophilic vasculitis syndromes. Am J Dermatopathol 2006;28(6):486–506.
85. Fiorentino DF. Cutaneous vasculitis. J Am Acad Dermatol 2003;48(3):311–44.
86. Holder SM, Joy MS, Falk RJ. Cutaneous and systemic manifestations of drug-induced vasculitis. Ann Pharmacother 2002;36(1):130–47.
87. Carlson JA, Chen KR. Cutaneous vasculitis update: neutrophilic muscular vessel and eosinophilic, granulomatous, and lymphocytic vasculitis syndromes. Am J Dermatopathol 2007;29(1):32–43.
88. Marzano AV, Vezzoli P, Berti E. Skin involvement in cutaneous and systemic vasculitis. Autoimmun Rev 2013;12(4):467–76.
89. Howard T, Ahmad K, Swanson JAA, et al. Polyarteritis nodosa. Tech Vasc Interv Radiol 2014;17(4):247–51.
90. Chen KR, Sakamoto M, Ikemoto K, et al. Granulomatous arteritis in cutaneous lesions of Churg-Strauss syndrome. J Cutan Pathol 2007;34(4):330–7.
91. González-Gay MA, García-Porrúa C, Salvarani C, et al. Cutaneous vasculitis and cancer: a clinical approach. Clin Exp Rheumatol 2000;18:305–7.
92. Stone JH, Nousari HC. "Essential" cutaneous vasculitis: what every rheumatologist should know about vasculitis of the skin. Curr Opin Rheumatol 2001;13(1): 23–34.
93. Ryan TJ. Common mistakes in the clinical approach to vasculitis. Clin Dermatol 1999;17(5):555–7.
94. Carlson JA, Cavaliere LF, Grant-Kels JM. Cutaneous vasculitis: diagnosis and management. Clin Dermatol 2006;24(5):414–29.

Common Cutaneous Infections

Patient Presentation, Clinical Course, and Treatment Options

Ana Preda-Naumescu, BS[a], Boni Elewski, MD[b],
Tiffany T. Mayo, MD[b],*

KEYWORDS

- Cutaneous infections • Bacterial infections • Herpesvirus • Superficial fungal

KEY POINTS

- This review is an evidence-based outline of the cutaneous manifestations of common bacterial, viral, and fungal pathogens.
- Within this review, the clinical presentations and treatment options available for cutaneous bacterial, viral, and fungal infections, as they might be encountered in clinical practice, are discussed.
- The scope of this article is to serve as a reference to guide clinicians in the treatment of common cutaneous infections.

INTRODUCTION

Bacterial, viral, and fungal skin-structure infections are common chief complaints, prompting patients to seek care in outpatient medical clinics. Between 2005 and 2010, approximately 4.8 skin or soft tissue infections (SSTIs) requiring medical attention occurred per 100 person-years annually among those aged 64 years and younger.[1] Although this number has remained relatively stable, the high incidence of SSTIs, if properly treated, has enormous potential to reduce disease morbidity and health care utilization.[1] The most common bacterial skin pathogens are *Staphylococcus aureus* and group A β-hemolytic streptococci (GAS); herpes simplex virus (HSV) is the most common viral skin disease.[2] Regardless of the pathogen, the first

Conflicts of interest: The authors have no financial nor commercial conflicts of interest to declare.
[a] School of Medicine, University of Alabama at Birmingham, 1670 University Blvd, Birmingham, AL 35233, USA; [b] Department of Dermatology, University of Alabama at Birmingham, 510 20th Street South, FOT Suite 858, Birmingham, AL 35233, USA
* Corresponding author.
E-mail address: tmayo@uabmc.edu

clue to cutaneous infection is often erythema. In skin of color, this diagnostic clue may not be obvious. Providers require a high degree of clinical suspicion, as well as an appreciation for differences in skin infection presentations to avoid missing a diagnosis among different patient populations. In addition to identifying cutaneous infections as they affect different skin types, clinicians require an understanding of normal skin microbiome in order to distinguish between contaminants and pathogens.

The composition of cutaneous microflora on the human skin varies depending on the microenvironment.[2] For example, different bacterial microflora characterizes each of 3 following regions of skin:

1. Axilla, perineum, toe webs
2. Hand, face, trunk
3. Upper arms, legs

Differences in microbiota composition depend on the physiology of the skin site. This physiology of the skin site includes moisture levels, temperature, and concentration of skin surface lipids.[2] For example, the axilla, perineum, and toe webs are frequently colonized by gram-negative bacilli when compared with drier areas of skin.[2] An appreciation for the bacterial diversity of skin, including regional variability, is essential when selecting sites for culture. **Table 1** outlines major inhabitants of skin.[2]

In addition to bacterial and viral pathogens, dermatophyte fungal infections, the most common pathogen of which is *Trichophyton rubrum*, are prevalent in the

Table 1 Common bacterial inhabitants of the skin	
Staphylococcus epidermidis	An aerobic inhabitant of the skin, making up 90% of the resident flora in some areas
S aureus	Although often implicated in skin infections, *S aureus* may also be found on normal skin. Common sites of colonization include • The nose, perineum, and vulvar skin • The skin of patients with certain dermatologic conditions, such as atopic dermatitis
Micrococcus	*Micrococcus luteus* is the predominant species encountered, accounting for 20%–80% of micrococci isolated
Diphtheroid (of the genus Coryneform)	Classification of diphtheroids includes • Lipophilic: common in axilla • Nonlipophilic: common in glabrous skin • Anaerobic: common in areas rich is sebaceous glands
Streptococci	• β-Hemolytic streptococci are rarely seen on normal skin • α-Hemolytic streptococci, exist primarily in the mouth, from where they may, in rare instances, spread to the skin
Gram-negative bacilli	A very small proportion of skin flora mainly found in moist, intertriginous areas, such as toe webs and axilla. The predominant organisms encountered include • *Enterobacter* spp • *Klebsiella* spp • *Escherichia coli* • *Proteus* spp • *Acinetobacter* spp

community and are frequently encountered in clinical settings as causes of both skin and nail infection.[2] Like the skin, understanding the nail's normal microbiome aids physicians in identifying pathogens. Although the microbiology of the nail is mostly similar to that of the skin, extraneous materials, such as dust particles and exogenous fungal and bacterial flora, are also encountered. Clinicians should be aware of fungal contaminants found under nails, as these should not be confused with virulent pathogens. Commonly encountered fungal contaminants include *Aspergillus*, *Penicillium*, *Cladosporium*, and *Mucor* species.[2]

The scope of this article is to describe common cutaneous infections with a focus on evidence-based treatment options, in hopes of providing clinicians with accessible information for the best medical care.

BACKGROUND

Pathogenic bacteria evade normal host defense and cause disease. Of these, the most widely recognized and well-studied are S aureus and GAS.[3] S aureus can colonize, and subsequently invade into, mammalian cells.[3] Colonization of the human host occurs on newborn skin, the anterior nares in up to 40% of healthy individuals, the skin of patients with atopic dermatitis (AD), and the skin of HIV-infected patients.[3]

Streptococcal species, although rarely cutaneous residents, are well-described commensal pathogens of the human skin. They are categorized into different groups based on their respective M-protein, a virulence protein that confers resistance to phagocytosis.[3] Groups A, B, C, D, and G are the most frequently involved in cutaneous skin infections.[3]

DISCUSSION OF EPIDERMAL INFECTIONS

Categorization of bacterial skin infections may be based on depth and extent of skin involvement. Superficial (ie, epidermal) soft tissue skin infections include impetigo and ecthyma.[4]

Impetigo

Impetigo is the most common bacterial infection in children. Categorized as bullous or nonbullous, the most common bacterial culprits are methicillin-sensitive S aureus (MSSA) or GAS.[4] Infection occurs via direct invasion of intact skin or invasion of compromised skin.[4] Predisposing conditions include warm, humid environments and lack of hygiene.[4]

Nonbullous impetigo makes up approximately 70% of cases and presents with painless erythematous papules, pustules, or vesicles covered with honey-colored crust.[4] The main culprit is S aureus: either with GAS or alone. It may occur at any age, and it most commonly affects the limbs and face following minor trauma.[3] Associated lymphadenopathy or leukocytosis may occur.[3] Of note, impetigo caused by GAS can cause glomerulonephritis.[5]

Bullous impetigo is characterized by flaccid bullae that easily rupture, leaving behind a thin collarette of scale. It is caused almost exclusively by S aureus and generally affects children ages 2 to 5 in regions such as the diaper area, axillae, and neck.[4] Regional lymphadenopathy is rare.[4]

Ecthyma

Ecthyma is a deeper form of impetigo that commonly involves the lower extremities and is characterized by circumscribed crusted plaques, beneath which ulcers may form.[3] The bacterial culprits are the same as those of impetigo.[3] Scarring is common.[3]

Summary and Therapeutic Options

Gram stain and culture of exudate from skin lesions of impetigo/ecthyma may identify the causative organism; however, empiric treatment is appropriate in typical cases.[6] Pharmacologic strategies involve topical antibiotics if the lesions are local (<5 lesions).[3] Saline soaks for the removal of the crusts are an appropriate adjunctive measure.

Topical antibiotic of choice for bullous/nonbullous impetigo[5,6]

- Mupirocin
- Fusidic acid
  - Used widely throughout the world, although not currently approved in the United States.[7] Awareness of this agent as a treatment option is necessary, as efforts are made for its approval as a safe and effective topical and oral alternative for treatment of acute bacterial skin and skin structure infections.[7]
- Retapamulin
- Neomycin
- Bacitracin

If there is widespread involvement of the epidermis or the presence of systemic signs of infection, oral antibiotics are appropriate.[6] Options include the following[6]:

- A 7-day course of an agent with activity against MSSA:
  - Dicloxacillin
  - Cephalexin
- If methicillin-resistant *Staphylococcus aureus* (MRSA) is suspected:
  - Clindamycin
  - Trimethoprim-sulfamethoxazole
- If culture or gram-stain data suggest streptococcal infection alone:
  - Oral penicillin

Clinics care points

1. Use topical antibiotics if lesions are local (<5 lesions)
2. Use oral antibiotics for severe infection. Agents should have activity against MSSA.

INTRODUCTION TO DERMAL INFECTIONS

Deeper cutaneous infections caused by *S aureus* and GAS include erysipelas, which affects the upper dermis, and cellulitis (this topic is covered in depth in another article in this issue), which classically involves the deeper dermis and subcutaneous fat.[4] Along with wound infections and abscesses, erysipelas and cellulitis are sometimes grouped as acute bacterial skin and skin-structure infection.[8] The reasoning behind this selective grouping is explained by the causative organism. For these infections, the most commonly implicated organism is *Streptococcus*, although others, including *Staphylococcus*, *Haemophilus influenzae*, *Aeromonas hydrophilia*, and *Pseudomonas aeruginosa*, fungi, and Gram-negative rods, have been isolated.[8] Empiric treatment regimens should be tailored to the most common culprit as culture data are collected.

Erysipelas

Erysipelas is an acute infection involving the dermis and dermal lymphatics.[3] Caused almost exclusively by GAS, infection is characterized by sharply demarcated, tender, erythematous plaques with elevated borders.[3] It commonly occurs on the lower extremities and/or face following a traumatic insult or inflammatory dermatosis.[3]

Constitutional symptoms and leukocytosis are common.[3] Erysipelas may be confused with angioedema or allergic contact dermatitis but can usually be distinguished by extreme skin tenderness and systemic symptoms.[5] Complications may include fatal streptococcal septicemia in debilitated patients, guttate psoriasis, acute glomerulonephritis, or lymphatic damage after recurrent attacks.[5]

Summary and Therapeutic Options: Erysipelas

Prompt treatment of erysipelas is crucial, and topical treatment is not appropriate.[5] Resolution requires systemic penicillin or erythromycin if penicillin allergy exists.[5] In a 60-patient study, there was no appreciable benefit from intravenous (IV) compared with oral penicillin therapy; therefore, oral therapy is recommended in the absence of coexisting complications with the infection.[9–13]

Clinics care points

1. Erysipelas is caused almost exclusively by GAS. Treatment requires oral penicillin, or, in the case of allergy, macrolides.
2. Topical treatment is not appropriate.

Necrotizing Fasciitis

Necrotizing fasciitis (NF) is a potentially life-threatening cutaneous infection involving the subcutaneous fascia and deeper dermis. Characterized by the acute onset of erythema and edema, it quickly progresses to violaceous, dusky plaques that may necrose and cross fascial planes.[3]

There are 2 types of NF. Type I is a polymicrobial infection caused by facultative bacteria and anaerobes (generally a mixture of gram-positive and gram-negative organisms). Type II, or streptococcal gangrene, is caused by GAS.[14] Management of both relies on surgical debridement, with antibiotics playing a secondary role.[14]

Type I commonly involves the legs, abdominal wall, perineal area, postoperative wounds, and umbilical stump in newborns.[14] Patients with diabetes mellitus, morbid obesity, and alcohol abuse are predisposed. Infection begins with a swollen, erythematous area of skin without distinct margins that is warm and tender to the touch.[14] As the infection progresses, the affected area changes color from red-purple to darker patches of blue-gray before progressing to the development of frank cutaneous bullae and gangrene, with soft tissue gas often detectable.[14] Cutaneous hypoesthesia and systemic toxicity may precede skin necrosis.[14] Characteristically, the infection dissects and crosses tissue planes, which may produce a compartment syndrome requiring prompt decompression to avoid frank myonecrosis.[14]

Type II (Streptococcal gangrene) occurs following minor trauma/surgery, and most commonly involves the fascia.[14] A hallmark is quick progression of erythema with distinct borders to gangrene and frank myonecrosis.[14] Even when *S aureus* is isolated from the necrotic tissue, it usually contributes little to the pathogenesis.[14]

Therapeutic Options and Recommendations: Necrotizing Fasciitis

Prompt surgical consultation is required for patients with suspected NF.[6] In polymicrobial infections, deep tissue specimens should be cultured for aerobes and anaerobes to guide antibiotic treatment.[14] Empiric antibiotic treatment should be broad.[6] Therapeutic options include[6] the following:

1. Vancomycin or linezolid *plus*
   - Piperacillin-tazobactam
   - Carbapenem

○ Ceftriaxone and metronidazole

In documented type II streptococcal gangrene, antibiotic therapy relies on high-dose penicillin and/or clindamycin.[14]

Clinics care points

1. Prompt surgical consultation is required.
2. Deep tissue specimens should be collected.
3. Empiric antibiotic treatment should be broad in case the cause is polymicrobial.
4. In documented type II NF, treatment relies on high-dose penicillin and/or clindamycin.

DISCUSSION OF FOLLICULITIS AND RELATED CONDITIONS

Common infections of the hair follicle include folliculitis, abscesses, furuncles, and carbuncles. The most common pathogen is *S aureus*.[5] Predisposing conditions include obesity, diabetes mellitus, and occlusion from clothing.[5]

Folliculitis is a pustular infection involving multiple hair follicles often found in heavy hair-bearing areas, such as men's faces (*sycosis barbae*) or women's legs, following hair removal.[5] Furuncle refers to abscess or boil formation in adjacent hair follicles.[5] They present as tender, erythematous, and suppurative pustules on the face, neck, scalp, axillae, and perineum that heal with scarring.[5] In contrast, carbuncles are deep abscesses formed in a group of follicles that result in a painful suppurating mass.[5] Distinction from hidradenitis suppurativa, a chronic inflammatory condition characterized by a painful, reoccurring abscesses and deep-seated nodules affecting mostly apocrine gland-bearing skin, is important for proper diagnosis and management of folliculitis and related conditions.[5]

Therapeutic Options for Follicular Conditions

Bacterial culture and Gram stain may be taken from the lesion and carrier sites.[5,6] Empiric treatment without this data is reasonable.[5,6] Initial treatment should include incision and drainage (I&D) in the case of abscess, furuncle, or carbuncle.[6]

The use of antibiotics depends on systemic signs of infection.[6] Treatment usually includes systemic (ie, flucloxacillin or erythromycin) and topical (eg, fusidic acid, mupirocin, or neomycin/bacitracin) antibiotic coverage.[5] Treatment of carrier sites with a topical antibiotic and improved general hygiene can reduce recurrence rates.

Clinics care points

1. Management of follicular infections should include:
   a. I&D in the case of abscess, furuncle, or carbuncle
   b. Antibiotic therapy if systemic signs of infection present

INTRODUCTION TO HERPESVIRUS INFECTIONS

HSV-1 and HSV-2, members of the Herpesvirus family, cause either primary (self-limited, immunocompetent host) or secondary (reactivation of latent virus, immuno-compromised host) cutaneous infections.[15] Following primary infection, the viruses establish latent infection in ganglionic neurons, which allows for reactivation and secondary infection later on.[15] In the case of severe or recalcitrant infection, antiviral therapy may be used.

Herpes Labialis

Herpes labialis is an infection of the buccal and gingival mucosa (gingivostomatitis) that manifests as orolabial lesions. Although usually caused by HSV-1, HSV-2 has been implicated.[15] The virus infects the skin and mucous membranes, damaging keratinocytes and causing inflammation that manifests at the vermilion border of the lips as small groups of vesicles that may become pustular, ulcerative, or crusted.[15,16]

Although both primary and secondary episodes of Herpes labialis are usually self-limiting, treatment options do exist. Soothing self-help remedies include alcohol-based tinctures, surface dressings, and antiseptic creams.[16] Topical and systemic antiviral options include acyclovir, valaciclovir, and foscarnet.[16]

Acyclovir reduces the duration of healing time when initiated early during acute infection. In patients with frequent reactivation, prophylactic treatment may be effective. The following different formulations exist[16–18]:

1. Acyclovir buccal patch
   - Shown to reduce healing time by 1 day compared with placebo
2. Acyclovir 5% in combination with 1% hydrocortisone cream applied 5 times daily
   - Shown to reduce the risk of ulceration
3. Oral acyclovir therapy (200 mg 5 times daily)
   - More effective than topical treatment in reducing healing time and pain

Alternative treatment options include valaciclovir, a prodrug of acyclovir, and famciclovir, a prodrug of penciclovir.[16] These medications have improved bioavailability and require less frequent dosing (1–2 times daily) when compared with acyclovir. Oral valaciclovir has been shown to be as efficacious as IV acyclovir treatment.[16–19]

Prophylactic antiviral therapy should be considered in immunocompromised patients or those with recurrent relapses. Acyclovir 400 mg twice daily is efficacious in reducing frequency and severity of attacks.[16,19] In persistent infection, especially in immunosuppressed individuals, IV acyclovir therapy may be required. In such cases, more toxic therapeutic options, such as foscarnet or cidofovir, should be considered.[16]

Herpes Genitalis

Herpes genitalis, a common sexually transmitted disease, is most commonly caused by HSV-2.[15] HSV-1 is estimated to cause roughly 20% to 40% of primary infections.[15] Primary infection usually occurs in young adults and is more severe than recurrent disease. Recurrence rates are higher when the infection is due to HSV-2.[15] Primary genital herpes manifests with lesions involving the vulva, cervix, vagina, urethral or perianal skin, and other areas, such as the buttocks, thighs, or perineum in women.[15] Men develop lesions on the glans penis or penile shaft, with extragenital infections in the same region as women.[15] Presenting lesions may appear as skin splits, fissures, minor abrasions, furuncles, erythema, and pain.[15] These less obvious epidermal manifestations require a high degree of clinical suspicion to diagnose.[15] Primary infection lesions typically last 2 to 3 weeks during which time they progress from grouped papules on an erythematous base to vesicles and ulcers with eventual crusting.[20] In 79% of primary infections, constitutional complaints (ie, fever, headaches, malaise) are present.[20] Recurrent infection generally lacks constitutional symptoms; lesions are fewer, and there is less viral shedding.[15]

No cure exists, and treatment strategies are aimed at reducing the number/severity of recurrences, reducing infectivity, and decreasing complications (namely, aseptic meningitis and urinary retention).[20] Antiviral therapy should be initiated within 72 hours of primary infection and continued for 7 to 10 days.[20] Acceptable treatment choices for primary infection include acyclovir, valacyclovir, and famciclovir.[20] The following regimens may be considered:

- Acyclovir 400 mg 3 times daily or 200 mg 5 times daily
- Valacyclovir 1000 mg twice daily
- Famciclovir 250 mg 3 times daily

Topical acyclovir is less effective than oral therapy and is generally avoided.[20] For recurrences, oral treatment regimens include[19] the following:

- Acyclovir 200 mg 5 times daily for 5 days
- Acyclovir 400 mg 3 times daily for 5 days
- Acyclovir 800 mg 3 times daily for 2 days
- Acyclovir 800 mg twice daily for 5 days

Treatment regimens with less frequent dosing include[20] the following:

- Valacyclovir 500 mg twice daily for 2 days or 1000 mg once daily for 5 days[20]
- Famciclovir 1000 mg twice daily for 1 day or 125 mg twice daily for 5 days

Management of immunocompromised individuals is similar; however, higher doses and longer periods of treatment are indicated.[20] Depending on the severity of infection, IV therapy may be necessary.

Clinics care points

1. Herpes labialis: Acyclovir, valacyclovir, and famciclovir reduce duration of healing time if initiated early.
2. Herpes genitalis:
   a. Start antiviral therapy within 72 hours of primary infection and continue for 7 to 10 days.
   b. Acceptable treatment choices include acyclovir, valacyclovir, and famciclovir.
   c. Topical therapy is less effective than oral therapy.

Eczema Herpeticum

Eczema herpeticum (EH), a cutaneous viral (commonly HSV) infection of preexisting dermatoses, most commonly occurs in young patients with AD.[15] Patients develop extensive clusters of tender, umbilicated, dome-shaped vesicles in areas of diseased skin.[21] Vesicles progress to hemorrhagic, crusted erosive pits or punched-out ulcers.[21,22] Systemic dissemination and multiple organ viremia are possible.[21] Polymerase chain reaction of vesicle fluid can aid diagnosis.[23]

EH is considered a dermatologic emergency, and acyclovir is the treatment of choice.[24] Treatment regimens include[24] the following:

- For pediatric patients:
  ○ Oral acyclovir 25 mg/kg/d, divided into 5 equal doses, for 5 to 10 days is appropriate.
- For adults:
  ○ Oral acyclovir 400 mg 5 times daily for 5 to 10 days in less severe disease is appropriate.
  ○ Hospitalization and IV acyclovir at 15 mg/kg/d for a minimum of 5 days in the case of severe disease or immunosuppression is recommended.

Clinics care points

1. Acyclovir is the treatment of choice for EH.
2. Patients with disrupted epidermal barrier (ie, AD) are at the greatest risk.

Erythema Multiforme

Erythema multiforme (EM) is a relatively rare condition characterized by erythematous papules that develop into targetoid lesions. Although not a true infection, EM occurs in patients following a variety of stimuli, the best documented of which is HSV-1/2 infection.[14] EM is recognized by 3-zone target lesions with a predominantly acral distribution.[25] Of note, EM major is a specific variant with mucosal lesions only.[25]

Acute episodes of EM are self-limiting and require only symptomatic treatment. Options include[25] the following:

- Oral antihistamines
- Mild- to moderate-potency topical corticosteroids

For mucosal lesions, mouthwashes, topical anesthetics, and topical corticosteroids provide relief.[25] In more severe disease, oral prednisone and strict eye care to reduce secondary infections may be required.[25,26] Recurrent attacks may respond to long-term, continuous acyclovir.[25–27]

Clinics care points

1. EM is commonly triggered by HSV.
2. Symptomatic treatment is the mainstay of therapy.
3. Recurrent attacks may respond to acyclovir.

Herpetic Whitlow

Herpetic whitlow is a painful cutaneous infection caused by HSV-1/2 that involves the pulp of the finger on the distal phalanx.[28] Classically associated with health care or occupational workers that come into contact with infected mucous membranes or secretions, herpetic whitlow may also occur in children.[28]

Patients may experience a prodrome of burning, pruritus, or tingling in the affected digit, followed by the appearance of painful vesicles with clear or serosanguineous fluid.[28] Vesicles may coalesce and resemble a pyogenic bacterial infection.[28] Systemic signs of infections can occur, although they are more common in the immunocompromised.

In the immunocompetent, infection is usually self-limited.[28] Severe infection is managed with acyclovir, valacyclovir, or famciclovir.[28] Immunocompromised patients or those suffering from recurrent infection may benefit from daily use of oral acyclovir.[28] A double-blind, placebo-controlled, crossover study found that treatment with oral acyclovir during the prodromal stage of recurrent HSV-2 herpetic whitlow reduced symptom duration significantly.[28] Topical acyclovir has not been shown to provide clear benefits in treatment.[28]

Clinics care points

1. Herpetic whitlow is generally self-limited.
2. Severe infection is managed with acyclovir, valacyclovir, or famciclovir.
3. Recurrence is managed with prophylactic oral acyclovir.

INTRODUCTION TO SUPERFICIAL FUNGAL INFECTIONS

Superficial fungal mycoses are limited to the outer, keratinized skin layers (ie, the stratum corneum).[29] These superficial fungal infections are most commonly caused by dermatophytes *Microsporum*, *Trichophyton*, and *Epidermophyton*.[30] These organisms reside on keratin found in skin, hair, and nails and very rarely cause deeper infection or elicit a cellular response.[29] Colloquially, infections caused by these organisms are referred to as tinea, followed by the Latin term delineating the anatomic location of infection (**Table 2**).

Diagnostic Tests

Collection of skin scrapings or nail clippings with subsequent KOH (potassium hydroxide) microscopy provides rapid diagnosis.[28] Fungal culture provides diagnosis as well as fungal identification; results may take up to 6 weeks to return.

Therapeutic Options

Treatment depends on the location, severity, and extent of infection. Topical therapy is appropriate for most cutaneous dermatophytoses (ie, tinea corporis, pedis, or cruris).[31] Commonly used therapeutic agents include the allylamine and benzylamine class (ie, butenafine, terbinafine) and the -azole class of medications.[31] Butenafine and terbinafine are more generally considered more efficacious when compared with azole antifungals.[31] In vitro studies demonstrated butenafine as 10 to 100 times more effective, whereas terbinafine therapy proved 2 to 30 times more effective.[31] Topical antifungal agents are usually applied twice a day until resolution of symptoms, usually for 1 to 4 weeks.[31]

Onychomycosis

Although superficial dermatophytoses usually respond to topical antifungal agents, fungal infection of the hair or nails generally require systemic therapy.[31] In the case of onychomycosis, the following regimens are recommended:

- Oral terbinafine[30–33]
  - ○ Terbinafine comes in 250-mg tablets and 125-mg or 187.5-mg packets of granules. Oral granules are taken after sprinkling on a nonacidic, nonfruity, soft food and are indicated for tinea capitis infections.
  - ○ *Dosage* recommendations for oral terbinafine (tablets) in the treatment of onychomycosis include the following:
    - ■ *Adults:* minimum 250 mg daily
    - ■ *Duration:* 6 weeks for fingernails; 12 weeks for toenails
    - ■ For children, weight-based pediatric dose regimens are required:
      - • Less than 20 kg: 62.5 mg daily
      - • 20 to 40 kg: 125 mg daily
      - • Greater than 40 kg: 250 mg daily
- Oral azoles (fluconazole, itraconazole):
  - ○ Fluconazole, although not Food and Drug Administration (FDA) approved, is approved for off-label use in the treatment of onychomycosis.[34]
  - ○ *Dosage* recommendations include
    - ■ Itraconazole[30–33]
      - • Pulsed versus continuous therapy may be considered. Efficacy is similar.
      - • *Pulsed therapy:* 200 mg twice daily for 1 week and then 3 weeks without treatment, repeated twice or more for a total of 3 pulses of therapy for toenails (3–4 months). For fingernails, 200 mg twice daily for 1 week and then

Table 2
Common cutaneous dermatophyte infections

Dermatophyte Infection	Risk Factors	Subtypes & Clinical Manifestations
Tinea pedis	• Occlusive footwear • Sweating • Communal spaces • Occurrence increases with age • Untreated onychomycosis	Interdigital subtype: • Maceration, erosion, & scaling between the toes Chronic hyperkeratotic (moccasin) subtype: • Chronic plantar erythema • Scaling of lateral and plantar surfaces of the foot • Dorsal foot surface generally spared Vesicular subtype: • Clusters of vesicles/pustules on the plantar surface
Tinea unguium (onychomycosis)	• Increasing age • Underlying nail disease • Immunocompromise • Diabetes	Distal lateral subungual subtype: • Yellow or brown discoloration with associated onycholysis and subungual hyperkeratosis White superficial subtype: • White spots on nail plate; may coalesce
Tinea capitis	• Prepubescence	• Scaly patches with alopecia • Diffuse scaling of the scalp with mild alopecia characterized by black dots at follicular opening • Cervical lymphadenopathy Kerion: • Severe form; painful • Pustules and crusting of the scalp with plaque formation
Tinea corporis	• Younger age, childhood	• Tinea at sites other than feet, face, hands, or groin • Annular plaques with central clearing and leading scale • Single vs multiple lesions • Varying size • May coalesce • Active edge may exhibit pustules or vesicles
Tinea cruris	• Adult men	• Located in the groin fold • Annular erythematous plaques with central clearing and leading scale • Single vs multiple lesions • Varying size • May coalesce • Active edge may exhibit pustules or vesicles
Tinea incognito	• Misdiagnosed or mistreated tinea infection	Term given to tinea infection that has been misdiagnosed or inappropriately treated leading to masking of classic clinical features • Development of attenuated scale, erythema, and poorly defined border • Exacerbation of infection with folliculitis

3 weeks without treatment followed by another week of 200-mg tablets, twice daily. This should be repeated twice, for a total of 2 pulses (approximately 2 months).
- *Continuous therapy*: 200 mg daily for 6 weeks for fingernails, 12 weeks for toenails
- Fluconazole[31,34]
  - 150 to 450 mg once weekly. Treatment should continue until resolution of infection. For fingernails, this is approximately 12 to 24 weeks, whereas toenails require between 24 and 52 weeks of treatment.

If systemic therapy cannot be tolerated, 3 FDA-approved topical therapies for mild to moderate onychomycosis exist.[31] These treatments have been shown to have cure rates after daily application for 48 weeks.[31] They include[31] the following:

- Tavaborole 5%
- Ciclopirox olamine 8% nail lacquer
- Efinaconazole 10% solution

Although the cure rate with ciclopirox and tavaborole is often inadequate, efinaconazole 10% solution, a relatively new triazole treatment, has been shown to have increased efficacy and a statistically significant, positive impact on patient satisfaction and quality of life.[35,36]

Systemic therapy for superficial dermatophytoses becomes first line when topical treatment has failed, when skin involvement is severe or extensive, and in cases of tinea capitis.[30] For these indications, first-line therapy and dosage recommendations remain equivalent to that of onychomycosis.[32] Treatment duration depends on location of infection. Tinea capitis requires a minimum 4 weeks of therapy. Cases involving areas other than the scalp or nails require 2 weeks.[32] Dosage reductions should be considered in patients with chronic renal insufficiency; alternative treatment methods need to be considered in cases of liver impairment.[32]

Tinea Capitis

In the case of tinea capitis, identifying the causative organism is important. Although terbinafine is first line in infections caused by *Trichophyton*, Griseofulvin is superior in the case of *Microsporum* infection.[30–32] Of note, in the United States, the most common cause of tinea capitis is *Trichophyton tonsurans*.[31]

- *Griseofulvin microsize*
  - Available as 125-mg/5-mL suspension; 250- and 500-mg tablets.[30–32]
  - *Dosage:* Although prescribing information on package inserts recommends 10 mg/kg per day for pediatric patients, and 500 mg day for adults, these doses are generally inadequate.[37] Rather, the following doses are recommended[31]:
    - Pediatric: 20 to 25 mg/kg daily
    - Adults: 750 to 1500 mg/per day
    - Duration: 6 to 12 weeks
- Oral terbinafine (granules)[30–32]
  - *Dosage* by body weight
    - Less than 25 kg: 125 mg/d
    - 25 to 35 kg: 187.5 mg/d
    - Greater than 35 kg: 250 mg/d
    - *Duration:* once a day for 3 to 6 weeks

Patients should also be encouraged to maintain personal hygiene and to avoid sharing personal items or walking barefoot in moist areas. Prophylactic topical treatment may be considered. Topical antifungal therapy (ie, ciclopirox, amorolfine, bifonazole, terbinafine) can be used weekly for prophylaxis and has significant evidence supporting a lower recurrence rate.[38]

Clinics care points

1. Topical therapy (terbinafine, -azole class) is appropriate for tinea corporis, cruris, or pedis.
2. Systemic therapy is necessary for onychomycosis and tinea capitis.
3. Duration of treatment depends on the location of infection.

SUMMARY

Cutaneous bacterial, viral, and/or fungal infections are frequently encountered in the medical setting. To provide high-quality care, all clinicians require a strong medical understanding of the most common pathogens, presentations, and best treatment options available. This review provides an accessible and thorough outline covering the cutaneous manifestations of commonly encountered infections, including their presentation, patient morbidity, and treatment options. Rooted in evidence-based medicine, the authors hope this article will serve as a useful guide for clinicians as they formulate treatment plans.

DISCLOSURE

No author has a financial or proprietary interest in any material or method mentioned.

REFERENCES

1. Miller LG, Eisenberg DF, Liu H, et al. Incidence of skin and soft tissue infections in ambulatory and inpatient settings, 2005-2010. BMC Infect Dis 2015;15:362.
2. Aly R. Microbial infections of skin and nails. In: Baron S, editor. Medical microbiology. 4th edition. Galveston, TX: University of Texas Medical Branch at Galveston; 1996. Chapter 98.
3. Chiller K, Selkin BA, Murakawa GJ. Skin microflora and bacterial infections of the skin. J Investig Dermatol Symp Proc 2001;6(3):170–4.
4. Ibrahim F, Khan T, Pujalte GG. Bacterial skin infections. Prim Care 2015;42(4): 485–99.
5. Gawkrodger D, Ardern-Jones M. Bacterial infection – Staphylococcal and streptococcal. In: Dermatology: an illustrated colour text. 6th edition. Elsevier; 2017. p. 50–1.
6. Stevens DL, Bisno AL, Chambers HF, et al. Practice guidelines for the diagnosis and management of skin and soft tissue infections: 2014 update by the Infectious Diseases Society of America. Clin Infect Dis 2014;59(2):e10–52.
7. Fernandes P. Efforts to support the development of fusidic acid in the United States. Clin Infect Dis 2011;52(7):S542–6.
8. Heagerty A, Harper N. Cellulitis and erysipelas. In: Lebwohl M, Heymann W, et al, editors. Treatment of skin disease: comprehensive therapeutic strategies. 5th edition. Elsevier; 2018. p. 139–42.
9. Jorup-Rönström C, Britton S, Gavlevik A, et al. The course, costs and complications of oral versus intravenous penicillin therapy of erysipelas. Infection 1984; 12(6):390–4.

10. Raff A, Kroshinsky D. Cellulitis. JAMA 2016;316(3):325.

11. Golan Y. Current treatment options for acute skin and skin-structure infections. Clin Infect Dis 2019;68:206–12.

12. Moran G, Krishnadasan A, Gorwitz R, et al. Methicillin-resistant S. aureus infections among patients in the emergency department. N Engl J Med 2006; 355(7):666–74.

13. Brindle R, Williams O, Barton E, et al. Assessment of antibiotic treatment of cellulitis and erysipelas. JAMA Dermatol 2019;155(9):1033.

14. DiNubile MJ, Lipsky BA. Complicated infections of skin and skin structures: when the infection is more than skin deep. J Antimicrob Chemother 2004;53(2):37–50.

15. Toney J. Skin manifestations of herpesvirus infections. Curr Infect Dis Rep 2005;5: 359–64.

16. Sterling J. Herpes labialis. In: Lebwohl M, Heymann W, Berth-Jones J, editors. Treatment of skin disease: comprehensive therapeutic strategies. 5th edition. Elsevier; 2018. p. 337–9.

17. Bieber T, Chosidow O, Bodsworth N, et al. Efficacy and safety of aciclovir mucoadhesive buccal tablet in immunocompetent patients with labial herpes (LIP trial): a double-blind, placebo-controlled, self-initiated trial. J Drugs Dermatol 2014;13:791–8.

18. Arain N, Paravastu S, Arain M. Effectiveness of topical corticosteroids in addition to antiviral therapy in the management of recurrent herpes labialis: a systematic review and meta-analysis. BMC Infect Dis 2015;15(1):82.

19. Spruance S, Jones T, Blatter M, et al. High-dose, short-duration, early valacyclovir therapy for episodic treatment of cold sores: results of two randomized, placebo-controlled, multicenter studies. Antimicrob Agents Chemother 2003; 47(3):1072–80.

20. Ramya V, Karas L, Sharghi K, et al. Herpes genitalis. In: Lebwohl M, Heymann W, Berth-Jones J, editors. Treatment of skin disease: comprehensive therapeutic strategies. 5th edition. Philadelphia, PA: Elsevier; 2018. p. 333–6.

21. Hasegawa K, Obermeyer Z, Milne L. Eczema herpeticum. J Emerg Med 2012; 43(5):e341–2.

22. Cooper B. Eczema herpeticum. J Emerg Med 2017;53(3):412–3.

23. Wollenberg A, Zoch C, Wetzel S, et al. Predisposing factors and clinical features of eczema herpeticum: a retrospective analysis of 100 cases. J Am Acad Dermatol 2003;49:198–205.

24. Mackley C, Adams D, Anderson B, et al. Eczema herpeticum: a dermatologic emergency. Dermatol Nurs 2002;14:307–10.

25. Revuz J. Erythema multiforme. In: Lebwohl M, Heymann W, Berth-Jones J, editors. Treatment of skin disease: comprehensive therapeutic strategies. 5th edition. Elsevier; 2018. p. 342.

26. Ting HC, Adam BA. Erythema multiforme – response to corticosteroid. Dermatologica 1984;69:175–8.

27. Schofield JK, Tatnall FM, Leigh IM. Recurrent erythema multiforme: clinical features and treatment in a large series of patients. Br J Dermatol 1993;128:542–5.

28. Wu IB, Schwartz RA. Herpetic whitlow. Cutis 2007;79(3):193–6.

29. Dorr P. Fungi and fungal disease. In: Taylor J, Triggle D, editors. Comprehensive medicinal chemistry II. 7th edition. Elsevier; 2007. p. 419–43.

30. Kovitwanichkanont T, Chong AH. Superficial fungal infections. Aust J Gen Pract 2019;48(10):706–11.

31. Carley AC, Stratman EJ, Lesher JL, et al. Antimicrobial drugs. In: Bolognia J, Schaffer JV, Cerroni L, editors. Dermatology. *4th edition*. Elsevier; 2017. p. 2231–6.
32. Expert Group for Dermatology. Tinea. In: eTG complete. Melbourne: Therapeutic Guidelines Limited; 2015.
33. Kreijkamp-Kaspers S, Hawke K, Guo L, et al. Oral antifungal medication for toenail onychomycosis. Cochrane Database Syst Rev 2017;(7):CD010031.
34. Scher RK, Breneman D, Rich P, et al. Once-weekly fluconazole (150, 300, or 450 mg) in the treatment of distal subungual onychomycosis of the toenail. J Am Acad Dermatol 1998;38(6):S77–86.
35. Gupta AK, Fleckman P, Baran R. Ciclopirox nail lacquer topical solution 8% in the treatment of toenail onychomycosis. J Am Acad Dermatol 2000;43:S70–80.
36. LaSenna T. Patient considerations in the management of toe onychomycosis - role of efinaconazole. Patient Prefer and Adherence 2015;9:887–91.
37. Janssen Pharmaceutical Companies. Grifulvin V (Griseofulvin Tablet, USP (Microsize) and Griseofulvin Oral Suspension, USP (microsize) [package insert]. U.S. Food and Drug Administration; 2011. Available at: https://www.accessdata.fda.gov/drugsatfda_docs/label/2014/062279s022lbl.pdf. Accessed January 5, 2021.
38. Shemer A, Gupta AK, Kamshov A, et al. Topical antifungal treatment prevents recurrence of toenail onychomycosis following cure. Dermatol Ther 2017;30(5).

Printed and bound by CPI Group (UK) Ltd, Croydon, CR0 4YY

03/10/2024

01040468-0004